WILSON, JAMES GRAVES
ENVIRONMENT AND BIRTH DEFECTS
000346192

HCL   QL991.W74

KU-405-358

DENTAL SCHOOL LIBRARY

WITHDRAWN FROM STOCK
The University of Liverpool

DENTAL SCHOOL LIBRARY

ENVIRONMENT AND BIRTH DEFECTS

ENVIRONMENTAL SCIENCES

An Interdisciplinary Monograph Series

EDITORS

DOUGLAS H. K. LEE
National Institute of
Environmental Health Sciences
Research Triangle Park
North Carolina

E. WENDELL HEWSON
Department of
Atmospheric Science
Oregon State University
Corvallis, Oregon

DANIEL OKUN
Department of Environmental
Sciences and Engineering
University of North Carolina
Chapel Hill, North Carolina

ARTHUR C. STERN, editor, AIR POLLUTION, Second Edition. In three volumes, 1968

L. FISHBEIN, W. G. FLAMM, and H. L. FALK, CHEMICAL MUTAGENS: Environmental Effects on Biological Systems, 1970

DOUGLAS H. K. LEE and DAVID MINARD, editors, PHYSIOLOGY, ENVIRONMENT, AND MAN, 1970

KARL D. KRYTER, THE EFFECTS OF NOISE ON MAN, 1970

R. E. MUNN, BIOMETEOROLOGICAL METHODS, 1970

M. M. KEY, L. E. KERR, and M. BUNDY, PULMONARY REACTIONS TO COAL DUST: "A Review of U. S. Experience," 1971

DOUGLAS H. K. LEE, editor, METALLIC CONTAMINANTS AND HUMAN HEALTH, 1972

DOUGLAS H. K. LEE, editor, ENVIRONMENTAL FACTORS IN RESPIRATORY DISEASE, 1972

H. ELDON SUTTON and MAUREEN I. HARRIS, editors, MUTAGENIC EFFECTS OF ENVIRONMENTAL CONTAMINANTS, 1972

RAY T. OGLESBY, CLARENCE A. CARLSON, and JAMES A. MCCANN, editors, RIVER ECOLOGY AND MAN, 1972

LESTER V. CRALLEY, LEWIS T. CRALLEY, GEORGE D. CLAYTON, and JOHN A. JURGIEL, editors, INDUSTRIAL ENVIRONMENTAL HEALTH: The Worker and the Community, 1972

MOHAMED K. YOUSEF, STEVEN M. HORVATH, and ROBERT W. BULLARD, PHYSIOLOGICAL ADAPTATIONS: Desert and Mountain, 1972

DOUGLAS H. K. LEE and PAUL KOTIN, editors, MULTIPLE FACTORS IN THE CAUSATION OF ENVIRONMENTALLY INDUCED DISEASE, 1972

MERRIL EISENBUD, ENVIRONMENTAL RADIOACTIVITY, Second Edition, 1973

JAMES G. WILSON, ENVIRONMENT AND BIRTH DEFECTS, 1973

In preparation

RAYMOND C. LOEHR, AGRICULTURAL WASTE MANAGEMENT: Problems, Processes, and Approaches

Environment and Birth Defects

James G. Wilson

CHILDREN'S HOSPITAL RESEARCH FOUNDATION
AND DEPARTMENTS OF PEDIATRICS AND ANATOMY
UNIVERSITY OF CINCINNATI COLLEGE OF MEDICINE
CINCINNATI, OHIO

ACADEMIC PRESS   *New York and London*   *1973*

A Subsidiary of Harcourt Brace Jovanovich, Publishers

COPYRIGHT © 1973, BY ACADEMIC PRESS, INC.
ALL RIGHTS RESERVED.
NO PART OF THIS PUBLICATION MAY BE REPRODUCED OR
TRANSMITTED IN ANY FORM OR BY ANY MEANS, ELECTRONIC
OR MECHANICAL, INCLUDING PHOTOCOPY, RECORDING, OR ANY
INFORMATION STORAGE AND RETRIEVAL SYSTEM, WITHOUT
PERMISSION IN WRITING FROM THE PUBLISHER.

ACADEMIC PRESS, INC.
111 Fifth Avenue, New York, New York 10003

United Kingdom Edition published by
ACADEMIC PRESS, INC. (LONDON) LTD.
24/28 Oval Road, London NW1

Library of Congress Cataloging in Publication Data

Wilson, James Graves, DATE
      Environment and birth defects.

        (Environmental sciences)
        "Selected references on embryology and reproduction
of laboratory animals": p.
        Bibliography: p.
        1.   Environmentally induced diseases.   2.   Deformi-
ties—Causes and theories of causation.   I.   Title.
II.   Series.   [DNLM: 1.   Abnormalities—Etiology—
Collected works.   2.   Environment—Collected works.
QS675 E61 1973]
RB152.W5   616'.043   73-800
ISBN 0-12-757750-5

PRINTED IN THE UNITED STATES OF AMERICA

*To the men and women in government and industry
who share in the responsibility of evaluating
the hazards of the environment to as yet
unborn generations—may they do their job well!*

CONTENTS

Chapter 4   Mechanisms of Teratogenesis

Chapter 5   Manifestations of Abnormal Development

Chapter 6   Access of Environmental Factors to Developing Tissues

Chapter 7   Normal Development and Susceptible Periods

Chapter 8   The Assessment of Teratologic Risk

Chapter 9   Collection and Interpretation of Results

FOREWORD

Morbid curiosity, mixed with a modicum of human sympathy, has from ancient times focused attention upon errors in development and abnormalities in the newborn, but it is only in this century that their acceptance as inescapable hazards of procreation has yielded to scientific inquiry into root causes and that a hope has been engendered of significantly reducing the risk. Ironically, if human suffering can be discussed in such delicate terms, it was man's capacity for making things worse that did most to direct inquiry into causes and thus spark the hope of prevention.

With increasing use of radiography for abdominal and pelvic examination in the 1920's and 1930's, particularly in the resolution of obstetric and gynecological problems, it came to be realized that the fetus could be damaged thereby functionally as well as morphologically. In the 1940's it was established that a rubella infection in the mother during the first three months of pregnancy could result in severely affected infants. In the 1950's adverse effects of chemotherapeutic agents were noticed. But it was left to the 1960's for man to demonstrate in dramatic and shocking fashion that a drug, given with the best of intentions for the benefit of the mother, could have disastrous consequences for the developing embryo.

The wide interest and the spate of research currently devoted to deficiencies in the newborn undoubtedly owe a lot to the shocked reaction that followed the thalidomide disclosures, but the foundation was already laid. It had been shown earlier that substances akin to thalidomide could produce fetal abnormalities, and there are those who believe that adequate information systems could have alerted the manufacturers to possible consequences. It is possible that such a system, coupled with stringent requirements for exhaustive pretesting, could have forestalled events, but be that as it may, the current interest in the whole problem should do much to make a repetition of such an incident much less likely.

In an atmosphere of rising concern about possible health effects of various environmental pollutants, the clear demonstration that a specific chemical administered to a pregnant woman can have adverse effects on the embryo naturally raised the question whether numerous substances other than drugs present in our food, water, or air might also give rise to malformations. In fact, one could not help wondering if the long-accepted instances of "naturally occurring" malformations might not, in part at least, be attributable to environmental agents that could be identified and countered. Investigative techniques are too new and the number of agents to be considered too great for any quick answers to such questions. But current inquiries illustrate a widespread concern. At the present time, for instance, there is much discussion about the apparent association of anencephaly and spina bifida with the consumption of moldy potatoes. The problems of a retrospective analysis are enormous. Only in the most general terms can variation in the diet of pregnant women forty years ago be related to variations in a phenomenon of relatively low incidence. Good experimental models have yet to be devised and the results interpreted for man.

A further difficulty lies in the overlapping action of what are basically three different sets of processes. The effects of genetic changes in the parents brought about by the action of environmental mutagens may make their appearance at any time from the moment of conception, through intrauterine development, and on through the entire life of the offspring. The results of exposure of the embryo, through the mother, to teratogenic agents may appear in the course of intrauterine development and on through life. The effects of postnatal exposure of the offspring to environmental agents may appear at any time through its life. The defect or disturbance that is actually seen may be the result not merely of one but of two or more of these processes interacting with each other. It is not always easy to sort out the agents responsible just by examining the end result.

The purpose of this book is to present the current state of our knowledge on the causation of malformations and deficiencies in the newborn, not as a set of obiter dicta, but as a guide to practical application of what we now know and as an encouragement to improve our understanding of phenomena and mechanisms that are still obscure. This it does in logical and straightforward fashion. But this is not the book's only virtue. To the delight of the Editors, and no doubt to that of future readers, the style is clear, direct, and eminently readable. It is not often that scholarship is combined with lucidity, but this time we have that eminently desirable product, an authoritative book that does not confine itself to the arcane language of a particular "in" group. Dr. Wilson's status as an expert and as a teacher will be greatly enhanced, and perhaps some of that communication gap referred to earlier has been bridged. The Environmental Sciences Series is happy to have this volume on its list.

DOUGLAS H. K. LEE
National Institute of Environmental
Health Sciences

PREFACE

The aim of this book is to provide information that will be needed in evaluating environmental factors that may represent risks to unborn generations. These involve two areas of special concern, mutagenesis and teratogenesis. The risks from mutagenesis and teratogenesis are somewhat different, as will be discussed. Nonetheless, they share the disturbing characteristic of being among the most insidious of all environmental hazards. As such they must be dealt with objectively by informed persons who are capable of making scientific and social judgments without being swayed by emotion and popular opinion. This will not be easy because the mere words "mutagenesis" and "teratogenesis" conjure images not only of suffering and death but, more pathetically, of deformed children, of lifelong invalids, and of whole families blighted by heavy financial and emotional burdens.

An effort is made in this book to direct the discussions of facts and concepts particularly to those persons who will set policies and make decisions about environmental risks to human development rather than to either the enlightened public or the scientific specialist. This objective was made difficult by the fact that persons who set such policies and make such decisions are likely to have had diverse backgrounds, probably ranging between the extremes of orthodox science and practical politics. The subject, however, is mainly scientfic and therefore requires for the sake of precision that some specialized language and ideas be employed. A seemingly reasonable compromise has been to introduce the necessary biological concepts, but in doing so to avoid technical jargon as much as possible and to provide explanatory comment wherever it seemed to be needed.

This book was initially planned for those professionals in government and industry who are perhaps best designated as scientific administrators. In due course, however, efforts to organize the subject into a logical and coherent whole pointed up the fact that this had not previously been undertaken in a comprehensive way. Since the needs of the scientific administrator who may not be an expert in the relevant disciplines of embryology, genetics, and toxicology are not greatly different from those of the student or the young scientist in training, it was decided to broaden the coverage of the book sufficially so that it would serve as an introduction to the field of teratology for all who had such a need. Accordingly, some material has been included that exceeds the original utilitarian purpose. I will be pleased if these additions have in any measure extended the scope of the book so that it may serve as a text or source book for students at the advanced undergraduate, graduate, or professional school levels or for young scientists considering a career in this or related fields.

An apology is offered to those investigators whose research has contributed to the elucidation of the principles contained herein but whose work has not been fully credited in the reference citations. Bibliography in the field of teratology now far exceeds the possibility of exhaustive review in a book of this dimension. Selection of representative experiments was necessary, and I readily admit that the selection was not always the best owing to my personal biases, limited linguistic skills, and inability to read and assimilate all of the accumulated literature. Nevertheless, considerable effort has been made to provide through reference citations an entrée to all aspects of the subject except the strictly clinical.

Appreciation is warmly expressed to many people who contributed knowingly and otherwise to this book. Among these are several professional colleagues and a whole generation of graduate students at several institutions. Through discussions and collaborations they helped to formulate and substantiate the ideas presented here. Deserving of special mention are my good friend and wife, Harriet Chamberlain Wilson, who prepared the index and read galley proof; my dependable research associate, Rochelle Fradkin, who supervised data collection and analysis; and my efficient secretary, Janice Hagedorn, who cheerfully retyped several versions of the manuscript and tirelessly tracked down references.

JAMES G. WILSON

CHAPTER 1

IS THE UNBORN AT RISK IN THE ENVIRONMENT?

I. Introduction

Living things during early developmental stages are more sensitive than at any other time in their life cycle to adverse influences in the environment. This is not to say that embryos and other formative stages are always exposed directly to the environment. Most species have evolved protective devices that tend to insulate their early stages from the commoner harmful influences in the surroundings. The best protection is achieved by those animals whose young reside during their vulnerable early stages within the body of the maternal animal. This arrangement not only provides physical insulation from many potentially harmful outside factors such as mechanical impact, temperature fluctuations, and some radiations; it also enables the maternal animal to modulate other factors of a chemical nature so that if they reach the embryo at all, it is in a less damaging form, or at least in reduced concentration. The sharks and a few reptiles possess this advantageous system of maternal incubation; but it reaches its most efficient development in mammals, those animals that nidate their early offspring in a uterus by means of a placental attachment.

Because of its sequestered position in the uterus, surrounded by the maternal body, the mammalian embryo might seem to be protected from all of the adversities of the environment. In fact, during the first half of the present century this view was given considerable credence among scientists. This was perhaps a natural consequence of the rediscovery around the turn of the century of the laws of heredity, formulated some 36 years earlier by Gregor Mendel, the father of genetics. As this new science was accepted, it

1

was taken for granted that deviations from as well as adherence to the normal patterns of embryogenesis could be ascribed to the genes.

An opposite but equally unrealistic view seems to have arisen in the modern climate of increasing concern about the rate at which the environment is being changed. Indeed there is reason to wonder whether man is altering his surroundings faster than he is able to adapt to the changes, and it is certain that the changes are occurring faster than he can critically evaluate their effects on his health and general well-being. An irresponsible writer or lecturer can take the facts that (1) the early embryo is potentially susceptible to many outside influences and that (2) the maternal body is incapable of protecting against these in all conceivable doses, and by ignoring the adaptive and homeostatic functions of the maternal organism and assuming that exposure to large doses of detrimental factors is commonplace, he can easily conjure up a truly alarming picture.

A. Nature of the Risk

The actual situation is somewhere in between, hopefully somewhat closer to the side of complete protection than of complete vulnerability. In most instances the maternal organism, together with the function of the placenta in slowing passage of many chemicals, is able to protect against doses of outside influences that would otherwise be detrimental to early development. This generalization, however, does not give carte blanche assurance when pregnant women are exposed to new drugs or other environmental chemicals, for there is no reliable way to make blanket predictions about the safety of untested factors. Even if it were possible to evaluate in general terms all such factors, absolute safety would remain an elusive goal because of varying susceptibilities from one individual to another. Many aspects of our present surroundings have never been critically examined for effects on development, although a degree of security can be derived from the fact that a few of these have been present for some time and have never been implicated in abnormal development. Such logic is not entirely satisfying but it is an alternative to hysteria or hopeless resignation. There is, however, a better alternative.

B. Recourse

Sufficient information and technical know-how are already available to make possible a fairly reliable estimation of the more obvious risks to developmental processes, and intensified efforts and improved capability could lead to much better evaluation of potentially damaging factors in the environment than is currently undertaken. The information and methodology that can make this possible are embodied in the science of teratology. It is the objective of this book to assemble and organize the pertinent facts of teratology so that they may be applied to the problems of evaluating risks which confront the unborn child in today's environment.

II. Some Essential Concepts

A. THE UNBORN

The unborn is not only the embryo and the fetus *in utero* but also the as yet unconceived individuals whose potential for future development is represented in the germ cells residing in the parental gonads. Also of interest here, because they too are still at some risk, are those who have already been born but who are incompletely developed and consequently remain more vulnerable to certain adverse factors than are more mature individuals. In the following pages reference will be made to developing organisms as encompassing all immature stages, whether germ cells, embryos, fetuses, infants, or children. All of these share the common characteristics of being at some stage in the developmental span and of being generally more vulnerable to environmental influences than are most of the tissues in postpubertal human beings.

B. ENVIRONMENT

For the present purpose, environment is defined as all influences from outside the developing organism. To the embryo or the fetus the environment is everything outside his own skin, namely, the amniotic fluid in which he floats; the enclosing membranes, amnion and chorion, the placenta being a localized specialization of the latter; the uterus; the remainder of the maternal body; and finally the total physical and chemical surroundings of the mother. Despite the considerable insulation afforded by the maternal body, a few physical and most chemical factors in these surroundings are transmitted in some fractional dosage to the embryo or fetus. Thus, substances normally mediated by the mother, such as nutrients and oxygen, as well as many foreign chemicals of extramaternal origin, are all from the environment.

For the germ cells, whether as undifferentiated stages or as gametes ready to participate in fertilization, the environment begins at their cell walls. Germ cells of both sexes during most of their existence reside in the gonads of the parents; but their relationship to the surroundings differs according to sex, in that the male gametes in the testes are more exposed to extraparental influences owing to the more superficial location of the gonad.

Furthermore, to effect fertilization the male gametes must traverse the length of the paternal genital tract, be deposited in the lower part of the maternal tract and then find their way to the female gamete in the upper reaches of the maternal tract. There is no evidence that this greater exposure to diverse environments is detrimental to male germ cells.

C. Teratology

In simplest terms, teratology is the study of the adverse effects of environment on developing systems, that is, on germ cells, embryos, fetuses, and immature postnatal individuals. A more comprehensive definition is that teratology is the science dealing with the causes, mechanisms, and manifestations of developmental deviations of either structural or functional nature. If the deviations occur in the germ cells and are transmissible from one generation to another, they are called germinal mutations. The genetic material (DNA) of ordinary somatic cells can also be damaged in the same ways as the DNA of germ cells, but these defects are only transmitted to descendant cells within the same individual and are called somatic mutations. Damage during development to the DNA of somatic cells, however, is rarely recognized and it is thought that somatic mutations account for only a small fraction of abnormal development. Damage is more likely to affect groups of cells in more general ways; if these groups of cells have undergone differentiation toward filling a specialized role in embryogenesis, the damage may be manifested as a developmental defect.

Developmental defects are variously designated as terata, malformations, anomalies, birth defects, or congenital defects. Actually these terms are not all synonymous. Terata and malformations historically and literally refer to structural abnormalities. There are no overall designations for functional abnormalities, although the descriptive term inborn errors of metabolism encompasses an important group of functional disorders that have a developmental origin. Anomalies, birth defects, and congenital defects are more general terms that may be applied to most types of developmental abnormality, although the latter two imply that the defect is present at birth. This is not always the case, as will be explained presently. Thus, anomalies and developmental defects would seem to be the most widely applicable terms for all deviations of development.

III. Overview of Modern Teratology

Teratological studies in the past have in large part dealt with the developmental history of anomalies before birth or with description of the defects as seen after birth. Like other sciences, it was first necessary to define the subject matter as to its varied phenomena and their frequency of occurrence. Accordingly the descriptive phase of teratology has dwelt on the classification, incidence, and other characteristics of abnormal development. Increasingly during the past 30 or 40 years, however, interest in the causes as well as the manifestations of deviant development has become evident. The recent concern about the effects of the rapidly changing environment on life processes generally has naturally intensified interest in how these changes affect development.

A. ALL CAUSATION FROM THE ENVIRONMENT

It is probable that all abnormal development has its causation in some aspect of environment. Even hereditary defects that can be traced back through several generations presumably were initiated as mutations at some time in the past; modern geneticists assume that mutations are triggered by extrinsic factors, although these usually cannot be identified. The realization that most anomalies may be traceable to adverse influences in the environment, however, has not given much insight into how these actually bring about deviations in developmental processes. Cause-and-effect relationships in teratology are not always apparent and when they are they are often imprecise; for example, radiations can cause both hereditary and nonhereditary defects, each of quite diverse types. Certain chemicals may cause one type of developmental error in one species of animal, a different type of abnormality in another, and have no appreciable effect in a third. Many maternal infections during pregnancy have little effect on the offspring; some cause embryonic death or growth retardation, but a few such as rubella are highly teratogenic. Thus, although knowledge of causes has increased, little still is known about what really happens when normal development is disrupted and why this is able to lead to such varied manifestations.

B. CAUSES ACTIVATE MECHANISMS

Clearly more is involved than simply an agent in the environment producing a stereotyped pattern of abnormality by interfering with development in some direct way. Information is still meager but there is increasing evidence to indicate that a causative agent may produce more than one type of initial reaction in developing cells and tissues. These initial reactions are inapparent and may bear little specific relationship to the final defect, except in the sense of being the first in a series of changes that ultimately leads to the final defect. Thus, an initial action followed by a chain reaction seems to be the course of events in teratogenesis: not the cause alone, but the cause together with the particular sequences of responses it elicits in cells and tissues determines how development will be diverted. These early reactions in response to the environmental cause are here called *mechanisms*.

C. Three Aspects of Teratology

The three aspects of teratology are causes, mechanisms, and manifestations, which are sequentially related as diagramed in Scheme 1-1. They will be discussed more fully in later chapters, but a few explanatory comments are appropriate here. The summary of causes in this diagram includes all of the major categories known in mammals, perhaps excepting certain variable conditions best designated as altered maternal physiologic states. The probability of interactions between the individual agents that make up these categories must also be recognized. Chemical agents comprise by far the largest group of causes, both as regards individual entities and in the variety of subgroups, e.g., drugs, industrial chemicals, pesticides, food additives and preservatives, and environmental pollutants. Of the nine categories listed,

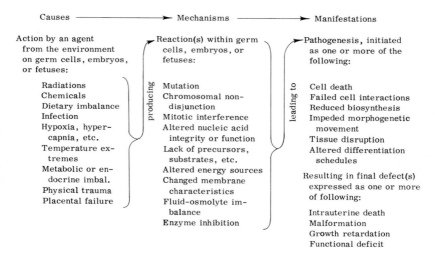

Scheme 1-1. Teratology is schematically summarized in three categories: causes, mechanisms, and manifestations. Causes are from the environment and act directly or indirectly on developing tissues (germ cells, embryos, or fetuses). Mechanisms are the early determinative reactions within the conceptus or the germ cells and are at present poorly understood, although the existence of those listed here is supported at least by inferential evidence. One or more mechanisms activates the sequence of abnormal developmental events which leads to the final defect. These intervening events, collectively called pathogenesis, and the final defect are the manifestations or demonstrable aspects of teratogenesis.

only four contain agents clearly implicated as teratogenic in man, namely, (1) ionizing radiations, (2) chemicals in the form of a few drugs and one known pollutant, (3) a few infectious agents, and (4) a small number of endocrine and metabolic inbalances.

Mechanism as a term has been broadly used in teratology to designate some or all of the events that intervene between the embryo's first response to a causative agent and the final manifestation of abnormal development; thus it lacks precise meaning. It is used in Scheme 1-1 in a more restricted sense to designate the early, presumably determining, reactions of the developing system to the causative agent. A single cause can activate more than one mechanism; for example, radiation is capable of producing point mutations, mitotic interference, and enzyme inhibition. Dietary deficiency, in addition to producing lack of substrates and precursors, may also result in reduced energy sources and fluid–osmolyte imbalances.

The list of mechanisms proposed in Scheme 1-1 is tentative. The first two and the fourth are probably supported by ample evidence to establish them as mechanisms in the sense defined above. Some evidence can be marshaled in support of most of the others, but in every case it is not clear that these are the initial biological reactions to the inciting agent. For example, mitotic interference may be secondary to some primary effect concerned with the formation or maintenance of the microtubular system needed in the mitotic spindle. In other instances it is difficult to determine which of two possible mechanisms is primary, e.g., either changed membrane characteristics or fluid–osmolyte imbalance could equally well lead to changes in osmotic pressure and abnormal fluid accumulations.

Manifestations, that is, the types, degrees, and incidences of abnormal development, have been the subject of a vast literature and to attempt to review it would exceed the scope of this book. The author is pleased to defer in this matter to his teacher and colleague, Dr. Josef Warkany, who has recently completed a monumental review of the final manifestations of abnormal development (Warkany, 1971). For the present purpose only brief comment on the events leading up to the final defect is needed. The initial reactions of a developing system to an environmental cause, the mechanism, must be translated into either morphogenetic or biochemical events that will lead ultimately to structural or functional abnormality. Information is limited but it is probable that all of the mechanisms listed in Scheme 1-1 could lead to a limited number of demonstrable deviations of embryogenesis, such as cell death, failed cellular interactions, altered biosynthetic rates, impeded morphogenetic movements, and perhaps a few other conditions that would interfere with the schedules of differentiation. Through intermediate steps that are poorly understood, abnormal development proceeds to its eventual expression as structural or functional defects. This sequence of abnormal events between the initiating mechanism and the final expression constitutes the pathogenesis of a defect. The later events in the pathogenesis of many structural defects have been described in histogenetic and organogenetic terms and comprise much of the literature of descriptive teratology. Less well known is the pathogenesis of most functional abnormalities, although some metabolic errors have been traced to specific enzyme or transport deficiencies.

There are four types of final manifestations of abnormal development, namely, death, malformation, growth retardation, and functional deficit. Teratology was defined earlier only in terms of structure and function, that is, malformation and functional abnormality, without specific mention of death and retarded growth. It is assumed that in most instances intrauterine death and growth retardation are secondary to structural or functional abnormality or to some combination of the two, but the true nature of these relationships is usually not known. There is no collective term for all four manifestations of abnormal development. Of the broader terms that have been applied, such as embryotoxic, fetotoxic, and embryopathic, all have the limitation of designating a single period rather than the entire span of development. Perhaps a general descriptive phrase such as developmental toxicity would be adequate.

IV. A Quick Look Backward

The usual order of presentation in introductory sections has been reversed here so that the reader is made aware of the meaning of modern teratology before contemplating the remarkably diverse attitudes that man in the past has entertained about his own developmental variability. Clues to some of his thoughts on the matter are seen in the derivation of the word teratology, from the Greek, *teras,* meaning monster, and in the origin of the English word monster from the Latin, *monstrum,* having a connotation of something that demonstrates or provides foreknowledge of coming events.

Man's early pictorial and written records give evidence of his awareness that some of his fellowmen were afflicted from birth with physical features that were unusual. The Chaldeans in ancient Babylon made lists that assigned specific meanings to the birth of particular types of defective infants. They were taken as messages from the gods foretelling events in the affairs of man, much as these people also used the flights of migratory birds, the disposition of the entrails in sacrificial animals, and the positions of heavenly bodies to obtain foresight into the future.

The Greeks doubtless held to some of these views, but there is reason to believe that they used the birth of defective babies in a more romantic connection, namely, as models for some of the fabulous creatures that populate Greek mythology, the sirens, cyclops, etc. Another attitude rooted in classical antiquity is the belief that the mental impressions and emotions of a pregnant woman could influence the physical development of her child. The women of Greece were encouraged to gaze upon beautiful statuary of the human figure with the expectation that it would cause their unborn children to be well formed. Many versions of the belief that maternal impressions could influence intrauterine development arose at widely separated places and times in man's cultural history. Accordingly one is not greatly surprised to find a Biblical account of the use of sensory stimuli during pregnancy to achieve a desired end in the breeding of livestock *(Genesis:* 30).

The interbreeding of man with animals has at times been blamed for the birth of monstrous offspring, a notion that may have originated in India or Egypt where certain animals were regarded as at least the equals of man. Such offspring were sometimes accorded reverence by the established religion (an anencephalic infant is said to have been found among the mummies of sacred animals in an Egyptian tomb); and the centaurs, minotaurs, satyrs, and other part-animal, part-human beings come to mind. An even more fanciful view held that malformations resulted from cohabitation of human beings with demons and witches, and many pamphlets were circulated in fifteenth and sixteenth century Europe describing imagined and real birth defects that were attributed to this cause. From this it was only a short stretch of the imagination to what might be called the theory of divine retribution, in which the divine hand was thought to have diverted development in punishment for some wrongdoing of the parents, or perhaps of society in general, recalling the stern Biblical promise that "the sins of the father shall be visited . . . ," etc.

With the emergence of biological sciences during the seventeenth and eighteenth centuries, explanations with some basis in scientific fact were formulated, although they by no means replaced those based on fancy and superstition. Important among the more rational new theories was one holding that birth defects resulted from an arrest in an embryological process at some stage prior to its normal completion: the theory of developmental arrest, first clearly stated by William Harvey in 1651. Much earlier both Hippocrates and Aristotle were aware that direct injury to the embryo or increased pressure on or within the uterus could cause malformation. The French surgeon, Ambrois Paré, in particular expounded this idea in the sixteenth century when he wrote that there were three causes of monstrosities: (1) narrowness of the uterus, (2) faulty posture of the pregnant woman, and (3) external violence, such as a fall. St.-Hillaire the Elder in the nineteenth century contended that strands, bands, and fusions between the embryo and the overlying amnion were important causes of birth defects, and efforts to defend this notion against the criticisms leveled by his contemporaries led him and his son into the first attempts at experimental teratology in animals.

Then in 1900, 36 years after the Austrian monk Gregor Mendel first enunciated them, the principles of genetics were rediscovered. It was quickly assumed that the genes that control normal development could also determine abnormal development. In the ensuing 50 years the tendency to attribute all human developmental error to this cause became deeply ingrained in medicine. Like many another generalization with some basis of fact, this one offered the convenience of ready explanation without requiring rigorous proof. Thus teratology during the early part of the present century again found itself with less than an objective outlook, this time not under the sway of superstition and fancy but owing to the overextension of a scientific principle. (The reader interested in a fuller account of the fascinating history of teratology than was attempted in this brief summary should consult Hickey, 1953; and Warkany, 1959, 1971.)

Modern teratology has taken shape in the last 35 years under the impetus of three significant events. In 1940 Warkany and his associates (1940, 1944, 1947, 1948) began a long series of experiments in which it was shown that maternal dietary deficiencies in rats could cause predictable types and percentages of malformations in the offspring. Soon thereafter it was reported by Gregg (1941) that a high proportion of children born to women infected with rubella virus during the first third of pregnancy gave birth to defective infants. Thus in short order it was demonstrated that the embryos of mammals, including man, are susceptible to such commonplace environmental influences as inadequate diet and infection during intrauterine development. The immediate impact of these observations was not great but in time the implications began to be accepted in biomedical circles. Full realization that factors in the environment must be regarded as potential risks to the unborn child, however, was not forcefully brought to the attention of the informed public, governmental regulatory agencies, and the pharmaceutical and chemical industries until 1961. After Lenz (1961) and McBride (1961) established an association between the taking by pregnant women of the presumably nontoxic sedative, thalidomide, and the birth of severely malformed infants, the literate world was quickly aware of the problem. If a single drug could cripple some 8000 children in a span of two years, there might indeed be reason to question the effects of other environmental factors on development.

CHAPTER 2

PRINCIPLES OF TERATOLOGY

The series of animal experiments begun in 1940 by Warkany and his associates (Warkany and Nelson, 1940; Warkany and Schraffenberger, 1944; Wilson *et al.,* 1953b) first forcefully called attention to the fact that environmental factors such as deficiency in the maternal diet could adversely affect intrauterine development. Since then hundreds of other such factors also have been shown to cause developmental abnormality in animals. They have been adequately reviewed (Gruenwald, 1947; Giroud, 1955; Kalter and Warkany, 1959; Nishimura, 1964; Wilson, 1964a; Karnofsky, 1965a; Cahen, 1966; Chaube and Murphy, 1968; Tuchmann-Duplessis, 1969), and need not be enumerated here.

Realization that mammalian embryos were subject to environmental influences was not for long limited to laboratory animals. In 1941 Gregg showed that maternal rubella infection could cause malformation in man and in 1961 McBride (1961) and Lenz (1961) found the human embryo to be highly susceptible to thalidomide. Other types of extrinsic agents are now also known to cause disturbances in human intrauterine development (see Chapter 3); although the number of proved agents is far fewer than in animals, there is no doubt that the early stages of man are vulnerable to adverse factors from the environment.

From this considerable accumulation of observations over the past 30 years, certain generalizations about the nature of the teratogenic susceptibility of mammalian embryos have emerged. A list of five such "principles" of teratology was first tentatively proposed in 1959 (Wilson, 1959). These were accepted with some modification by subsequent authors (Nishimura, 1964; Beck and Lloyd, 1965). Although still basically valid today, recent

11

experience and new information require that the original five be restated in
more precise terms and that a sixth generalization relative to dosage effects
be added. The principles are not intended to encompass all of the basic facts
in teratology; rather they describe the usual or seemingly typical occurrences. Very likely with increased understanding of teratogenic mechanisms,
it will be necessary to formulate additional principles and to revise those
now formulated.

I. Susceptibility to Teratogenesis Depends on the Genotype of the Conceptus and the Manner in Which This Interacts with Adverse Environmental Factors

A. SPECIES DIFFERENCES

This principle may be broadly illustrated by the often demonstrated fact
that some species respond more readily to certain teratogenic agents than do
others. For example, mice are generally susceptible to the induction of cleft
palate by cortisone; hamsters and guinea pigs are less so; rats are rarely so;
and most other mammals are refractory to this action. Man and other higher
primates are highly vulnerable to thalidomide during early embryogenesis,
showing characteristic limb and facial malformations; rabbits react in a
somewhat similar fashion but larger dosage is required; a few strains of mice
react to the drug but the defects do not typically involve the limbs, whereas
most other animals including rats and some lower primates are resistant to
thalidomide teratogenesis. Many other examples of divergent reactions
among animals are known but this is adequate to illustrate the point that
species is, in a gross way, a genotypic determiner of whether teratogenesis
will occur with a given agent. It must be admitted, however, that the metabolic characteristics of the maternal animal, also genetically determined,
may be the controlling factor in species differences such as those noted
above.

B. STRAIN AND INTRALITTER DIFFERENCES

The frequent observation that different strains or stocks of animals of the
same species may respond in differing degrees to the same agent is also explained in terms of unlike genotypes. Fraser and Fainstat (1951) noted
varying incidences of cleft palate in different strains of mice similarly treated with cortisone. Gunberg (1958) reported striking quantitative differences in mortality and malformation among the offspring of three strains or
substrains of rats treated during pregnancy with trypan blue; great diversity

in the reaction of rabbits of different genetic background to thalidomide was observed by Sawin *et al.* (1965); and variations in teratogenic response to hypervitaminosis A in three strains of rats were reported by Nolen (1969). Zimmerman and Bowen (1972) have recently related differences among three strains of mice in their sensitivity to triamcinolone-induced cleft palate to differing rates of metabolism of the drug by the maternal animals; embryos of the resistant strain were shown to receive appreciably lower doses than those of the sensitive strains.

It is well known that, even in homogeneous strains of animals, all individuals in a litter do not react alike to teratogenic treatment. An agent applied during the susceptible period often causes some embryos to die and resorb soon after treatment, others to be stillborn at term, others to survive with varying degrees of malformation, while some may develop normally. Intralitter variation in developmental stage could account for some of these differences after short duration treatment, but exposure to the agent for more than a few hours would tend to negate this explanation. There is no proof that the remaining unaccounted variability is attributable to genotypic differences, but in the absence of other known causes it is assumed that subtle genetic differences account for most of intralitter variation.

C. INTERACTION OF GENOME AND ENVIRONMENT

An interplay between the genome and the immediate environment of the embryo is often evident. For example, Kalter (1954) gave the same dose of cortisone to two strains of pregnant mice and noted that strain A produced offspring 100% of which had cleft palate, while only 19% of the young from strain C57BL showed this defect. When these strains were crossbred so that the maternal animal was of the A strain, 43% of young had cleft palate; but when the dam was of the C57BL strain the incidence of defective young dropped to 4%. Some maternal characteristic, probably ability to metabolize cortisone, as well as the genotype of the embryos which should have been identical in both hybrid groups, were both shown to be involved in determining teratogenesis. Trasler (1960) observed that a stock of mice, prone to have cleft lip spontaneously, showed the defect significantly more often in embryos implanted near the ovaries than at other sites in the uterus, whether or not the maternal animals were treated with a teratogen. Similarly, Warkany and Schraffenberger (1947) found that rat embryos in the cephalic end of the uterine horns were more susceptible to the teratogenic effects of x-irradiation than their more caudally situated littermates. Thus, maternal phenotype and implantation site within the uterus, and undoubtedly extramaternal environmental factors as well, act in an unknown way with the genotype of the embryo to cause deviations from normal development.

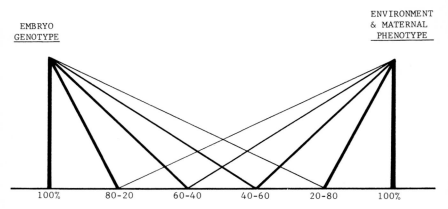

FIG. 2-1. Diagram suggesting varying degrees of interaction between genotype of the embryo and the environment, including the maternal body, that are thought to account for most deviations in development. Proabably relatively few such deviations are caused solely by either genetic or environmental influences, most are thought to result from an interplay between the two. (From Wilson, 1972a.)

Fraser (1959) has suggested that a minority of malformations have major environmental cause and a minority have major genetic cause, but that most probably result from complex interactions between genetic predispositions and subtle factors in the environment, as suggested in Fig. 2-1. Well-documented examples are not numerous, but Hurley (1969), in reviewing the subject of interaction between maternal nutritional deficiency and the genotype of the offspring, describes a striking instance of reciprocal interplay between a gene and the metabolism of manganese. The congenital ataxia of a mutant strain of mice *(pallid)* was mimicked by maternal manganese deficiency in nonmutant animals, and the ataxia of mutant mice was prevented by manganese therapy of the pregnant mother. A possible human example of interacting genetic and environmental factors may be the condition among certain Mediterranean peoples known as favism, which is related in a complex way to both genetic background and the eating of the Mediterranean broad bean (Sartori, 1971).

The nature of the interaction between the genes of an embryo and a teratogenic agent is not clear, but certain possibilities seem likely. In discussing phenocopies (induced abnormalities that simulate naturally occurring ones), Goldschmidt (1957) concluded that ". . . the hypothesis can hardly be avoided that all phenocopies are due to a bringing into light of already present, non-penetrant, subthreshold . . . mutants." Landauer (1957) expresses a similar thought in other words: ". . . our evidence leads us to conclude that specific defects as well as experimental phenocopies are the results of events through which ordinarily hidden weaknesses of developmental equilibria become manifest and that these weaknesses have a definite, if complex, genetic basis." This hypothesis receives support from experiments in which animals without treatment exhibit spontaneously a low incidence of a given malformation, but show a marked increase in incidence of the defect when teratogenic treatment is given. Runner (1959) observed that the 129 strain of mice regularly showed a 2% occurrence of axial skeletal defects, but that when a folic acid antagonist, insulin, starvation, or iodoacetate was given during pregnancy, the occurrence of these abnormalities was increased 10 to 15 times. Similar examples have been described by Andersen (1949), Ingalls and Curley (1957), Landauer (1957), and others. Russell and Russell (1954) pointed out that the converse is also true: that a feature which shows little or no natural variability is likely to be resistant to change under the influence of extrinsic factors.

D. MULTIFACTORIAL CAUSATION

It has been proposed by Fraser *et al.* (1957) and Kalter (1957) that a majority of spontaneously occurring malformations are the result, not of single genetic or single extrinsic factors, but of a combination of many genetic and many environmental factors. Although this hypothesis is not easily investigated in the laboratory, a few experiments involving the use of multiple extrinsic factors in small doses have been undertaken. The effects of combined treatments were often additive but with surprising frequency there was potentiation, that is, a greater-than-additive effect, even when similarity of mode of action among the agents seemed unlikely (see Wilson, 1964b for review). It is now recognized that maternal metabolic patterns may be involved in apparent interactions between chemical agents (Burns, 1970). The probability of multifactorial causation, whether involving interaction of genetic loci and adverse factors in the environment, or multiple factors within either category, should not be lightly regarded, despite the paucity of good examples at this time. Several investigators have expressed the view that many of the human developmental defects now designated as being of unknown causation (see Table 3-1) are the result of multifactorial interactions too complex to be identified by present methods.

II. Susceptibility to Teratogenesis Varies with the Developmental Stage at the Time of Exposure to an Adverse Influence

A. SUBDIVISIONS OF THE DEVELOPMENTAL SPAN

A remarkable series of changes is displayed by the human conceptus during the first few weeks of intrauterine life, as summarized in Chapter 7. The

Pre differentiation Period

Usually Not Susceptible
to
Teratogenesis

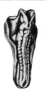

Period of Early Differentiation

Highly Susceptible
to Teratogenesis

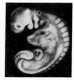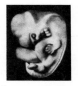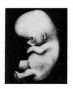

Period of Advanced Organogenesis

Increasingly Resistant
to Teratogenesis
With Increasing Age

FIG. 2-2. Variable susceptibility to teratogenesis during the embryonic period. An initial refractory phase includes cleavage and blastocyst stages and probably continues up to the time when the primitive streak is established (about 17 days postconception in man, see Fig. 7–8). The embryo becomes highly susceptible during the early stages of tissue and organ differentiation (probably days 18 or 20 to 30 in man) and thereafter shows increasing resistance to teratogenesis as organogenesis advances (mainly completed by days 55 to 60 in man). (From Wilson, 1965a.)

most dramatic of these occur during the period of organogenesis, that is, from gestation days 20 to 55, but some aspects of development, e.g., histogenesis, growth, and functional maturation, continue throughout fetal life and are not completed until after birth. There is a degree of vulnerability to induced developmental deviation throughout the total span of development; but experimental studies in animals have clearly demonstrated that the greatest danger is associated with a relatively short period of critical embryogenesis between germ-layer differentiation (gastrulation) and completion of major organ formation. Susceptibility varies even within this period of embryogenesis (Fig. 2-2). There is an initial refractory period from fertilization through cleavage, blastocyst, and early germ-layer stages, when little teratogenesis, but appreciable lethality, may occur. This is followed by a pe-

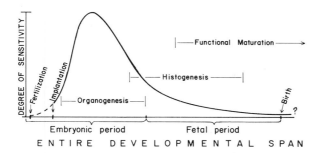

FIG. 2-3. Curve approximating the susceptibility of the human embryo to teratogenesis from fertilization throughout intrauterine development. The highest sensitivity, at least to structural deviation, occurs during the period of organogenesis, from about days 18 to 20 until about days 55 to 60, although as noted in Fig. 2-2 the absolute peak of sensitivity may be reached before day 30 postconception. As organogenesis is completed susceptibility to anatomical defects diminishes greatly, but probably minor structural deviation is possible until histogenesis is completed late in the fetal period. Deviations during the fetal period are more likely to involve growth or functional aspects because these are the predominant developmental features at this time. (From Wilson, 1972a.)

riod of maximal susceptibility to teratogenesis that coincides with differentiation and early organogenesis. Appreciable embryolethality also occurs during this period if dosage is at high teratogenic levels. As organogenesis advances during the latter part of the embryo period, both teratogenicity and lethality steadily decline, although both still can occur if dosage is elevated sufficiently.

Teratogenic susceptibility is represented in Fig. 2-3 as a hypothetical curve in relation to various developmental processes. It is seen that some degree of response can be elicited throughout the intrauterine part of development and may continue at a diminished level for a time after birth. As suggested above, the nature and the degree of embryotoxic manifestations change as the times of their inception coincides with different developmental processes. During organogenesis when the major processes within the embryo are differentiation, mobilization, and organization of cell and tissue groups into organs, interference with development causes gross structural defects of the type usually designated as malformations. As the end of the embryonic period approaches, but before organogenesis is complete, histogenesis begins and by means of successive cellular and tissue specializations converts the primordial organs into definitive ones. While histogenesis proceeds, functional maturation also begins and both continue throughout the fetal period. The fetal period is further characterized by growth toward the size and proportions typical of the newborn infant. Interference with development during the fetal period would, therefore, be expected to result primarily in growth retardation and in functional disturbances, although less conspicuous structural defects at the tissue level might also result if the progress of histogenesis were disturbed. Such segregation of the types of defects according to the times of their inception has often been noted in animal experiments (see Section II, B–F) and now has been observed among infants born to women infected at different times during pregnancy with rubella (Sever, 1970).

B. THE EARLY REFRACTORY PERIOD

That the mammalian embryo is usually refractory to teratogenesis during cleavage, blastocyst, and early germ-layer stages has been repeatedly shown with a variety of agents such as irradiation (Hicks, 1953; Russell, 1950; Wilson, 1954a), vitamin deficiencies (Cheng et al., 1957; Nelson et al., 1955), vitamin excess (Cohlan, 1954), and many others. The rare exceptions include a few ocular defects seen in newborn rats subjected to hypoxia on days 1 to 8 of gestation (Werthemann and Reiniger, 1950), and monstrous development in a litter of hamsters subjected to hypothermia on day 2 of gestation (Smith, 1957). There is evidence that drugs inhibiting RNA biosynthesis may act earlier than other types of teratogenic agents, e.g., actinomycin D is teratogenic on day 5 in the rat, well before visible embryonic differentiation begins (Wilson, 1966).

The exact nature of the phenomenon that makes these early embryonic stages more refractory to teratogenesis is not known. Very likely it has something to do with whether individual cells in the embryos have become predetermined (induced) to form specific parts of the future organism, or whether they retain a degree of the original totipotency of the fertilized egg. The change in cellular potentiality that occurs about the time of first mesoderm formation in mammals, or gastrulation in lower forms (Gross, 1967), is probably the time at which the new varieties of RNA needed for organogenesis begin to be synthesized in embryo cells. In any event, when a teratogenic agent acts before such chemical differentiation begins, specific tissue or organ defects are not produced because cells have not yet been chemically induced to form specific tissues and organs. Before differentiation all cells are probably alike in having the same susceptibilities and metabolic needs and, therefore, would be expected to react alike to a teratogenic insult. A stimulus adequate to kill or damage a portion of such a homogeneous population of cells would kill the embryo or retard its growth, but ordinarily would not cause specific malformations (Wilson et al., 1953).

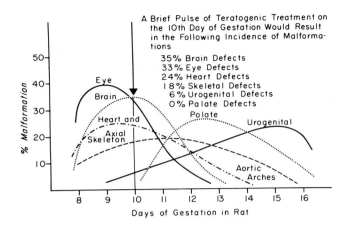

FIG. 2-4. Group of curves representing the susceptibility of particular organs and organ systems in rat embryos to a hypothetical teratogenic agent given on different days of gestation. If the agent were applied on day 10, a syndrome comprised of organs the curves of which are intersected by the vertical line would result, with percentages of incidence corresponding to the points at which the curves were crossed. Shifting the time of treatment from day 10 to another day would alter the composition of the syndrome both qualitatively and quantitatively. (From Wilson, 1965a.)

C. The Highly Susceptible Period of Organogenesis

Abruptly, as organogenesis begins, the embryo becomes susceptible to most teratogenic agents (Fig. 2-3) and at or soon after this time many agents produce their highest incidence of malformations (Ingalls and Curley, 1957; Hicks, 1953; Russell, 1950; Cheng *et al.,* 1957; Nelson *et al.,* 1955; Cohlan, 1954; Wilson, 1957). Visible differentiation of tissue and organ primordia at this time is thought to be preceded by several hours by chemical differentiation or, as noted above, synthesis of the appropriate RNA's to code for the enzymatic and structural proteins characteristic of specific tissues and organs. Although malformations are often most easily produced soon after the structural differentiation of the target organ begins, it is by no means always the case that overt developmental events can be correlated with the time an agent is active. For example, renal anomalies were induced by irradiating rat embryos on day 9 of gestation, but the earliest primordium of the metanephros does not appear until day 12 (Wilson *et al.,* 1953). Skeletal abnormalities have been produced by a variety of means many hours before even rudimentary skeletal structures are recognizable (Murphy, 1959; Russell, 1956).

Most organs, nevertheless, have a period of particular susceptibility to extrinsic teratogenic influences during the early developmental events in that organ, although the total period of organ-specific sensitivity may extend over several days (Fig. 2-4). The high point and usual duration of this susceptible period are best studied with minimal doses of the agent (Russell, 1950; Wilson, 1954a; Landauer, 1954). Excessive doses cause individual defects to appear on days other than those of greatest susceptibility (Warkany and Schraffenberger, 1947; Russell, 1950). Many organs show more than one susceptible period, reflecting the fact that their embryogenesis is multiphasic, with vulnerable stages at different times (Russell and Russell, 1954; Landauer, 1954).

D. DIMINISHING SUSCEPTIBILITY IN FETAL PERIOD

Teratogenic susceptibility decreases as organogenesis proceeds (Fig. 2-3). The proliferative and morphogenetic activities characteristic of early or-

TABLE 2-1

CHANGING TYPES AND INCIDENCES (%) OF MALFORMATIONS IN RAT EMBRYOS IRRADIATED ON DIFFERENT DAYS OF GESTATION[a]

Gestation day	Dose (R)			
	25	50	100	200
8	None	None	None	No survivors
9	Eye (6)	Eye (72), brain (9), spinal cord (3)	Eye (90), brain (41), spinal cord (27), heart (20), face (14), situs inversus (13), aortic arch (10), urinary (5)	Eye (100), brain (78), spinal cord (67), situs inversus (55), heart (22), face (11), aortic arch (11)
10		Eye (11)	Eye (75), urinary (11), brain (3)	Eye (94), feet (33), brain (19), urinary (11), aortic arch (11)
11			None	Eye (100), urinary (77), brain (54), spinal cord (31), aortic arch (23), ear (23), tail (23), heart (15), jaw (15), feet (7)

[a] From Wilson (1954a).

gan formation become less evident and increasing structural specialization becomes more evident as the embryo grows older; accompanying these signs of advancing differentiation is increasing resistance to teratogenic agents (Fraser and Fainstat, 1951; Kalter, 1954; Dagg and Karnofsky, 1955; Wilson, 1954a; Wilson *et al.,* 1953). Larger doses of an agent are required to produce comparable degrees of abnormality than were needed earlier and, indeed, comparable degrees and types of defects may become impossible to induce during fetal life. With individual organs collectively becoming more resistant, naturally the embryo as a whole also becomes more resistant to teratogenesis (Hicks, 1953; Nelson *et al.,* 1955). This was exemplified by an experiment in which exposure of rat embryos to 100 R of x-rays on day 9 of gestation caused many types of malformations in virtually all fetuses; the same treatment on day 10 caused somewhat fewer malformations in 75% of the animals, whereas the same treatment on day 11 did not produce any malformations (Table 2-1).

The syndrome of malformations changes when the same agent is applied at different times in gestation, as has been shown in experiments with short-term vitamin deficiencies at various times in gestation (Nelson *et al.,* 1955, 1956; Skalko *et al.,* 1971). Such changes relate to the fact that the various organs pass through susceptible periods at different times; hence an induced vitamin deficiency extending from days 11 to 14 affects other organs than one extending from days 7 to 9 (Table 2-2). The duration of action of an agent also affects the composition of the syndrome. Vitamin A deficiency terminated on day 10 by large doses of the vitamin resulted only in heart abnormalities, whereas allowing the deficiency to continue to day 15 produced abnormalities of the eyes, aortic arches, diaphragm, lungs, and

TABLE 2-2

TIME SPECIFICITY RELATIVE TO ORGANS AFFECTED BY TRANSITORY FOLIC ACID DEFICIENCY DURING RAT GESTATION[a]

Days deficient	No. abnormal young	Percentage with specific abnormality						
		Cleft palate	Fore-limb	Hind-limb	Kidney	Heart, aortic arch	Abdominal hernia	Brain
11–14	124	48	60	92	—	—	—	—
10–13	126	100	90	88	66	29	—	—
10–12	115	61	—	61	11	32	—	—
9–11	125	86	5	48	49	58	22	—
7–9	39	—	—	—	8	53	21	49

[a] From Nelson *et al.* (1955).

several genitourinary organs (Wilson *et al.,* 1953). Short-term treatments tend to cause only a portion of the total syndrome that would result from long-term treatment (Fig. 2-4).

E. BIRTH AND AFTERWARD

Birth transfers the fetus from the relatively stable intrauterine environment to the more variable, usually more stressful, extramaternal environment. Since full development is not complete in some systems (e.g., the nervous and endocrine systems) until after birth, it would appear *a priori* that the shock of birth or subsequent events might occasionally impair unfinished developmental processes. There is only limited evidence that this occurs, aside from birth injuries such as torn blood vessels and nerves, and it can be concluded that many of the more vulnerable aspects of development are complete before birth. Several studies, however, indicate that older fetuses or postnatal infants may have certain aspects of their functional development diverted or arrested by drugs (Apgar, 1964; Sutherland and Light, 1965) or possibly by nutritional deprivation (Yaktin and McLaren, 1970). The postnatal period has only recently begun to be examined critically for situations that might adversely affect subsequent development, particularly of growth and mental maturation. As more attention is focused on this subject and as better methods for critical evaluation become available, it is probable that further examples will be found.

F. WHAT ABOUT THE GERM CELLS?

Germ cells and the germinal epithelium from which they derive are subject to damage by such varied environmental influences as dietary deficiency (Mason, 1933) and a variety of drugs (Fox and Fox, 1967), but it has not been definitely established whether certain stages of gametogenesis are more susceptible to lasting damage than others. Oocytes and mature ova were readily destroyed by irradiation of adult rodents (Genther, 1934; Ingram, 1958); a single exposure of the ovaries of rhesus monkeys with 600 R of x-rays not only reduced the number of ova, but also resulted in early abortion in virtually all treated females (van Wagenen and Gardner, 1960). The latter suggests that surviving ova, although capable of fertilization and of proceeding to implantation, were defective in some way that contributed to early death of embryos. The more mature stages of spermatogenesis have long been known to be inhibited by abrupt elevation of environmental temperature (Bowler, 1972), or simply by the slight elevation of mean temperature that occurs when the testes remain in the pelvis instead of descending into the scrotum. There is little information to indicate whether germ cell mutations are more likely to be induced by such environmental changes at one time than another in the spermatogenic cycle. Russell (1951) induced mutations in mice by irradiating spermatagonia at doses that killed intermediate stages in spermatogenesis. Ehling *et al.,* (1968) reported that dominant lethal mutations in mice were more often induced by alkane sulfonate esters in mature sperm then in the earlier spermatids.

III. Teratogenic Agents Act in Specific Ways (Mechanisms) on Developing Cells and Tissues to Initiate Sequences of Abnormal Developmental Events (Pathogenesis)

Early studies in experimental teratology demonstrated that particular agents often produced characteristic patterns of malformations (Ancel, 1950; Landauer, 1954). The term "agent specificity" was applied to situations wherein the agent was thought to be associated with a recognizable pattern of defects (Wilson, 1957). This belief received considerable support from the repeated demonstration by Landauer and associates (1954, 1958, 1960, 1963, 1964, 1968, 1970) that precise relationships existed between chemical teratogenic agents and the metabolic needs of chick embryos. Attempts to protect embryos against the effects of known teratogens by administering specific supplements revealed that riboflavin protected against 6-aminonicotinamide and 3-acetylpyridine; nicotinamide against insulin, sulfanilamide, and eserine; and 1-proline against nicotine. It was concluded not only that abnormal embryogenesis followed interference with localized metabolic needs, but also that many, if not all, such interferences were with enzymatic processes.

A. MECHANISMS OF TERATOGENESIS

Experimental approaches to the problem of how teratogenic agents initiate abnormal development are still limited in number, but the conviction has grown that there are several ways, in addition to the one suggested by Landauer, by which adverse environmental influences may attack developing cells. A recent attempt to summarize information on this subject (Wilson, 1972a) yielded a tentative list of nine ways in which extraneous influences were thought likely to affect cells in such a way as to change their prescribed course of development. These were called mechanisms of teratogenesis (Scheme 1-1) and were defined in Chapter 1 as early, presumably determining, reactions of developing cells to extraneous influences. They will be discussed fully in Chapter 4, but in the present context of teratogenic principles they are briefly mentioned as an important link between cause (agent) and final effect (defect). A particular cause from the environment probably is able to initiate one or several mechanisms; for example, ionizing radiations may cause point mutations, chromosomal nondisjunction, mitotic interference, and enzyme inhibition. Similarly, maternal nutritional deficiency

TABLE 2-3

COMPARISON OF MATERNAL LD$_{50}$ AND TYPICAL EMBRYOTOXIC DOSES IN RATS GIVEN SINGLE TREATMENT AT A TERATOGENICALLY SUSCEPTIBLE TIME IN GESTATION[a]

Agent	Approximate maternal LD$_{50}$ (mg/kg)	Typical embryotoxic dose (mg/kg)	Approximate ratio
Alkylating agents			
Nitrogen mustard	2	0.5	4:1
Cyclophosphamide	40	15	3:1
Triethylenemelamine	1.25	0.75	2:1
Triethylenethiophosphoramide	8	2	4:1
Chlorambucil	24	6	4:1
Myleran	60	18	3:1
Antimetabolites			
Azaserine	100	3	33:1
6-Mercaptopurine	250	25	10:1
6-Mercaptopurine riboside	2000–3000	50	50:1
Thioguanine	350	12	29:1
Thioguanine riboside	200–400	15	20:1
5-Fluoroorotic acid	300–400	75	5:1
5-Fluorouracil	230	30	8:1
5-Fluorouridine	400–800	20	30:1
5-Fluorodeoxycytidine	800–1600	2.5	500:1
5-Iododeoxyuridine	4000–8000	1200	5:1
5-Bromodeoxyuridine	1500–4000	500	5:1
Cytosine arabinoside	1000	100	10:1
6-Aminonicotinamide	15	8	2:1
Methotrexate	17	0.5	34:1
Antibiotics			
Actinomycin D	0.4	0.3	1.3:1
Mitomycin C	3	3	1:1
Streptonigrin	0.4	0.2	2:1
Miscellaneous			
Hydroxyurea	4700	500	9:1
Methylhydrazine	350	50	7:1
Thiadiazole	200	100	2:1
Triazene	180	60	3:1

[a] From Wilson (1968), based on data collected in the laboratories of Dr. Lois M. Murphy and of the author.

could result in lack of substrates and precursors or in osmolar imbalance. Whatever the nature of these early reactions, however, they undoubtedly lead to abnormal embryogenesis if present in sufficient amount.

B. PATHOGENESIS OF THE DEFECT

It is postulated that one or a combination of mechanisms could precipitate a sequence of abnormal developmental pathogenetic events that would lead to the final defect (Table 2-3). Strictly speaking, the first event of pathogenesis is the initiating mechanism itself, but in the interest of clarity it may be better to consider pathogenesis as beginning with the first readily demonstrable event. Accordingly, pathogenesis can usually be shown to begin as one or more overt occurrences, such as cell death (Gruenwald, 1958; Menkes *et al.,* 1970); reduced biosynthesis (Ritter *et al.,* 1971; Scott *et al.,* 1971); impaired morphogenetic movement (Trinkaus, 1965); failed tissue interaction (induction) (Saxén and Toivonen, 1962); or mechanical disruption, as by fluid accumulations (Grabowski, 1970). It is possible that these initially different types of pathogenesis may converge into a relatively narrow channel of abnormal development, for example, one that would lead ultimately to insufficient cells or cell products to carry out morphogenesis or to carry on function at the site of the final defect.

To propose such a final common pathway (Scheme 2-1) may be an oversimplification of pathogenesis, despite the fact most structural and many functional defects do indeed seem to be the result of too few cells or cell products. In the realm of malformations there are a few obvious exceptions including the structural defects that involve supernumerary parts, such as in polydactyly or duplication of segments of the digestive and urinary tracts,

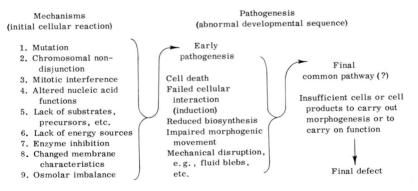

SCHEME 2-1. Schematic summary of initial cellular reactions and different types of pathogenesis converging into a final common pathway.

which appear to involve an excess rather than a deficiency of tissue. This subject will be discussed further in Chapter 5 and is mentioned here mainly to emphasize the fact that the earlier view of specificity, in the sense of one cause leading directly to one pattern of defects, may no longer be tenable. The bulk of evidence seems strongly to indicate that agents may activate more than one teratogenic mechanism and that mechanisms•may initiate pathogenesis in one or several ways but that these various early events often appear to converge into a few if not a circumscribed pathway to produce the final defect.

IV. The Access of Adverse Influences to Developing Tissues Depends on the Nature of the Influence (Agent)

A. PHYSICAL AGENTS

Developing tissues, whether germ cells, embryos, or fetuses, are more sensitive to environmental factors than are mature somatic tissues, but fortunately they are less often or less intensely exposed. The parental body affords a degree of protection by shielding formative tissues from extraneous influences, but the effectiveness of this shielding varies with the type of the agent. Physical agents, such as low-energy radiations, tend to be excluded from germ cells and the intrauterine occupant simply by the thickness and mass of parental tissues. Extreme variations in the concentrations of respiratory gases or in environmental temperatures are required to override the homeostatic mechanisms of the parental body sufficiently to cause abnormal development. The notable exception among physical factors is ionizing radiations which, although reduced in intensity by passage through parental tissues, nevertheless are able to penetrate to the developing tissues in some fraction of the air dosage. This may account for the fact that x-radiation was one of the first environmental agents to be implicated in both mammalian and in human teratogenesis, and it remains today as one of the most precise experimental tools.

B. CHEMICAL AGENTS

Chemical agents, on the other hand, probably always reach germ cells, embryos, or fetuses in some fraction of their concentration in the parental bloodstream, at least when the level is more than negligible. Whether developmental abnormality results depends on whether a critical dosage reaches or is able to accumulate in the developing tissues. The subject of modulation of the dosage of chemical agents by parental homeostasis and placental transport is discussed fully in Chapter 6 and is only introduced here because it is a basic principle and is one of the main determinants of teratogenesis.

The concentration of foreign substances in the parental bloodstream tends to be reduced by catabolic degradation (detoxification), excretion, protein binding, tissue storage, etc., but the reduction of the initial concentration by half (half-life) may require many hours. Depending on the nature of the compound, the placenta is often able to maintain a concentration gradient that is lower on the embryonic or fetal side than on the maternal side. Nevertheless, the placenta should not be regarded as a barrier in the sense of being impervious because it probably does not absolutely exclude any chemical agent (Villee, 1967). Even molecules of large size and of high electrical charge are known to cross, albeit at a slow rate. The critical determinant in chemical teratogenesis, therefore, is not whether but at what rate the substance traverses the placenta.

The amount of a chemical transported per unit of time depends on, in addition to molecular size and charge, lipid solubility, degree of ionization, whether complexed to other compounds, existence of a transplacental concentration gradient, and possibly metabolism of the compound by the placenta (Moya and Thorndike, 1962; Ginsburg, 1971). If in sum these conditions favor rapid transport from maternal blood to embryonic fluid compart-

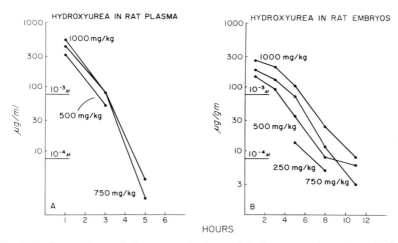

Fig. 2-5. Comparison of the concentrations of hydroxyurea in maternal plasma and in embryos from 12-day pregnant rats at varying hours after treatment. A. Concentration in maternal plasma after different IP doses. The ordinate is in log units. Each point is the mean of at least 3 animals. B. Concentration in embryos after different IP doses. The ordinate is in log units. Each point represents the mean of at least 3 animals with a minimum of 4 embryos from each animal. Molar concentrations *(M)* on the ordinate indicate the level at which DNA synthetic rate in embryos was resumed after being inhibited at higher concentrations and also corresponds with the inhibitory dose for cells in culture. (From Scott *et al.,* 1971.)

ments, the embryo may receive an embryotoxic dose. If, on the other hand, an effective level is not reached within a few hours after maximal concentration in maternal blood, an embryonic effect-level may not be reached because further maternal–embryonic transfer is increasingly unlikely after concentration of free compound in maternal blood falls to low levels. This does not mean that total concentration may not remain high on the embryonic side. Certain chemicals are known to traverse the placenta from embryo to mother more slowly than from mother to embryo, presumably as a result of incorporation or selective binding within the embryo (Fig. 2-5). Thus, because absorption, metabolism, and elimination by the parental organism, as well as transport by the placenta, are determined by the properties of a chemical agent, the particular agent may fail to be teratogenic or mutagenic in mammals regardless of its potential for affecting embryos or cells *in vitro*. It simply may never reach the *in vivo* embryo or germ cell in effective dosage.

V. The Four Manifestations of Deviant Development Are Death, Malformation, Growth Retardation, and Functional Defecit

An adverse influence at any time during the span of development is theoretically capable of producing one or more of four types of developmental deviations, namely, (1) death of the developing organism, (2) structural abnormality (malformation), (3) growth retardation, or (4) functional deficiency. In animal experiments, however, these have not been found equally likely to occur at all exposure times, as was particularly well demonstrated with radiation (Brent, 1969). Irradiation during cleavage and blastocyst stages has mainly caused death of the embryo (Russell and Russell, 1954), although growth retardation has also been induced by treatment after implantation but prior to differentiation (Wilson, 1954a). Malformations were rarely produced at such times even with high dosage. During early organogenesis both embryonic death and malformations have been readily induced by most teratogenic agents, and both manifestations tended to increase in dose-related fashion (Nelson *et al.,* 1952, 1955, 1956; Landauer, 1958; Giroud and Martinet, 1955; Grabowski and Paar, 1958; Waddington and Carter, 1952; Wilson, 1955). Strains of mice that were highly sensitive to the teratogenic effects of cortisone were also found to be highly susceptible to its lethal effects and, conversely, resistant strains were resistant to both effects (Fraser and Fainstat, 1951). As embryolethality has approached totality, however, the percentage of malformed young reaching term has decreased because many malformed conceptuses died early and were resorbed (Beck and Lloyd, 1963).

A. DEATH VERSUS MALFORMATION

This raises the difficult question of the relationship between intrauterine death and malformation. For the present it is sufficient to say that there is reason in many situations to regard them as separate manifestations rather than as different degrees of reaction on the part of the embryo to the same type of injury. Landauer (1958) assumed that a majority of the teratogenic agents he used in chicken eggs had "systemic effects," aside from the teratogenic ones, with which the recuperative powers of the embryo could not cope, thus resulting in death. Grabowski and Paar (1958) observed a high incidence of immediate death among chick embryos exposed to hypoxia which they felt had nothing to do with the malformations observed later, although they regarded many of the delayed deaths as owing to undetected classes of malformations. Johnson and Lambert (1968) noted that 20 mg/kg of N-nitroso-N-methylurea on days 8 or 10 of rat gestation produced only embryolethality, whereas the same dose on day 13 produced mainly malformation. Cohlan (1954) reported that the incidence of malformations resulting from hypervitaminosis A did not change when the dose of vitamin A was raised from 35,000 to 75,000 IU although this increase caused a considerable reduction in the number of litters reaching term. On the other hand, Zwilling and De Bell (1950) found that the teratogenic effect of sulfanilamide increased as dosage increased but that the lethal effect did not. Both malformations and mortality usually decrease as gestational age at the time of teratogenic treatment increases (Kalter, 1957; Wilson, 1954a).

In experimental situations, generally, death and deformity often occur together and respond to teratogenic stimuli in such a way as to suggest that they are only different degrees of response to the same type of injury. If embryonic stages are examined prior to term following teratogenic treatment, severe types of malformations are found which are rarely seen if the offspring are allowed to go to term (Beck and Lloyd, 1963; Kaven, 1938; Wilson and Warkany, 1949). This doubtless means that certain malformations themselves cause death *in utero,* but it does not exclude the likelihood that some induced mortality is independent of malformation.

B. GROWTH RETARDATION AND FUNCTIONAL DEFICIENCY

As intrauterine development progresses both death and malformation of the conceptus become less likely and the possibility of growth retardation and functional deficiency may increase (Hurley, 1968a). Although not widely investigated, the latter possibility is to be expected because growth and functional maturation are the primary developmental processes that remain at least theoretically vulnerable until birth. In fact these developmental parameters are not complete in any mammal until after birth and there is some evidence that nutritional deprivation during infancy is associated with chemical, functional, and growth rate changes in young animals and children (Winick, 1969, 1971; Yaktin and McLaren, 1970). There is a logical basis for regarding growth retardation as a mild expression of generalized functional retardation.

C. DOSAGE LEVEL AND TYPES OF MANIFESTATIONS

Because the different manifestations of deviant development are not induced with equal ease at different times in the developmental span, the dosage required to induce them is also variable. The susceptible early embryo is readily malformed or killed by a relatively small dose of suitable agents, but much larger doses of the same agents may be harmless to the fetus, as was frequently shown with thalidomide, or cause only moderate growth retardation, as was observed with malnutrition (Hurley, 1968b). The low dosage needed to induce malformation and intrauterine death, on the one hand, and the relatively higher dosage required to cause congenital functional disorder, on the other, undoubtedly account for the higher frequency of the former than of the latter types of developmental disorder. It is unwise, however, to generalize too broadly about the scarcity of functional deficits until more is known about the etiology as well as the detection of such disorders. It has only recently been realized that mental deficiency in children is frequently associated with phenylketonuria in their mothers (Hansen, 1970; Yu and O'Halloran, 1970). Mental retardation is one of the most common developmental defects but in the majority of instances its causation remains obscure.

VI. Manifestations of Deviant Development Increase in Frequency and Degree as Dosage Increases, from the No-Effect to the Totally Lethal Level

This principle is of major importance in relation to the safety evaluation of new drugs and other environmental agents. The focal issue is whether the demonstration of abnormal development at high dosage levels signifies that the substance in question is unsafe at all levels. In other words, is there a threshold below which no manifestation of abnormality is seen, i.e., a no-effect range of dosage, or does the probability of adverse effects simply become smaller as dosage is lowered toward the vanishing point?

A. THRESHOLDS IN TERATOGENESIS

Experimental teratologists have generally assumed that all embryotoxic agents do have a threshold below which no effect of any kind can be dem-

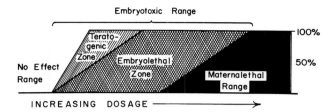

Fig. 2-6. Diagram of the toxic manifestations shown by the embryos and the maternal organisms as dosage of a teratogenic agent increases. Numerous teratological studies in animals have consistently shown that there is a no-effect range of dosage below the threshold at which embryotoxic effects begin abruptly to appear. Teratogenesis and increased embryolethality often have a similar threshold, and they may increase at roughly parallel rates as dosage increases up to the point that all conceptuses are affected. Increase in dosage beyond this point causes embryolethality to increase, but teratogenicity appears to decrease because increasing numbers of defective embryos die before term. Further increase in dosage eventually reaches the maternal lethal range.

onstrated. This is based on a large number of studies in animals using the easily quantitated criteria of intrauterine death and structural abnormality in near-term fetuses. When a suitable range of dosage has been given during sensitive periods of development, a no-effect range below the threshold at which embryotoxicity began (Fig. 2-6) has regularly been demonstrated. The argument that extremely large numbers of animals are necessary to establish the existence of no-effect levels is valid under two conditions: (1) when the slope of the dose–response curve is flat, and (2) when independent cells rather than organisms capable of regulation and repair are studied. As will be discussed below, dose–response curves in teratology are typically quite steep. Furthermore, embryotoxic responses depend on the reaction of integrated groups of cells, tissues, and organs, rather than on independent cells, as will be discussed in Chapter 3.

Thus, all evidence indicates that a dosage can always be found below which intrauterine death or malformation in excess of that seen in controls is not produced. The same is almost certainly true as regards growth retardation, although this has not been so exhaustively studied as death and malformation. The only area of embryotoxicity for which the existence of a no-effect range of dosage can reasonably be questioned concerns postnatal functional disorders, and this because there is only limited direct evidence on which to base a conclusion at this time. A definitive determination of whether small doses of adverse influences during development can cause permanent functional disorder would require that large numbers of animals be subjected to a comprehensive battery of physiologic tests for an extended

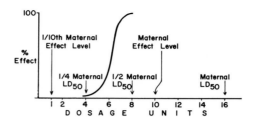

FIG. 2-7. Chart illustrating that embryotoxic effects are usually seen at some fraction of the dosage that causes maternal toxic or pharmacological effects. In this diagram the teratogenic range is represented by the curve and occurs between one half and one fourth of the maternal LD_{50} dose. The dose–response curve for teratogenicity is typically steep, sometimes rising from a no-effect level to a 100%-effect level by doubling the dose, as is represented in this diagram.

period after birth. Until such tests become practicable, the lack of evidence to the contrary permits a tentative assumption that functional disorder, like the other types of developmental toxicity, has a threshold of dosage below which it is not induced.

B. EMBRYOTOXICITY AND MATERNAL TOXICITY

As noted earlier, increased malformations and embryolethality often begin to appear at approximately the same dosage. Beyond this point these manifestations tend to increase in roughly parallel fashion for a time, although embryolethality eventually overtakes malformation and precludes any survivors at term. Further increase in dosage beyond that causing total embryolethality sooner or later reaches levels that are first toxic and then lethal to the maternal organism (Fig. 2-6). There is no standard ratio between maternal-effect levels and the embryotoxic ranges of dosage, except that the latter is almost always some fraction of maternal effect-levels (Fig. 2-7). When animal studies are undertaken without prior knowledge of the embryotoxic range, a convenient starting point for selecting dose levels is to make serial half-decrements of the adult LD_{50} dosage, which is easily determined if not already known. Three levels representing one half, one quarter, and one eighth of the maternal LD_{50} will often encompass the embryotoxic range, although embryotoxicity may occasionally not begin until a much smaller fraction of maternal effect-level is reached, as is illustrated in Table 2-3.

C. Dose–Response Curve in Teratogenesis

Typically the dose–response curve for embryotoxic effects has a steep slope, sometimes going from minimal to maximal effect levels by merely doubling the dose (Fig. 2-7). The well-known primate teratogen, thalidomide, seems to be an exception in that initial teratogenic effects are seen during the susceptible period of the embryo at surprisingly low dosage, but many multiples of this may be required to produce total embryolethality, and maternal toxicity is exceedingly difficult to demonstrate (Wilson, 1972b). A less dramatic disparity between embryotoxic and maternal toxic effects is evident in rubella teratogenesis in man, wherein severe malformations are seen among infants born to women who had inapparent or subclinical infection during pregnancy.

D. High Embryotoxicity, Low Maternal Toxicity

In addition to the foregoing human examples, high embryotoxicity associated with minimal maternal toxicity have frequently been observed in experimental teratology (Giroud *et al.,* 1951). Pregnant females have been mildly if at all affected by such potent teratogens as cortisone (Fraser and

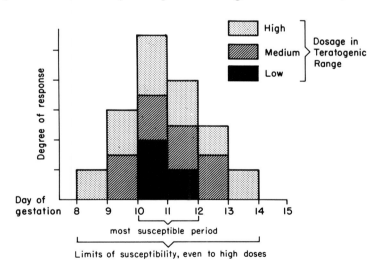

Fig. 2-8. Hypothetical graph to show how increasing dosage affects the degree of response on any one day in the sensitive period and, in addition, may increase the number of days on which a particular defect may be elicited; in other words, lengthening the susceptible period.

Fainstat, 1951), folic acid deficiency produced by PGA antagonist (Nelson *et al.*, 1952), pantothenic acid deficiency (Lefebvres-Boisselot, 1951; Nelson *et al.*, 1957), hypervitaminosis A (Cohlan, 1954), and riboflavin deficiency produced by the antagonist galactoflavin (Kalter and Warkany, 1959). The dams were not always spared, however; Murphy (1959) found that several teratogenic antimetabolites produced wide variables in LD_{50} responses by the mothers as compared with embryotoxicity in their progeny, ranging from a 1:1 ratio for thiadiazol to a 530:1 ratio for 1-norleucine.

E. Dosage Level and Degree of Response

Within the embryotoxic range of dosage it is axiomatic that increased dosage produces an increased degree of response; although, as indicated above, the type of response may change from growth retardation to malformation to intrauterine death. In addition to degree of response at any one time, however, increased dosage has often been observed to lengthen the period of gestation during which a particular defect may be elicited (Russell, 1956; Warkany and Schraffenberger, 1947). For example, a low dose within the teratogenic range might tend to induce a particular defect, mainly on day 10 of gestation, but might also cause a modest incidence on day 11 (Fig. 2-8). Raising dosage to a median level within the teratogenic range would be expected to cause a quantitative increase in the incidence of the defect on days 10 and 11, but in addition the defect might now occur on days other than these, e.g., days 9 and 12. Similarly, increasing dosage to high levels might further enlarge the span over which this defect could be induced, although it would probably also cause some increase in intrauterine death, so that the overall incidence of the defects among treated embryos could actually decrease owing to the attrition of death. As already emphasized, the composition of the syndrome in terms of varieties of defects would also be expected to expand as dosage increases.

CHAPTER 3

CAUSES OF DEVELOPMENTAL ABNORMALITY

Several categories of causation were mentioned in Scheme 1-1 including radiations, chemicals, dietary imbalance, infection, alterations in respiratory gases (hypoxia, etc.), extremes of temperature, metabolic and endocrine imbalances, physical trauma, and placental failure. Theoretically these apply equally to man and to other mammals, but some of these categories are not at this time known to be teratogenic in man. For example, maternal deficiencies of any one of a number of nutritional factors are well known to cause predictable types of developmental defects in laboratory animals but not in man, although the possibility that deficient maternal or infant diets in man may lead to permanent impairment of growth or mental function in the child is at present controversial. It has never been shown that alterations in respiratory gases or extremes of temperature are teratogenic in man, whereas numerous experimental studies have shown that these may divert normal development in animals. Thus the categories of known causation in man are not only fewer but are usually less well substantiated, often being based on incompletely documented case reports and epidemiologic surveys. Because of this difference in the nature of supporting evidence, the causation of developmental deviation in laboratory animals and that in man are discussed separately.

I. In Animals and in General

The individual agents now known to produce deviations in mammalian development number in the hundreds. In recent years these have been variously listed and classified in several reviews (Cahen, 1966; Fave, 1964;

Kalter and Warkany, 1959; Karnofsky, 1965a; Lenz, 1966; Tuchmann-Duplessis, 1965; Wilson, 1964a). Many of the types listed above are also capable of producing alterations in the genetic material of germ cells in postnatal
animals, in addition to acting on embryos and fetuses *in utero;* accordingly,
they are mutagenic (Fishbein *et al.,* 1970) as well as teratogenic in the
usual sense. All mutagenic agents, however, cannot be regarded as teratogenic because by conventional usage a teratogen has a detrimental effect on
development, but all mutations are not detrimental. It is thus necessary to qualify comparisons between mutagenesis and teratogenesis by
noting that only mutagens that produce genetic changes of a detrimental nature are teratogenic. Other aspects of the relationship between mutagenesis
and teratogenesis have been discussed elsewhere (Kalter, 1971; Wilson,
1972c).

To present a catalog of the agents shown to date to be teratogenic in
mammals would be of questionable value in this book. In fact, the publication of lists of toxic agents of any type introduces the dangers of rigidity and
of unquestioning acceptance that are inherent in all static lists. It can be
misleading to categorize a substance as teratogenic or nonteratogenic without considering such experimental variables as animal stocks, dosage, methods of ascertainment, competence of the investigator, etc. The chance that
useful substances uncritically tested may be unjustly restricted from use and
the possibility that others involving an element of risk will be misrepresent-
ed as safe without adequate testing should cause all undocumented catalogs
of teratogenic agents to be regarded with skepticism.

A. Radiations

Ionizing radiation, particularly x-rays, was the first environmental influence shown experimentally to be capable of interfering with intrauterine
development by traversing the mammalian body and acting directly on the
embryo *in utero.* It was also the first agent shown to induce heritable changes
in the germ cells of any animal. The facts that radiations act directly on developing tissues, both germ cells and embryos, with only a reduction of dosage by intervening parental tissues and with sharply delineated duration of
dosage, has made them precise tools in studies of mutagenesis and of teratogenesis generally. Several of the basic principles of teratology were first
clearly elucidated in irradiation experiments (Chapter 2).

1. *Threshold and Radiation Effects*

A striking difference exists in the dosage of radiations required to produce different types of biological effects (Brent, 1972b). Gene mutations,
chromosomal aberrations, and perhaps cancer can be induced by compara-

tively small doses, and several investigators have argued that there may be no threshold (i.e., dosage below which no effect occurs) for the production of these effects. In contrast, malformation, growth retardation, intrauterine death, and postnatal functional deficit generally require larger dosage and are thought by most investigators to have thresholds of dosage below which these effects are not seen. A threshold for production of malformations by radiation has been seriously questioned only by Jacobsen (1970), who reported that doses of x-ray as small as 5 R occasionally were associated with a higher incidence of certain minor skeletal variations than was observed in controls. The minor nature of the defects and the inconsistent dose–response relationships suggest that this dose was itself at or near the threshold, and the study certainly does not rule out the existence of a threshold at lower dosage.

Radiation effects provide excellent illustrations of the conditions which determine the presence or absence of thresholds in biological systems. As noted, such biological effects of radiations as gene mutations, chromosome breaks, and possibly cancer induction may have no or a very low threshold, while most other biological effects exhibit a threshold. A basic difference between the systems that do and those that do not exhibit a threshold is illustrated in Fig. 3-1. Effects that seem not to show a dosage threshold occur in independent or individual cells such as germ cells or cells in culture. Ef-

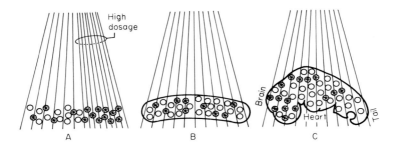

Fig. 3-1. Diagrammatic representation of the threshold phenomenon in relation to cell death caused by radiations or other cytotoxic agents. A. Independent cells such as those in cultures or the germ cells in the gonads do not exhibit a threshold as far as the population as a whole is concerned, cells are killed in proportion to dosage and some may be killed even at extremely small doses. B. Associated cells, such as those comprising an early embryo before organogenesis has begun, can tolerate some cell death without lasting effect, if the lost cells are later replaced by proliferative activity of surviving cells. A threshold for embryo death is evident when cell death exceeds the capacity of surviving cells to restore the loss by later proliferation. C. Associated cells, as in an embryo that has begun organogenesis, show thresholds for teratogenesis when critical numbers of cells in particular organs are affected, otherwise regeneration may occur. (The darker circles represent "hit" cells which are presumed to die.)

fects that appear only after a threshold of dosage is reached occur in organized or associated groups of cells such as comprise an embryo. When radiation or other cytotoxic agents are applied to nonassociated cells, each presumably reacts independently of what may happen in surrounding cells. The total number of cells affected, probably tantamount to the number killed (Hollaender and Stapleton, 1959), is proportional to dosage and in the case of radiations depends on how many individual cells are "hit." The probability of hitting any one cell diminishes as dosages decreases but theoretically does not disappear as long as any ionizing radiation reaches the chromatin of any cell.

Effects in multicellular organisms, death, growth retardation, and malformation, depend on the destruction of critical numbers of cells out of the total of those making up the organism, or embryo. Although the initial effect may be on the chromatin of individual cells (Dewey et al., 1971), probably leading to cell death, the final effect on the embryo depends on the proportion of the total number of cells in vital parts destroyed. It has been reported by a number of investigators (Brent, 1969; Russell and Russell, 1954; Wilson, 1954a; Wilson et al., 1953) that irradiation of embryos prior to the beginning of organogenesis produces very few malformations but may cause embryonic death and growth retardation if the dosage is above a threshold level (25–100 R). Cells are undoubtedly killed at subthreshold doses (Fig. 3-1B), but embryos of all species are thought capable of tolerating the loss of a limited number of cells without lasting effect, owing to their regulative or regenerative capacity.

After organogenesis begins (Fig. 3-1C) different groups of cells acquire different potentialities for future development. Nevertheless, a certain number of cells may still be killed without causing a lasting effect. If a critical number of cell deaths occurs in a differentiating tissue, however, the organ derived from this tissue may be malformed, as has been demonstrated with chemical cytotoxic agents as well as radiations (Hicks, 1954; Ritter et al., 1971; Scott et al., 1971). Thus the regenerative or regulative powers of the embryo make possible the repair of organ primordia up to a point, beyond which repair is inadequate and malformation is likely to be the result. Such a threshold phenomenon probably exists in all organisms that have retained appreciable regenerative capacity.

2. Varied Effects of Radiations on Development

Radiations are capable of affecting developing systems in a variety of ways as indicated above. In addition to mutagenesis and the familiar types of embryotoxicity, e.g., intrauterine death, malformation and growth retardation, ionizing radiations can cause lasting effects on postnatal growth, neural functions and biochemical maturation (Baker, 1971; Hicks, 1954;

Nair, 1969; Yamazaki, 1966). Although radiations are capable of affecting all cells undergoing proliferative activity, it nevertheless is evident that certain tissues are more susceptible than others to radiation induced damage during development. The central nervous system including the eyes has long been known to be particularly susceptible, but the axial skeleton, appendages, and such organs as the heart and kidneys are occasionally rendered structurally or functionally abnormal by radiations during intrauterine development. These effects are fully described in several references already cited in this chapter.

B. Chemicals and Drugs

Unquestionably the largest category of teratogenic causes is that of chemicals, including drugs, some pesticides, and a few solvents and industrial effluents. Table 3-1 lists several classes of chemicals with representative examples of each that have been shown to be embryotoxic in one or more species of laboratory mammal. Certain of these classes, such as antibiotic, antineoplastic, and antimalarial drugs, and all types of pesticides, would automatically be suspect of having teratogenic potential because they were originally formulated for the express purpose of suppressing growth and metabolism in living tissues or organisms. Until proved otherwise, it should be

TABLE 3-1

Some Types of Drugs and Other Chemicals That Have Been Shown to Be Tetatogenic[a] in One or More Species of Laboratory Mammal

Drug type	Examples
Salicylates	Aspirin, oil of wintergreen
Certain alkaloids	Caffeine, nicotine, colchicine
Tranquilizers	Meprobamate, chlorpromazine, reserpine
Antihistamines	Buclizine, meclizine, cyclizine
Antibiotics	Chloramphenicol, streptonigrin, penicillin
Hypoglycemics	Carbutamide, tolbutamide, hypoglycins
Steroid hormones	Triamcinolone, cortisone, testosterone
Alkylating agents	Busulfan, chlorambucil, cyclophosphamide, TEM
Antimalarials	Chloroquine, quinacrine, pyrimethamine
Anesthetics	Halothane, urethane, nitrous oxide, pentobarbital
Antimetabolites	Folic acid, purine and pyrimidine analogs
Solvents	Benzene, dimethylsulfoxide, propylene glycol
Pesticides	2,4,5-T, carbaryl, captan, folpet
Industrial effluents	Some compounds of Hg, Pb, As, Li, Cd
Miscellaneous	Trypan blue, tryparanol, diamox, etc.

[a] Teratogenic effects were usually seen only at doses well above therapeutic levels for the drugs, or above likely exposure levels for the environmental chemicals.

assumed that all of these substances in sufficient dosage are capable of impairing the rapid growth and high metabolic activity of mammalian embryos and fetuses. As will be emphasized in Chapter 6, however, maternal homeostatic mechanisms and placental transport rates tend to modify this risk.

It is impossible to generalize about the teratogenic mechanisms through which the varied chemical agents initiate their actions within developing systems, except to say that there is great diversity in the ways different chemicals act on living systems. Some are capable of causing mutations and chromosomal aberrations (Kalter, 1971; Fishbein *et al.,* 1970) as well as the more usual teratogenic manifestations. Others interfere with various aspects of the mitotic cycle (Malowista *et al.,* 1968) or interfere with nucleic acid synthesis or function (Schumacher *et al.,* 1969). In other words, virtually all of the teratogenic mechanisms (Scheme 1-1 and Chapter 4) can be activated by one or more types of chemical agents. Once access is gained to the parental bloodstream, it must be assumed that some fraction of the concentration of all foreign chemicals reaches the germ cells and probably also the embryo or fetus *in utero.* Thus the critical question may not be whether developing tissues are exposed to environmental chemicals, but rather at what dosage and for what duration does exposure occur. In other words, are the parental homeostatic system and the embryonic and fetal placentae able to reduce the concentration soon enough to avoid mutagenic or teratogenic effects in developing tissues?

The great majority of safety evaluation testing for both teratogenic and mutagenic potential is now and will doubtless continue to be directed toward chemical agents. This is not necessarily because these agents inherently involve greater risk than other agents, but mainly because among the various types of potential causative agents (Scheme 1-1), new chemicals are probably being introduced into the environment faster than all of the other kinds of agents combined. Numerous lists of chemicals and drugs known adversely to affect mammalian development are available in the literature (Cahen, 1966; Kalter and Warkany, 1959; Nishimura, 1964; Tuchmann-Duplessis and Mercier-Parot, 1964a; and others); the subject is discussed in some detail as regards man in Sections II, F and G of this chapter.

C. DIETARY IMBALANCE

Giroud (1971) has emphasized the importance of nutritional balance as well as caloric intake during pregnancy in determining the condition of the offspring. For the most part, however, nutritional causes of abnormal development in animals have involved several specific deficiencies of vitamins such as vitamin A, riboflavin, folic acid, vitamin E, and pantothenic acid (Asling, 1969; Hurley, 1967; Warkany, 1952–1953). In addition, deficiency of vitamin B$_6$ or pyridoxine has recently been shown to cause functional (Körner and Nowak, 1971) as well as structural (Davis *et al.,* 1970) abnormalities in young rats. Less striking developmental abnormalities have been reported in rats after deficiencies of protein (Zeman, 1967; Nolen, 1971), vitamin D (Warkany, 1943), methionine (Sims, 1951), tryptophan (Pike, 1951), and biotin (Giroud *et al.,* 1956). By use of specific antagonists to normal dietary factors, malformations have been produced with the niacin analog 6-aminonicotinamide (Chamberlain and Nelson, 1963), the riboflavin analog galactoflavin (Nelson *et al.,* 1956), folic acid antagonists (Nelson, 1963), and the near-analog of vitamin A, retinoic acid (Kochhar, 1967).

The manifestations of such nutritional deprivations in animals have typically involved intrauterine death, many types of malformations, and growth retardation, but recent evidence indicates that permanent behavioral and biochemical deficiencies also result from inadequate maternal nutrition prenatally or postnatally (Hurley, 1968b), particularly as regards protein (Platt and Stewart, 1968; Pond *et al.,* 1969). Thus, although specific dietary deficiencies have been identified as teratogenic in laboratory animals, none has been proved in man, excepting those situations involving use of folic acid antimetabolic drugs (see Sections II, F and I, C.).

This apparent difference in susceptibility to nutritional deficiency in animals and in man is very likely more apparent than real. In the animal experiments in which dietary deficiency was shown to be teratogenic, great care was necessary to insure that the diet was adequate in all other respects except a single factor, i.e., a vitamin, otherwise pregnancy did not occur or was terminated prematurely. In human situations such isolated deficiencies of a single nutrient probably do not occur. The poor diets consumed by deprived peoples, alcoholics, and others suffering from inadequate nutrition are deficient in many specific nutrients as well as in total caloric content. When such multiple deficiencies become extreme, as they did during World War II in certain famine areas of Europe (Smith, 1947; Antonov, 1947), reproductive cycles ceased as evidenced by widespread amenorrhea. In cases of less severe restrictions of diet, however, children were delivered but birth weight was reduced and there were increased rates of prematurity and of stillbirth. According to more recent reports, severely restricted diets during human pregnancy have possibly led to impaired physical and mental development postnatally (Keys *et al.,* 1950; Yaktin and McLaren, 1970). The question of permanent impairment of human development associated with adverse influences, including nutritional imbalance, in the perinatal period will be discussed further in Section II, H.

Excesses of certain vitamins are also detrimental to development, such as vitamin A (Cohlan, 1953) and possibly vitamin D (Friedman and Roberts,

1966) and vitamin K (Okuda *et al.,* 1968). Furthermore, normal intrauterine development is known to be dependent on adequate intake of minerals and dietary trace elements, including zinc (Hurley *et al.,* 1971), manganese (Hurley *et al.,* 1958), magnesium (Hurley and Cosens, 1970), and copper (Di Paolo and Newberne, 1971). Thus it is evident that nutritional imbalance can have severe repercussions on several aspects of development. To produce frank malformations, however, a specific deficiency or in some cases, excess, of a particular dietary factor, usually a vitamin or mineral, must be maintained during organogenesis. During the perinatal period maternal diets low in protein may cause increased mortality, growth retardation, and possibly functional deficits.

D. INFECTIONS

In view of the tremendous number of microorganisms known to be pathogenic in man and animals, it is surprising that so few have been associated with developmental abnormalities. Only five infectious agents have been implicated in man (see Section II,D) and only a few others have been shown to interfere with intrauterine development in all other mammals combined. A preponderance of infectious agents known to affect the embryos or fetuses of animals are viruses, the only exception being the protozoan *Toxoplasma* which mainly causes intrauterine death in mice and rats.

Table 3-2 summarizes studies in which the effects of experimentally induced infection were investigated in pregnant mammals. Few of these experiments yielded frank malformations and none produced the broad range of structural defects seen in human infants from mothers infected with rubella during the first 60 days of gestation. As in human rubella infection, however, the pregnant female often was only mildly affected by infections that caused high rates of intrauterine death, together with some growth retardation and malformation. Apparently the teratogenicity of microorganisms depends on their ability to enter the embryo and kill or otherwise damage selectively certain types of cells (Töndury, 1969). Evidently viruses more readily traverse the placenta and invade the embryo or fetus than do bacteria or protozoa, but the question remains as to why relatively few viruses are known to cross the placenta and affect the embryo or fetus. One explanation is that many viruses are actually able to invade the developing organism *in utero,* but that the more virulent ones cause early intrauterine death. Only a few viruses of low virulence invade the embryo and cause such limited or selective damage as to allow survival of some fetuses with malformation (Eichenwald, 1965). In this connection it is of interest to note that two of the agents listed in Table 3-2 are teratogenic only in the attenuated state, and several others would certainly qualify as being of low virulence as far as maternal pathogenicity is concerned.

TABLE 3-2

EFFECTS OF INFECTIOUS AGENTS ON INTRAUTERINE DEVELOPMENT IN MAMMALS[a]

Infection	Species	Developmental effect	Author
Rubella virus	Monkey (*Macaca irus*)	Cataracts, osseous lesions, abortions	Delahunt and Reiser (1967)
	Baboon	Abortions	Hendrickx (1966)
Cytomegalovirus	Mouse	Intrauterine death	Madearis (1964)
Herpes simplex virus	Rabbit	Intrauterine death	Middlekamp et al. (1967)
Blue tongue virus (attenuated)	Sheep	Malformations of CNS	Schultz and Delay (1955)
Hog cholera virus (attenuated)	Swine	Malformed nose, kidneys, brain, congenital ataxia	Young et al. (1955)
Rhinotracheitis virus	Cattle	Abortion	Chow et al. (1964)
Equine abortion virus	Horse	Abortion	Domock (1940)
H-1, rat virus	Hamster and rat	Malformed brain and face, abdominal hernia	Ferm and Kilham (1963); Kilham and Ferm (1964)
Feline ataxia virus	Cat	Cerebellar hypoplasia, congenital ataxia	Kilham and Margolis (1966)
Mumps virus	Hamster	Hydrocephalus	Johnson et al. (1967)
Toxoplasma	Mouse	Intrauterine growth retardation, death	Cowen and Wolf (1950)
	Rat	Intrauterine death, cataracts	Giroud et al. (1954)

[a] Based in part on Sever (1969).

E. EXTREMES OF RESPIRATORY GAS LEVELS

Hypoxia equivalent to high altitude (28,000 ft) during mid-organogenesis is known to cause some brain and varous skeletal malformations in mice (Ingalls and Curley, 1957; Murakami and Kameyama, 1963) and rabbits (Degenhardt and Knoche, 1959), but only cardiac defects were reported in rats (Clemmer and Telford, 1966). Hypoxia failed to produce abnormalities in hamsters but hyperbaric oxygen (3 to 4 times atmospheric) caused a few malformations and some increase in resorptions in this species (Ferm, 1964). Increased CO_2 tension or decreased O_2 tension in respired air was reported to cause a moderate number of heart malformations in rats (Haring and Polli, 1957). Thus, extreme alterations in the concentrations of respiratory gases breathed by pregnant females for a few hours daily during organogenesis can cause disturbances in embryonic development in rodents and rabbits.

More complex physiologic stress that also involved alterations in respiratory gas levels in blood available to the embryos have produced variable results. Severe hemorrhagic anemia in pregnant rats at various times during organogenesis failed to cause appreciable malformations even at levels sufficient to cause some maternal death and increased rates of intrauterine resorption and growth retardation in near-term fetuses (Wilson, 1953). Complete occlusion of the uterine blood flow by clamping the vessels for as long as 1 hour on day 9 of pregnancy in rats caused only moderate increase in embryolethality above control levels, and even longer periods of occlusion produced surprisingly few malformations, although intrauterine death and growth retardation increased rapidly (Brent and Franklin, 1960). Admittedly anemia and ischemia as illustrated in experiments such as those just cited involved a great deal more than alterations in respiratory gas tensions, but whatever other physiologic changes were present also appeared to have relatively low potential for causing malformations in surviving fetuses.

There is no substantial evidence that alterations in respiratory gas tensions are associated with defective prenatal development in man. There are, however, some indications that high altitude (Alzamora-Castro et al., 1960) and asphyxia in the neonatal period (Polani and Campbell, 1960) predispose to failure of normal closure of the ductus arteriosus postnatally. This malformation is not dependent on any known anatomic fault but rather appears to result from abnormal physiologic relationships after birth.

F. EXTREMES OF TEMPERATURE

The effects of extremes of temperature on development have been extensively studied in fish (Stockard, 1921) and chicks (Ancel, 1958; Nielsen, 1969; and others), doubtless because of the ease with which abnormally high or low temperatures can be imposed on the embryos of these submammalian forms. Typical of such studies were those of de la Cruz *et al.* (1966), who maintained chick embryos throughout incubation at higher than optional temperatures and observed increased mortality, eye and central nervous system defects, and torsions of the body axis. In mammals hyperthermia has also been shown to cause malformations and intrauterine death in rodents (Meniro and Barnett, 1969; Edwards, 1968, 1969) and rabbits (Brinsmade and Rübsaamen, 1957). Hypothermia has not been widely studied in mammals, although one report indicated that it has limited teratogenic potential in hamsters; cooling pregnant animals for 45 minutes at a temperature estimated to freeze 30% of body water caused scattered teratogenic effects and high mortality among the offspring (Smith, 1957). No instance of developmental abnormality is known to have been attributed to extremes of body temperature during human pregnancy.

G. MATERNAL METABOLIC OR ENDOCRINE IMBALANCE

Dosage with more than physiologic amounts of steroid sex hormones during pregnancy has long been known to be teratogenic. During the 1930's a series of experiments (Greene *et al.,* 1939, 1940; and others) demonstrated that injection of androgenic or estrogenic sex hormones into pregnant rodents prior to or during differentiation of the genitalia led to ambiguous development of these organs. The heterologous hormones caused males to be feminized and females to be masculinized. Somewhat earlier Lillie (1917), in his classic study of the free martin, concluded that in cattle twins of unlike sex sexual differentiation could be diverted by abnormal amounts of the heterologous gonadal hormones.

Sex hormones may be among the few universal teratogens in that they seem to result in a degree of hermaphroditism in a great variety of vertebrate species from amphibians to man. In contrast, adrenal steroids of the glucocorticoid variety, although shown to cause cleft palate in mice by Baxter and Fraser (1950) and subsequently in a number of other rodents and in rabbits (Hoar, 1962; Walker, 1966), have little or no teratogenic effects in other mammalian groups including man.

Other endocrine related metabolic states have been reviewed for teratological effects by Takano (1969), who found that many of the studies in experimental animals have yielded inconclusive results. The administration of antithyroid agents to pregnant animals has caused increased intrauterine death and a few assorted malformations but no consistent pattern of defects. The effects of hyperthyroid states during pregnancy are conflicting, some reporting teratogenic effects (Beaudoin and Roberts, 1966) while others found thyroxine antagonistic to other teratogenic agents (Woollam and

Millen, 1960). A number of experiments involving treatment of pregnant mice, rats, and rabbits with alloxan indicates that this diabetogenic compound causes high rates of fetal or neonatal death and a low level of teratogenicity (Takano, 1969). Insulin has been found mainly to cause intrauterine death in pregnant rodents, but other hypoglycemics of the sulfonylurea type have been shown to have appreciable teratogenic activity (Tuchmann-Duplessis and Mercier-Parot, 1958). Several altered physiologic states in the pregnant woman are known or strongly suspected to be associated with abnormal intrauterine development (see Section II, E).

H. PHYSICAL TRAUMA AND MECHANICAL FACTORS

Physical and mechanical factors in the environment impinge directly on the embryos of lower forms, but in mammals few such agents reach the embryo because of shielding by the maternal system. Holtfreter (1945) embedded fertilized amphibian eggs in agar for several days and found that size and external shape were greatly altered, although cytologic differentiation and the processes of gastrulation and neurulation were little affected. The simple expedient of jarring chicken eggs during incubation was shown by Stiles and Watterson (1937) to cause fatal hemorrhages or malformations. Neurath (1968) has reported that the hatchability of developing frog's eggs was reduced by placing them in a strong magnetic field but no malformations among survivors were reported. Inert particulate matter applied directly to the surface of chick embryos was shown by Williamson *et al.* (1967) to sink into internal tissue layers where necrosis and sloughing were seen in areas later affected by malformation. The remarkable capacity of the embryo to repair and regulate after some types of mechanical injury was demonstrated by Rickenbacker (1968), who found that extensive necrosis produced in chick limb buds by electrocautery subsequently caused malformation in only 20% of wings and 10% of legs when the treated animals were examined several days later.

The mammalian embryo is buffered from such extramaternal physical factors, but on occasion it may be affected by physical conditions within the uterus. An association has long been known to exist between an excess of amniotic fluid, polyhydramnios, and such malformations as anencephaly and atresias of the upper digestive tract, but most authors have concluded that the excess of amniotic fluid was secondary to malformation rather than the cause of it. A deficiency of amniotic fluid, oligohydramnios, is not known to have occurred during the early, teratogenically susceptible period of human pregnancy, but the possibility of such a state may be inferred from animal experiments. Trasler *et al.* (1956) found that puncture of the amniotic sac and subsequent leakage of the amniotic fluid in mice caused an increase in the incidence of cleft palate and intrauterine death. It was assumed that the space restriction that followed escape of the fluid resulted in crowding of the lower jaw against the chest region in such a way as to interfere with normal withdrawal of the tongue from between the palatal folds. Kendrick and Field (1967) produced oligohydramnios experimentally in pregnant rats and noted limb abnormalities in the offspring, including malrotation, syndactyly, and agenesis of various parts.

There is some evidence that the location of the initial implantation site within the uterus influences the normality or abnormality of subsequent development. Hertig *et al.* (1956) noted that a majority of the abnormal human embryos in a series of 26 were implanted on the anterior wall, while most of the normal embryos were implanted on the posterior wall. Trasler (1960) found that mouse fetuses with spontaneous cleft lip were significantly more often seen in sites nearest the ovary. Beck (1967) reported that trypan blue treatment of pregnant rats resulted in more abnormal fetuses at the ovarian end of the uterus, but a higher rate of fetal mortality occurred at the cervical end. The actual factors underlying such position effects are not known, but it has been suggested that they might be related to the adequacy of vascular supply. The experiments of Brent and Franklin (1960) have shown that acute ischemia induced by clamping the blood supply to individual embryo sites for 1 to 3 hours caused increased mortality and malformation. It is doubtful, however, that the abrupt metabolic changes attendant on occluded blood supply bear much resemblance to regional variations in blood supply proposed to explain position effects within the uterus.

I. PLACENTAL FAILURE AND ANTIBODIES

Numerous attempts have been made to demonstrate that immune substances against specific tissues could cross the placenta and selectively damage tissues within the embryo. Brent (1964a, 1971a) has critically reviewed this complex subject and found little evidence that maternal immunoproteins crossed the placenta in amounts and at times likely to cause specific developmental abnormalities in the offspring. Brent and Averich (1961, 1971), however, have shown that rabbit antisera to rat kidney and placenta do produce a dose-related spectrum of malformations in the offspring of female rats treated between days 7 and 10 of gestation. This procedure has been successfully repeated in other laboratories (David *et al.*, 1963) and extended to antisera of heart and lung (Barrow and Taylor, 1971). It has been clearly established, however, that these antibodies do not reach the embryo but instead are accumulated in the yolk sac epithelia, which comprise an accessory placental structure peculiar to rodents and rabbits.

These antibodies seem to act by interfering with the function of this specialized placental structure. Trypan blue and other teratogenic azo dyes also appear to interfere with transport functions of the yolk sac placenta but in this instance there is no indication that immunologic phenomena are involved (Beck *et al.,* 1967b). There is presumptive evidence that the heterologous antibodies are localized in the membranes of the yolk sac in such a way as to interfere with the transport or other nutritive functions of these membranes, resulting in what might be tantamount to a nutritional deficiency in the early embryo. Favoring this view are the facts that (1) the antisera do not reach the embryo proper but are localized in the yolk sac membranes, and (2) antisera have for the most part been shown to be teratogenic in animals that possess the inverted yolk sac placenta typical of rodents and rabbits, although the ferret has recently been reported to show similar effects (Brent *et al.,* 1972).

J. COMBINATIONS AND INTERACTIONS

Substances which are not in themselves teratogenic have been shown in laboratory animals to enhance greatly the effectiveness of threshold or subthreshold doses of known teratogens (Härtel and Härtel, 1960; Kalter, 1960; Landauer and Clark, 1964; Miller, 1958; Runner and Dagg, 1960; Smithberg, 1961; Wilson, 1964b; Wilson *et al.,* 1969; Woollam *et al.,* 1959). Such potentiation of two or more marginally teratogenic substances in man is not known to occur but there is some basis for assuming that it does, as will be discussed presently. It should be noted in the present context that two or more concurrently acting environmental agents may interact in other ways than by potentiation: their combined effects may be additive, may yield a nil effect, or may actually result in interference (Runner and Dagg, 1960; Wilson, 1964b). Clearly potentiation is the type of interaction of greatest concern because it is a mechanism by which a nonteratogen, or a low dose of known teratogen, can magnify the effects of another teratogen, or combine with another nonteratogenic agent, to produce unexpected effects (Gibson and Becker, 1968). The insidiousness of this situation for human teratology is the possibility that an observed developmental defect could be the result of potentiative interaction between agents, one or more of which is present in such low dosage as to elude suspicion as a causative factor.

II. Causes of Developmental Defects in Man

Table 3-3 summarizes the known causes of developmental abnormality in man. The percentage assigned to each category of causation is only a crude estimate intended to provide some indication of the relative contribution of

TABLE 3-3

<small>KNOWN CAUSES OF DEVELOPMENTAL DEFECTS IN MAN[a,b]</small>

Known genetic transmission	20%
Chromosomal aberration	3–5%
Environmental causes	
Radiations	<1%
Therapeutic	
Nuclear	
Infections	2–3%
Rubella virus	
Cytomegalovirus	
Herpesvirus hominis	
Toxoplasma	
Syphilis	
Maternal metabolic imbalance	1–2%
Endemic cretinism	
Diabetes	
Phenylketonuria	
Virilizing tumors	
Drugs and environmental chemicals	2–3%
Androgenic hormone	
Folic antagonists	
Thalidomide	
Organic mercury	
Some hypoglycemics (?)	
Some anticonvulsants (?)	
Potentiative interactions	?
Unknown	65–70%

[a] From Wilson (1972a).
[b] Estimates based on past experience.

each to the total. According to these estimates the sum of all environmental causes does not exceed 10%, but this is almost certainly an understatement. Some of the less well understood categories of causation are environmental in nature, and it is possible that other categories of this type have not yet been recognized. The contributions of genetic and chromosomal causes, although not precisely known, have nevertheless been studied intensively, and it is likely that these estimates more nearly approximate reality than do those for environmental factors. The class designated in Table 3-3 as "potentiative interactions" cannot at this time be documented with a known instance of interacting environmental agents in man. In view of the numerous examples of teratogenic potentiation demonstrated in laboratory animals, it is not unreasonable to suppose that a significant portion of human defects now listed as of unknown causation may eventually be shown to be the result of combinations and interactions of factors.

Interaction between genetic and environmental influences in the genesis of abnormal development has been accepted for many years. This was clearly stated by Fraser (1959), who emphasized that a minority of malformations have major environmental cause and a minority have major genetic cause, but most probably result from complex interactions between genetic predisposition and subtle factors in the environment. Although this is regarded as a principle of experimental teratology (see Chapter 2, Section I) and has often been demonstrated in laboratory animals (Dagg, 1967; Fraser, 1969; Hamburgh *et al.,* 1970; Hurley, 1969; Kalter, 1965; Winfield and Bennett, 1971), examples in man are limited to a few less well-established situations such as congenital hip disease (Wollf *et al.,* 1968), certain familial types of congenital heart disease (Boon *et al.,* 1972), and possibly favism (Sartori, 1971). Hereditary conditions with variable penetrance and expressivity may also be attributed in part to interaction between genes and factors in the environment. Hereditary diseases which are diagnosable in the heterozygous state by application of an appropriate environmental stress, e.g., sickle cell trait by hypoxia, illustrate a degree of interaction, although the full-blown disease does not necessarily require the environmental stress.

A. GENETIC TRANSMISSION

This cause of abnormal development implies that the genetic material of the affected individual was changed by one or more nonlethal mutations in a prior generation. The original cause of mutation is assumed to have been environmental in nature (see Chapter 4, Section I); but once the acquired genetic defect is transmitted to a subsequent generation, the cause of abnormal development is then said to be hereditary. The subject is treated in numerous books and monographs and needs no elaboration here except to indicate the relative place of heredity in the overall picture of causation. Neel (1961) has estimated that about 20% of human developmental defects may be solely or largely attributable to known modes of heredity, and in a recent personal communication that investigator felt no compelling reason to change the estimate at this time.

B. CHROMOSOMAL ABERRATIONS

This category of abnormality also involves the genetic material but in a grosser way than applies to the point mutations that account for most hereditary defects. Chromosomal aberrations refer to visible excesses, deficiencies or translocation of chromatin material, i.e., extra whole chromosomes, deficiency of one X chromosome, or transfer or deletion of the arms of one or more chromatids. Actually such chromosomal abnormalities are not causes of abnormal development but rather are probably themselves an early reaction of developing cells to agents in the environment. As with mutations, then, chromosomal aberrations should in the strict sense be classed with mechanisms (see Chapter 4, Section II) and as such would depend on environmental causes to initiate them in germinal or embryonic cells. The causes of chromosomal aberrations are not clear but have been variously related to radiations, chemicals, viruses, heat shock, and genetically determined abnormalities in mitosis and meiosis (Feckheimer, 1972). Owing to their uncertain cause–effect status chromosomal abnormalities are listed in Table 3-3 with causes of developmental disease in man.

In view of the widespread attention given to chromosomal aberrations in recent years, it is well to emphasize the relatively small contribution they are thought to make to the total of human developmental defects. A recent survey (Jacobs, 1970) based on almost 10,000 newborn infants from three different populations yielded 51 or 0.5% with some chromosomal abnormality. At least 13 of these, however, were aneuploids of sex chromosomes which are not associated with an abnormal phenotype; thus the estimated percentage of these combined populations that presumably had developmental defects attributable to chromosomal abnormality was less than 0.4%. In one of the hospitals in which the survey was carried out 8% of all babies had some congenital defect recognizable in the first few days of life. If these figures are assumed for purposes of illustration to be applicable to all of the survey population, 8% or 800 of the babies might have been expected to have recognizable defects soon after birth. If 0.4% of total population (40) had chromosomal abnormality that caused phenotypically recognizable defects, then not more than 5% of all congenitally defective newborns might be supposed to have some chromosomal aberration. The impreciseness of such calculations, however, is pointed up by the fact that mental deficiency and other chromosome-related defects are not diagnosable at birth. Accordingly, 5% must be regarded as a very rough approximation. As already noted, chromosomal abnormalities will be discussed further under mechanisms in Chapter 4.

C. RADIATIONS

Ionizing radiation was the first environmental cause of developmental defects to be definitely established in man (Goldstein and Murphy, 1929). Despite this early recognition of the teratogenic risks, the medical literature contains several hundred case reports of infants born after intensive pelvic irradiation during pregnancy. Typically, infants irradiated *in utero* with more than a few 100 R during the early months of gestation bore serious central nervous system and ocular defects, often accompanied by mental retardation (Thalhammer, 1967). In view of the widely recognized risk, a question can reasonably be asked as to why therapeutic irradiation continued to be used during pregnancy. Doubtless it was used in many instances without ample efforts to rule out the possibility of pregnancy or to avoid treatment during the period when the existence of pregnancy could not be ascertained. Pelvic irradiation was justifiable in the cases treated for a life-threatening neoplasm during the early stages of undiagnosed pregnancy, but in the more liberal climate of today the problem would in most instances have been resolved by therapeutic abortion when pregnancy was diagnosed.

Nuclear radiations such as those emanating from the atomic bombs exploded at Hiroshima and Nagasaki caused microcephaly and mental retardation in children whose mothers were within 2000 meters of the hypocenters during early months of their pregnancies (Miller, 1956; Wood et al., 1967). A review of literature on all types of central nervous system disturbances following irradiation in utero (Yamazaki, 1966) has revealed that behavioral and performance deficits can also be demonstrated postnatally after moderate dosage administered prenatally in laboratory animals. Prenatal irradiation has also been implicated in increased cancer rates during childhood (MacMahon, 1962) and it has long been suspected of producing genetic effects in man similar to those known to occur in other species (Neel, 1963).

D. Infection

In view of recent progress in the control of infectious diseases, it may be unfortunate that a larger proportion of human developmental errors cannot be attributed to this cause. As noted in regard to infections in animals, a few viruses account for most of the developmental abnormality produced by infectious agents. Apparently teratogenicity caused by microorganisms depends on their ability to enter the embryo and kill or otherwise selectively damage certain types of cells (Töndury, 1969). Rubella, cytomegalovirus, and *Herpesvirus hominis* II are now recognized as teratogenic in man (Table 3-2) (Sever, 1971; Sever and London, 1969).

1. *Rubella*

In a recent summary Sever (1970) reported that rubella caused defective development in approximately 50% of infants when maternal infection occurred in the first month of pregnancy, 22% in the second month, and 6–10% in the third, fourth, and fifth months. Infection during the first trimester results in the familiar syndrome of congenital heart disease, cataracts, deafness, microcephaly, and mental retardation, and subsequent studies have shown that infection during the second trimester may lead to mental and motor retardation and deafness (Gumpel *et al.,* 1971). This illustrates that in man as well as in laboratory animals unfavorable influences tend to produce structural defects when applied early in gestation and functional ones when exposure occurs at a more advanced stage of fetal development.

2. *Other Viruses*

Viruses other than rubella are implicated in human teratogenesis relatively rarely. Maternal cytomegalovirus has been mainly related to congenital microcephaly in the offspring, but it may also produce hydrocephaly, microphthalmia, chorioretinitis, blindness, and seizures (Hanshaw, 1970). *Herpesvirus hominis* II infection during pregnancy is sometimes followed by microcephaly, microphthalmia, and retinal dysplasia in the newborn infants (Baron *et al.,* 1969). Other viruses described as having been transmitted to the embryo or the fetus from infected mothers are variola, vaccinia, varicella, rubeola, polio, hepatitis, western equine encephalitis, and possibly mumps and influenza; but none is regularly associated with developmental defects (Sever, 1971). An epidemic of Asian influenza in Finland has been positively correlated with increased incidence of central nervous system malformations (Hakosalo and Saxén, 1971), although several other studies have failed to confirm this correlation. A prospective study of 22,935 pregnancies yielded some evidence of association between the birth of anomalous infants and maternal infection with coxsackieviruses, B2 and B4 in particular, but not with echovirus infection (Brown and Karunas, 1972). To the contrary, echovirus 7 antibodies have been reported to be significantly higher ($P = < 0.005$) among mothers of malformed than of normal children, whereas coxsackie B1 and B5 antibodies were less frequent in mothers of malformed than normal children (Lapinleimu *et al.,* 1972). The possibility has already been mentioned that the more virulent viruses reaching the early embryo cause intrauterine death, and that only a few of low virulence are able to invade the embryo and produce selective damage sufficient to cause malformations (Eichenwald, 1965).

3. *Nonviral Organisms*

Nonviral agents are known to cause congenital infections, but for the most part the manifestations of disease in these instances are similar to those in postnatal life; in other words, they produce congenital pathology but not developmental deviation. An exception is the protozoan toxoplasma, fetal infection with which is frequently associated with hydrocephalus, microcephalus, microphthalmus, mental retardation, etc. (Farquhar and Turner, 1949; Lechner and Leinzinger, 1965).

The existence of a developmental component among the varied symptoms of congenital syphilis has been a matter of some controversy. The growth distortions and hydrocephalus sometimes seen, as well as the characteristic deformities of the teeth, would seem to qualify as truly developmental defects. Thus at least some cases of congenital syphilis display teratological manifestations, as well as the pathological signs associated with perinatal or postnatal infection.

E. MATERNAL METABOLIC IMBALANCE

In this category of causation the primary disorder is thought to be within the maternal organism, instead of within the embryo or fetus. In other words the conceptus reacts secondarily to a pathophysiologic state within the mother. The judgment as to what is primarily maternal as opposed to what is primarily embryonic or fetal in origin is not always easily made. Nevertheless, the following are conditions in which the developmental abnormality in the offspring seems in considerable part to be secondary to disease or altered physiologic state in the pregnant mother.

1. *Endemic Cretinism and Maternal Thyroid Disorders*

The long-known congenital disease, cretinism, which hardly exists in the civilized world today, may in the past have accounted for as many defective human beings as any other single environmental cause. In strictest terms it can be regarded as the result of maternal nutritional deficiency of iodine, because the availability of iodine to an affected population quickly eliminates the birth of cretins. As Warkany (1971) has made clear in an extensive review, however, other factors appear to be involved. For example, the risk of cretinism increases with the parity of the pregnancy, and there is some evidence of hereditary predisposition. Nevertheless, the mothers of cretins are always goiterous, but adequate iodine therapy of a goiterous woman during pregnancy generally removes the risk of cretinism. Although cretinism is not always diagnosable at birth, irreparable developmental damage is present at birth as evidenced by the fact that the mental, motor, and hearing deficits cannot be corrected by postnatal treatment with iodine or thyroxine. A recent study (Pharoah *et al.*, 1971) has reported that all of the neurological damage associated with cretinism can be prevented by the administration of iodized oil to the mother, preferably before conception.

Hypothyroid states involving myxedema (Hodges *et al.*, 1952) and simple goiter (Dean, 1927) have in a few instances been associated with various developmental defects other than cretinism, but the absence of a repeated pattern in the defects suggests the likelihood of coincidence. Maternal ingestion of iodides may cause congenital goiter and hypothyroidism, sometimes associated with postnatal death or mental retardation (Carswell *et al.*, 1970). The administration of thyroid suppressing drugs (Milham and Elledge, 1972; Piper and Rosen, 1954; Whitelaw, 1947) or radioactive iodine (Russell *et al.,* 1957; Valensi and Nahum, 1958) for treatment of hyperthyroidism during pregnancy has been reported to be followed by the birth of defective infants in a number of instances, but other studies have reported normal births under similar circumstances (Dailey and Benson, 1952; Lederer, 1952). One report from Russia claims a high incidence of microcephaly, heart disease, and other malformations among children born to women with hyperthyroidism (Orlova, 1966). Thus, several types of maternal thyroid disease are sometimes associated with developmental abnormality of the offspring, but the frequency and significance of these relationships are not clear.

2. Diabetes

The occurrence of higher than normal stillbirth and neonatal death rates among the offspring of diabetic women has been known for many years, but in spite of accumulated statistical indications, many investigators hesitated to accept the evidence that malformations also occurred more frequently in such offspring (Rubin and Murphy, 1958). An extensive survey in Denmark (Pedersen *et al.,* 1964), however, has convincingly shown that diabetic women do in fact produce about three times as many infants with developmental defects as do nondiabetic mothers. This was soon confirmed (Dunn, 1964; Lenz and Maier, 1964) and a prevailing pattern of defects, designated as the "caudal regression" syndrome, was recognized in many of the affected children. Together with an assortment of other defects, approximately two thirds of the abnormal children born to diabetic women had one or more missing sacral and/or lumbar vertebrae and conspicuous musculoskeletal abnormality of the lower extremities (Kučera *et al.,* 1965; Rusnak and Driscoll, 1965).

Of possible significance in this connection is the report that more than half of the mothers of a consecutive series of 152 malformed infants had abnormal glucose tolerance tests, as against 3.3% of abnormal tests among mothers of normal infants (Navarrete *et al.,* 1967). In another study women who delivered malformed children were found (Navarrete *et al.,* 1970) to be much more likely to develop diabetes later than were women who delivered normal babies, particularly those mothers who had high glucose tolerance tests at the time the defective infants were delivered. There now seems to be no doubt but that the increased neonatal death and malformation rate among offspring of diabetic and prediabetic women is related to the mother's blood sugar level (Karlsson and Kjellmer, 1972).

3. Maternal Phenylketonuria

A small percentage of individuals who develop phenylketonuria during infancy escape the mental retardation and other debilitating effects usually accompanying this disease, and go on to lead more or less normal lives in spite of high phenylalanine levels in their blood. A number of women with such atypical phenylketonuria (PKU) are now known to have delivered defective babies (Hansen, 1970; MacCready and Levy, 1972; Yu and O'Halloran, 1970). Mabry (1970) has surveyed available literature on maternal phenylketonuria during pregnancy and found that of 84 births to such women, 5 children were normal except for PKU, 55 were mentally retarded and without PKU, 7 were retarded with PKU, and 17 died in infancy. Five of the retarded infants also had congenital heart disease. A smaller group of 27 births to women with less pronounced symptoms of PKU (phenylalanine blood level less than 20 mg/100 ml and negative $FeCl_3$ reaction) yielded 14 mentally retarded children of which only half themselves had PKU. Thus, it is evident that a high phenylalanine level in maternal blood during pregnancy, or some associated metabolic disorder, strongly predisposes to defective development of the brain, regardless of whether the child has PKU.

4. Virilizing Tumors

Maternal virilizing tumors, such as arrhenoblastomas and possibly some maternal adrenal tumors, cause virilization of genetic female fetuses, resulting in pseudohermaphroditism (Jones and Scott, 1958). Hormones with androgenic properties are thought to be secreted by these tumors, with the result that sexual differentiation of female fetuses is modified in a way similar to that seen after administration of androgenic hormones during pregnancy (see Section II, F,1).

5. Other Maternal Factors

The existence of other less specific maternal influences that sometimes seem to predispose to developmental disease is suggested by several scattered observations. An interesting study has been made of children in 139 family units each consisting of women whose children were fathered by more than one man. Each such family contained at least two half-sibships with malformations or other abnormality of similar if not identical nature (Myrianthopoulos, 1969). Identical abnormalities among half-sibships included afebrile seizures, Rh immunization, congenital heart defects, mental retardation, club foot, polydactyly, specific abnormalities of extremities, severe squint, specific abnormalities of lungs, and pilonidal cysts. Recognized and possibly unrecognized genetic influence probably accounted for some of these concurrences, but maternal disease or physiologic state, e.g., Rh incompatibility, must also be considered as possibly contributing.

A retrospective survey by Landtman (1948) found that among the mothers of 93 malformed babies several factors were statistically more frequent than in a control group, namely, older age of the mother, history of abortion, antepartum hemorrhage, and acute infection during the first trimester.

Toxemia of pregnancy was not reported to be significantly increased among these mothers of malformed infants, but it is well known from other studies that toxemia does predispose to excessive perinatal mortality and intrauterine growth retardation (Naeye, 1966). A higher concentration of the amino acids threonine and glutamic acid was found in 43 of 51 women giving birth to malformed infants than in mothers of normal infants (Roszkowski *et al.,* 1969). Although individually these reports are not conclusive, collectively they indicate that there is need for more attention to the possible effects of maternal disease and altered physiologic states on intrauterine development.

F. Drugs

The implications of the thalidomide catastrophe notwithstanding, drugs are still taken therapeutically in appreciable numbers during pregnancy. A prospective study of 240 pregnancies revealed that a mean of 3.7 drugs reguarded by the authors (Nora *et al.,* 1967b) as potentially teratogenic were taken during the first trimester. More recently a survey in Scotland showed that over 97% of 1369 mothers took prescribed drugs and 65% self-administered drugs during pregnancy (Nelson and Forfar, 1971). It was found that significantly more mothers of infants with developmental abnormality took aspirin, antacid, dextroamphetamine, phenobarbitone, sodium amytal, other barbiturates, cough medicines, iron, sulfonamides, and nicotinamide than did mothers in the control group. The majority of mothers taking most of these substances, however, produced normal babies. The real meaning of such data is uncertain, because it is impossible without appropriate controls to separate influences on development that might be caused by the drug from those caused by the condition for which the drug was taken. An untreated control group with identical indications for taking the drug at comparable times in gestation would be needed to evaluate such situations, but these data are usually not available. Furthermore, the time during gestation when a drug is taken, particularly when it is first taken, may determine whether or what type of embryotoxicity will result.

There are four criteria by which a new teratogenic agent for man might be readily recognized (Table 3-4). These were in essence used in identifying the agent in the two major human teratologic catastrophes, namely, rubella and thalidomide. This method, however, depends on the occurrence of a distinctive defect or pattern of defects and of sufficient numbers of cases to draw attention to the possibility of a common cause. For these reasons it is probably not dependable for recognition of all human teratogens. It has been demonstrated in animal experiments that some teratogenic agents do not produce a discrete, easily recognized defect or syndrome, and the same also holds for man, as will be evident later in this chapter. Furthermore, the possibility that an unknown portion of human developmental defects may

TABLE 3-4

Criteria for Recognizing a New Teratogenic Agent in Man

1. An abrupt increase in the incidence of a particular defect or association of defects (syndrome)
2. Coincidence of this increase with a known environmental change, e.g., widespread use of a new drug
3. Known exposure to the environmental change early in pregnancies yielding characteristically defective infants
4. Absence of other factors common to all pregnancies yielding infants with the characteristic defect(s)

result from the interaction of two or more causative factors would compound the difficulty of relating effect to cause(s). These complications, together with incomplete surveillance and reporting, and the lack of appropriate control groups for comparison, have hampered efforts to identify and better define conditions of use of several drugs that appear to involve some risk to the embryo, fetus, or postnatal individual (Cahen, 1966; Cohlan, 1964; Lenz, 1964; Nishimura, 1964; Palmisano and Polhill, 1972; Slater, 1965; Smithells, 1966; Tuchmann-Duplessis, 1965).

The literature on drug effects during human pregnancy has been surveyed and when sufficient information was available drugs were classified according to the following four categories. A few drugs have been positively implicated as teratogenic. Others are suspected of some teratogenic potential on the basis of several more or less well-documented case reports but are yet to be clearly established in this regard. Still others must be regarded as possibly having teratogenic potential under some conditions, on the basis of scattered, usually not-well-documented evidence, or of having appreciable teratogenic activity in animals. Some, however, have been used widely enough in suitably controlled situations to warrant the conclusion that as ordinarily used these drugs involve little or no teratogenic risk.

1. Drugs Positively Implicated as Teratogenic

a. *Thalidomide.* In the ten years since the recognition of its devastating effect on the human embryo, thalidomide has assumed the status of a classic teratogenic agent (Lenz, 1964). It has proved to be almost invariably effective if taken in adequate dosage on a very few days, probably even a single day, during the susceptible period of the human embryo, from approximately the twentieth to the thirty-fifth days postconception. It produces a well-defined pattern of musculoskeletal deformities, affecting mainly the extremities and face, that is not precisely duplicated in any other syndrome, although infrequently certain of the characteristic malformations occur spontaneously. It is virtually nontoxic to young adults and consequently carries no risk of overdosage. Thus, at the expense of several thousand crippled children, and the loss of an otherwise safe and effective sedative, teratologists have learned some valuable lessons. The most important one is that the human embryo may be inordinately sensitive to a substance that causes little or no toxicity in human adults or in test animals. It is a disquieting fact that the animals most widely used today for the testing of teratogenic effects of drugs, i.e., mouse, rat, and rabbit, are relatively insensitive to the embryotoxic effects of this most potent human teratogen. They require larger doses to produce a comparable incidence of abnormality; the malformations do not closely parallel those of man; and several strains of these species (particularly of rats) fail to respond even to massive doses.

The only animals known to react teratogenically to thalidomide as does man are five species of macaque monkeys (Delahunt and Lassen, 1964; Wilson and Gavan, 1967; Hendrickx, 1971b; Tanimura *et al.*, 1971; Vondruska *et al.*, 1971), baboons (Hendrickx *et al.*, 1966), and marmosets (Poswillo *et al.*, 1972) (Fig. 3-2). This has resulted in an increasing tendency to consider the simian primates as more valid test animals for the evaluation of human teratologic risk than are the currently used rodents and rabbits (Wilson, 1971), but it must not be assumed that because man and other primates react teratologically in an almost identical manner to thalidomide, they necessarily react alike to other agents. Nevertheless, evidence from several disciplines is accumulating in support of the view that higher primates are more like man in more ways than any other laboratory animals. In addition to established similarity as regards embryogenesis, reproductive physiology, and placental function and structure, recent studies indicate that embryotoxic and fetotoxic responses to a variety of drugs and chemicals are comparable but not identical (Wilson, 1972b). The urgent need for more suitable test animals in which to evaluate teratogenic risk for man has raised important questions about which criteria are most reliable in extrapolating animal results to man (see Chapter 8).

b. *Steroid Hormones, Particularly Androgens.* An association between congenital adrenal hyperplasia and virilization of the genitalia in genetic female newborns has been known for many years (Biggs and Rose, 1947; Qazi and Thompson, 1972). It was known even earlier that treatment of pregnant mammals, including monkeys (van Wagenen and Hamilton, 1943), with male sex hormones produced pseudohermaphroditism in the female offspring similar to that occurring spontaneously in human infants. The concurrence of female pseudohermaphroditism with adrenal hyperplasia is taken to mean that abnormalities in adrenal metabolism result in the elaboration of larger than normal amounts of steroid with androgenic properties (Klevit, 1960).

Androgenic hormones injected as treatment for breast cancer has resulted

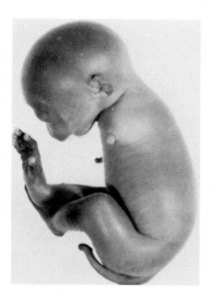 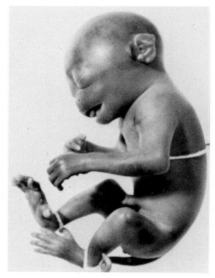

Fig. 3-2. The thalidomide syndrome in a 100-day rhesus monkey fetus (left) following treatment of the pregnant mother with 30 mg/kg thalidomide on day 26 of gestation. The malformations seen here, amelia of forelimbs, micrognathia, deformed ears, and abnormal tail, are typical of those produced by treatment during the first half of the susceptible period in this species (days 22–30). Similar malformations, excepting the tail, were observed in the children of women who took thalidomide during the early part of the human susceptible period (approximately days 20–35). The animal at the right is a normal 100-day monkey fetus. (From Wilson, 1972a.)

in the masculinization of a number of female fetuses when such treatment was commenced prior to the twelfth week of gestation (Grumback and Ducharme, 1960). The earlier practice of using progesterone from natural sources for treatment of threatened abortion led to the widespread use between 1950 and 1960 of synthetic progestins for the same purpose. Before it was realized that some of these synthetic compounds had appreciable androgenic activity, approximately 600 female babies with equivocal or frankly masculinized external genitalia were born (Cahen, 1966; Wilkins, 1960; Voorhess, 1967). Because differentiation of the external genitalia is largely completed by the twelfth week of gestation, treatment after this time is no longer able to cause irreversible modification of these organs.

Estrogenic hormones given at higher than physiologic levels are generally regarded as incompatible with pregnancy, therefore of little teratogenic risk. Their tendency to stimulate uterine contraction is thought sufficient usually to dislodge the conceptus, but this is not invariably the case (Bačić *et al.,*

1970). Three cases of malformed newborns have been attributed to maternal treatment with large doses of estrogen early in pregnancy (Uhlig, 1959), although no instances of feminization of genetic males is known. Paradoxically, treatment with the nonsteroidal estrogenic substance diethylstilbesterol during pregnancy has been associated with masculinization of the female fetus in four instances (Bongiovanni *et al.,* 1959). Another puzzling reaction to maternal treatment with diethylstilbesterol during pregnancy has recently been reported. A number of young women aged 16–22 years have developed adenocarcinoma of the vagina after a common history of having been exposed to this synthetic estrogen *in utero* when their mothers were treated for threatened abortion during the first trimester of pregnancy (Greenwald *et al.,* 1971; Herbst *et al.,* 1971). Although these neoplasms do not appear to represent deviations of normal developmental processes, and accordingly are not strictly teratic in origin, they seem to have been induced during early differentiation of the vagina, possibly as a somatic mutation. In any event, they raise interesting questions about the relationship between carcinogenesis and teratogenesis.

Adrenocortical steroids given during pregnancy in mice have produced cleft palate (Fraser and Fainstat, 1951) with such regularity as to cause concern about the use of these hormones during human pregnancy. Published reports on the administration of these substances to pregnant women indicate some increase in abortion, stillbirth, and prematurity above background levels (Reilly, 1958) but only 5 cases of cleft palate were observed in infants from more than 300 women treated for a variety of reasons (Bongiovanni and McFadden, 1960; Doig and Coltman, 1956; Harris and Ross, 1956; Popert, 1962). A few malformations other than cleft palate also have been attributed to cortisone treatment during pregnancy (Warrell and Taylor, 1968; Wells, 1953). Nevertheless, considering the extensive use of corticoids during human pregnancy and failure of any of the recent epidemiologic surveys to demonstrate statistical correlation, it is probable that these compounds under ordinary conditions of use have little or no adverse effects on intrauterine development (De Costa and Abelman, 1952).

c. *Folic Acid Antagonists.* Early reports of the use of folic acid antagonists in laboratory animals indicated that such compounds were almost invariably embryolethal, and this was the justification for using them as abortifacients in human pregnancies scheduled for therapeutic abortion (Thiersch, 1952, 1956). Of 24 pregnancies so treated, 8 failed to abort and 2 of these yielded malformed infants. In addition 2 of those that died *in utero* also appear to have been malformed. In another series of 20 cases treated with aminopterin during pregnancy (Goetsch, 1962), there was subsequent abortion of 15 and malformation in 1 of the 5 survivors. Combining these reports, 70% of treated pregnancies aborted and 23% of the survivors were malformed. Eight additional cases of malformed liveborn infants, making a total of 11, have now been attributed to antifolic compounds, mainly aminopterin (de Alvarez, 1962; Brandner and Nusslé, 1969; Emerson, 1962; Meltzer, 1956; Milunsky *et al.*, 1968; Shaw and Steinbach, 1968; Warkany *et al.*, 1959). Thus, although treatment with folic acid antagonists during the early months of human pregnancy usually results in intrauterine death, between 20 and 30% of the fetuses that reach term may be malformed. The types of malformations observed in the infants were varied and multiple, with no basic pattern or syndrome recognizable. This fact is in keeping with animal studies which have shown that almost any organ can be the site of abnormality depending on the time in gestation when a folic acid antagonist is applied (Table 2-2) (Nelson, 1963).

Attempts to reproduce these results in pregnant rhesus monkeys using large doses of methotrexate have been only partially successful (Wilson, 1971). Thirteen pregnancies so treated resulted in abortion in 3 instances and a minor malformation in 1. This is in sharp contrast to the relative ease with which 4-aminopteroylglutamic acid (Nelson, 1963) and methotrexate (Wilson, 1970) were shown to be teratogenic in rats. It appears that rat, monkey, and man differ appreciably in their teratogenic susceptibility to folic acid analogues, a fact probably related to differing rates of metabolism and excretion in these species.

2. *Drugs Suspected of Some Teratogenic Potential*

Several drugs are suspected of having some teratogenic potential because they are occasionally associated with malformations in the offspring of women treated during early pregnancy. These reports, however, constitute only a low percentage of the total number of women known or thought to have been treated, and consequently are subject to varied interpretations as (1) spontaneous occurrences only coincidentally related to drug treatment, (2) attributable in some part to the maternal disease for which the drug was given, or (3) manifestation of a low order of teratogenic potential of the drug. Reliance on voluntary reporting of individual cases generally does not provide the type or quantity of data needed to choose among these alternatives. Prospective epidemiologic surveys are sometimes able to rule out the possibility of drug-related causation, as was the case with meclizine (Mellin and Katzenstein, 1964), but more often such surveys provide suggestive rather than definitive data (Nelson and Forfar, 1971).

a. *Anticonvulsants.* Anticonvulsants are prominent in the group of drugs suspected of having some teratogenic potential in man. Meadow (1968, 1970) reported a total of 38 cases of cleft lip and/or cleft palate in infants born to epileptic women on anticonvulsant drugs throughout pregnancy; 8 also had congenital heart disease. In a preliminary account of a more recent retrospective study on 427 pregnancies in 186 epileptic women, Speidel and Meadow (1972) reported twice the expected frequency of major malformations, including congenital heart disease, facial clefts, microcephaly, and other defects. In a similar study of 65 babies born to epileptic mothers in Holland, Elshove and van Eck (1971) found that congenital anomalies were 8 times more frequent than in the control population and that facial clefts were 29 times more frequent. Four additional cases of facial clefts (Pashayan *et al.,* 1971) and one of equivocal genitalia (McMullin, 1971) have been reported after the taking of anticonvulsant drugs during pregnancy. Phenobarbital was most commonly used, but several other drugs were taken singly or in combination. Thus, although the incidence of defects in the above studies was substantially higher than would be found in an otherwise similar population that had not taken these drugs, in view of the bias inherent in retrospective surveys (see Chapter 8, Section I,A,2), these data must be taken as only suggestive.

Approaching the question differently, a survey of drug prescriptions issued to women giving birth to malformed babies reported that a significantly higher proportion of barbiturates was given to such mothers than to mothers of normal children (Crombie *et al.,* 1970). Mirkin (1971) followed prospectively three epileptic women on diphenylhydantoin (Dilantin) throughout pregnancy and reported that all gave birth to babies with cleft lip or palate.

Trimethadione, another antiepileptic drug, has been associated with malformation in 8 of 14 pregnancies of 4 women who received this compound during the early months of pregnancy (German *et al.,* 1970). Four of the defective children had facial clefts and four had cardiac defects, which, together with the above, strongly suggests a recurring pattern of malformations associated with anticonvulsant drugs.

The Report (6th Annual) of the Committee on Adverse Drug Reactions of New Zealand (1971) indicates that 11 of the 29 adverse effects attributed to various anticonvulsants in one year involved the birth of malformed children, and that 9 of the 11 mothers of these children were epileptic and were on continuous therapy throughout pregnancy; 7 of the children in the latter group had facial clefts and 3 had congenital heart disease. Kučera (1971a) in a large survey in Czechoslovakia has reported a marginally significant *(P* = 0.05) increase in facial clefts and congenital heart disease in infants born to epileptic women on anticonvulsant therapy, as compared with the general population. On the other hand, there are reports of many women on anticonvulsant therapy throughout pregnancy with no untoward effect (Bird, 1969) or in which the rate of malformations was only questionably elevated (Janz and Fuchs, 1964).

The foregoing data relate to use of several anticonvulsants, but they bring

TABLE 3-5

EMBRYOTOXIC EFFECTS OF DIPHENYLHYDANTOIN IN 100-DAY RHESUS MONKEY FETUSES[a]

Fetus No.	Maternal treatment		Weight (gm)	Condition of fetus		
	Daily dose (mg/kg)	Gestational days treated		External examination	Autopsy examination	Skeletal examination
♂3a	25 id	22–24	145	Normal	Normal	Normal
−29c	50 id	19–21		Aborted on day 29		
♀11c	25 bid	22–24	118	Normal	Normal	Small talus
♀90a	5 bid	25–45	141	Normal	Normal	Normal
♂13f	5 bid	25–45	129	Normal	Retrocaval right ureter[b]	Normal
♀73b	5 bid	25–45	141	Normal	Normal	Normal
♀71b	5 bid	25–45	136	Normal	Retrocaval right ureter	Normal
♀83b	10 bid	24–44	132	Normal	Normal	Normal
♀59d	10 bid	25–45	121	Normal	Normal	Normal
♂29f	10 bid	23–43	152	Normal	Normal	Normal
♂38d	10 bid	20–40	134	? Neck webbing	Normal	Normal
♂33e	20 bid	22–42	122	Normal	Retrocaval right ureter	Absent talus
♀50d	20 bid	24–44	144	Normal	Three cusps on mitral valve	Normal
♂13g	20 bid	20–40	146	Normal	Normal	Cervical ribs
−81c	20 bid	23–43		Aborted on day 44		
15 controls	Vehicle or none	—	143 ± 12[c]			Several skeletal variations[d]

[a] From dams given large doses early in pregnancy.

[b] Retrocaval right ureter has not been previously seen in rhesus monkeys.

[c] ±, standard deviation.

[d] Skeletal variants include 1 with no ossification of talus, 2 with extra pair ribs, 2 with extra rudimentary ribs, 1 with "knobby" ribs.

to a disturbing total the number of defective children attributed to the taking of drugs of this class during early pregnancy. It is noteworthy that a majority of the affected children had facial clefts and not a few had cardio-vascular defects, which tends to speak against a causative role for the folic acid deficiency known to be associated with some anticonvulsant therapy. Folic acid deficiency does not produce a characteristic syndrome of defects (see Section II,F,1,c). Of interest is that diphenylhydantoin in single doses is highly teratogenic in mice (Harbison and Becker, 1969). Because of the recurring suggestive reports in man the present author has undertaken to test the teratogenicity of Dilantin (diphenylhydantoin) in pregnant rhesus monkeys (Table 3-5). Using doses several times larger than recommended human dosage, the only embryotoxicity yet seen in this species was a minor urinary tract anomaly and possibly a slight increase in abortions. Neverthe-less, this class of drugs must continue to be watched closely.

b. *Neurotropic–Anorexogenic Drugs.* Such compounds as dexamphetam-ine and phenmetrazine have at times been held suspect, in part on the basis of results from animal experiments (Tuchmann-Duplessis and Mercier-Par-ot, 1964). For example, dexamphetamine sulfate readily produced malfor-mations when given during pregnancy in mice (Nora *et al.,* 1965), but retrospective analysis of 219 cases and prospective study of 52 cases involving use during human pregnancy yielded no teratogenic effects (Nora *et al.,* 1967a). The question was reconsidered, however, when a subsequent study of 184 mothers of infants with heart malformations showed a higher inci-dence of amphetamine ingestion than a control group (Nora *et al.,* 1970). Another study has found an elevated incidence of biliary tract atresia among offspring of mothers taking amphetamines (Levin, 1971). A recent ret-rospective survey of 458 mothers of children with various malformations (Nelson and Forfar, 1971) showed that a higher proportion of such moth-ers had taken dextroamphetamine for suppression of appetite during the early part of pregnancy than had the control mothers of normal infants. An-other neurotropic drug used as an appetite suppressant during pregnancy, phenmetrazine, was reported to have been associated with the birth of defective children in a few instances (Moss, 1962; Powell and Johnstone, 1962), but this was not confirmed by other reports (Notter and Delande, 1962). Neurotropic substances sometimes mentioned as possibly teratogenic are Dominal (Tuchmann-Duplessis and Mercier-Parot, 1964a) and bro-mine-containing compounds (Opitz *et al.,* 1972) but supporting evidence is meager.

c. *Oral Hypoglycemics.* Certain oral hypoglycemics must now be includ-ed in the suspect category. Since 1961, when 2 cases (Campbell, 1961; Larsson and Sterky, 1961) of malformed infants were reported as born to mothers taking tolbutamide or other sulfonylurea compounds throughout pregnancy to control diabetes, more than 10 similar cases have been described (Caldera, 1970; Campbell, 1963; Coopersmith and Kerbel, 1962; Dolger *et al.,* 1969; Schiff *et al.,* 1970). Generally malformed infants have occurred in a ratio of about 1 in 20 among all births to women taking tolbutamide during pregnancy; but there have been other reports of fairly large series of cases in which no abnormalities were observed (Sterne, 1963). The low incidence together with the absence of a syndrome of defects leaves the teratogenic status of the sulfonylurea hypoglycemics in man in some doubt. There is, however, no doubt but that these compounds are highly teratogenic in mice, rats, and rabbits (Tuchmann-Duplessis and Mercier-Parot, 1963).

d. *Alkylating Agents.* Because of their polyfunctional suppression of growth alkylating agents would be immediately suspect as teratogens. They are radiomimetic, cytotoxic, and highly teratogenic in laboratory animals (Chaube and Murphy, 1968; DiPaolo and Kotin, 1966; Tuchmann-Duplessis, 1969). Nevertheless, few instances of human maldevelopment have been attributed to use of these compounds during pregnancy (Sokal and Lessman, 1960), although intrauterine death and abortion may occur at high dosage. One woman given 6-mercaptopurine and busulfan (Myleran) during pregnancy produced a baby with multiple malformations (Diamond *et al.,* 1960), one given chlorambucil produced a fetus with urinary tract abnormalities (Shotten and Monie, 1963), and one given cyclophosphamide delivered a child with multiple musculoskeletal defects (Greenberg and Tanaka, 1964). A variety of cytotoxic, cancer chemotherapeutic agents have been administered to pregnant monkeys and were found to produce high rates of intrauterine death but relatively few outright malformations (Wilson, 1972b). The paucity of human cases may be attributed to (1) limited use during pregnancy because of high teratogenicity in laboratory animals (Hoskins, 1948; Murphy *et al.,* 1957; Thiersch, 1957), (2) probable high rate of treatment-induced death and abortion when used in man, and (3) easy justification of elective abortion because of the life-saving role of these drugs for the mother. In other words, the biologic effects of alkylating agents are such as to discourage their use during pregnancy except in the event of neoplasia. Apart from their direct teratogenic potential, several of these compounds are known to be mutagenic in mammals or mammalian cell cultures (Fishbein *et al.,* 1970).

3. *Drugs with Possible Teratogenic Potential*

This category includes several drugs that, in spite of widespread use, have only rarely been implicated in human teratogenesis. Some such as aspirin are not known to have produced embryotoxicity in man but have been demonstrated to have high teratogenicity in laboratory mammals. Others such as antibiotics are known to have adverse effects on most rapidly growing systems and it is supposed that they might possibly be teratogenic to man under certain conditions. Still others have been occasionally implicated in man but supporting data are meager or contradictory.

a. *Aspirin.* Since Warkany and Takacs (1959) demonstrated in rats and Larsson *et al.* (1963) in mice that large doses of salicylates were teratogenic, questions are sometimes raised about their possible embryotoxicity in man, particularly aspirin, in view of its widespread use as an analgesic and the high dosage used in rheumatic disease. Studies in pregnant rhesus monkeys have shown that doses of aspirin 5 or 6 times higher than the teratogenic level in rodents produced definite embryotoxicity in fetuses of this species (Wilson, 1971). Of 8 pregnant monkeys so treated, 2 aborted within 3 weeks of oral dosage, 3 produced malformed offspring (Fig. 3-3), 2 produced growth-retarded fetuses, of which 1 had unilateral cervical rib, and only 1 produced a normal fetus. It should be emphasized that the daily dose 500 mg/kg) was considerably in excess of that likely to be used therapeutically in pregnant women. This "margin of safety" has been made less secure, however, by the observation of Kimmel *et al.,* (1971) that the teratogenic potential of a given dose of aspirin in rats can be appreciably increased by concurrent administration of benzoic acid, a widely used food preservative (Fig. 3-4). Similar metabolic interaction of benzoic acid and salicylates is known to occur in man (Levy, 1965), but whether such interaction could raise the salicylate level in the maternal blood sufficiently to cause embryotoxicity remains a moot question.

There are no known instances of human teratogenicity directly traceable to the taking of large doses of aspirin during pregnancy, but there is epidemiologic indication of a relation between the taking of aspirin during pregnancy and the delivery of defective babies. In a retrospective survey of 833 pregnancies that yielded malformed infants (Richards, 1969), it was found that a significantly greater ($P = < 0.001$) percentage of women delivering defective babies had taken a salicylate preparation during the first trimester of pregnancy than had women delivering normal babies. This is well summarized in the author's words: "The results of this investigation suggest that either salicylates have a teratogenic effect or that the conditions for which they are given have such an action." In another retrospective study based on 458 mothers who gave birth to malformed infants it was reported (Nelson and Forfar, 1971) that analgesics (mainly aspirin) were taken by a significantly higher proportion, both throughout and during the first 56 days of pregnancy, than in the control mothers of normal babies. To the contrary, another survey of the types of drugs prescribed during early pregnancy to mothers of malformed children showed that significantly fewer aspirin-containing preparations were issued to such mothers than to women delivering

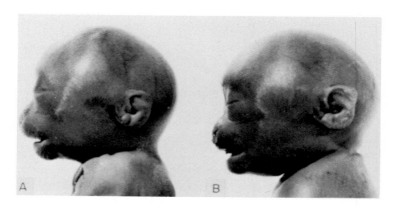

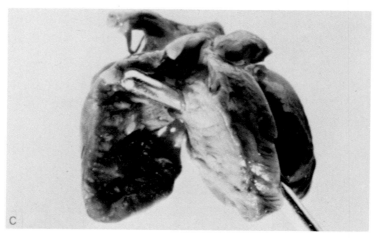

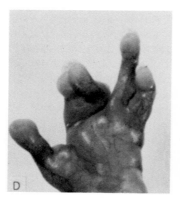
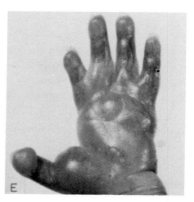

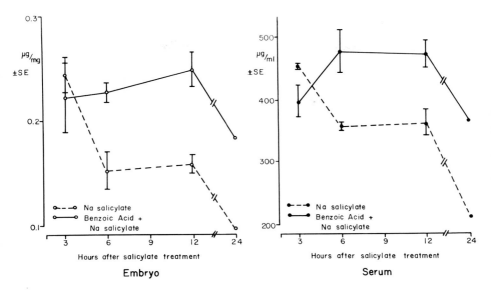

FIG. 3-4. Concentrations of free salicylate in embryos and maternal serum after treatment of maternal rats on day 11 of gestation with sodium salicylate alone at 500 mg/kg and treatment with the same dose of sodium salicylate 2 hours after benzoic acid at 510 mg/kg. (From Kimmel *et al.*, 1971.)

normal babies (Crombie *et al.*, 1970). Thus, by no means proved to have teratogenic potential, aspirin should not at this time be dismissed as involving no embryotoxic risk for man.

b. *Antibiotics.* This diverse group of drugs has been implicated in human teratology mainly by the reports of Carter and Wilson (1965), who made a retrospective analysis of the offspring of 85 women given an antibiotic during the first 12 weeks of pregnancy. Twelve of the infants were malformed, as against 2 that would have been expected in untreated pregnancies, and 13 aborted, whereas the expected number would have been 8. An additional 67 cases of antibiotic administration during the first 12 weeks of human gestation yielded approximately 25% of pregnancy wastage (the sum of abor-

FIG. 3-3. Malformations in a 100-day rhesus monkey fetus following treatment of the pregnant mother with aspirin at 500 mg/kg/day from days 19 to 22 of gestation. A. Micrognathia and moderate microcephaly in a fetus of the same weight as the animal in B, a normal control. C. Heart of fetus in A with a probe inserted through a moderate ventricular septal defect. D. Syndactyly in a hind foot (both were affected) compared with E, hind foot of a normal control of the same size. (From Wilson, 1972a.)

tion, malformation, stillbirth and neonatal death) as compared with 14% in the control group (Carter, 1965). Deafness has occasionally been reported in young children following streptomycin therapy of the mother during pregnancy (Boletti and Croatto, 1958; Robinson and Cambon, 1964). In two recent retrospective surveys (Nelson and Forfar, 1971; Richards, 1969), however, no indication was found of an increase in malformations after administration of antibiotics during pregnancy.

Several antibiotics have been shown to be teratogenic in rodents, e.g., tetracycline (Filippi, 1967), streptonigrin (Warkany and Takacs, 1965), hadicidin (Lejour-Jeanty, 1966), penicillin–streptomycin mixtures (Filippi, 1967), actinomycin D (Tuchmann-Duplessis and Mercier-Parot, 1960; Wilson, 1966), and mitomycin C (Nishimura, 1963). All antibiotics are not potent teratogens in animals, however. Those thought to act primarily by inhibiting protein synthesis, such as puromycin and lincomycin, have been found at high doses to be little, if at all, teratogenic but highly embryolethal (unpublished data, author's laboratory).

The widespread use during pregnancy of antibiotics over the past 20 years and the fact that appreciable embryotoxicity for man has not been reported probably mean that the teratogenic potential of these compounds is low under usual conditions of usage. Nevertheless, their known effects on rapidly proliferating cells in culture, together with demonstrated teratogenicity of some antibiotics on mammalian embryos *in vivo,* suggest that such potential under some conditions be regarded as a possibility in man.

c. *Antituberculous Drugs.* Of this assorted group some have been questioned as regards adverse effects on pregnancy or its outcome but no one or combination has been proved to have such effects in man. Ethionamide was reported to be teratogenic in one study of 22 women who received the drug during pregnancy (Potworowska *et al.,* 1966). Only 5 were known to have taken the drug during the early months of pregnancy, but of these 4 produced malformed children. There was no common defect or syndrome, but the central nervous system was involved in all. The simultaneous use of two or more antituberculous drugs (streptomycin, isoniazid, and p-aminosalicylic acid) in 123 pregnant women was reported (Varpela, 1964) to have increased the frequency of malformations among their offspring by a factor of 2 or 3 compared with controls. Other studies on the use of isoniazid during pregnancy reported "harmful effects" but no malformations (Monnet *et al.,* 1967) and studies on the use of various antituberculous drugs found "nothing to suggest that any of the drugs was teratogenic" (Lowe, 1964). Again the evidence is conflicting and too limited for a firm conclusion at this time.

d. *Quinine.* In high doses such as might be used in attempted abortion, this antimalarial drug has at times been mentioned as a possible human teratogenic agent. Winckel (1948) was able to collect only 17 cases in which some visual or auditory defects in the offspring were associated with the taking of quinine during pregnancy, but the evidence for a causal relationship was tenuous in several of these. Tanimura (1972) undertook to survey the literature and was able to find 20 cases of human malformation said to be associated with the taking of quinine to induce abortion, but there was no indication of the sample size from which these were taken and the details of dosage in such cases are often not reliable. Animal experiments reviewed by the same author reported frequent intrauterine death and growth retardation but few malformations among the offspring of treated animals, including several rhesus monkeys.

e. *Imipramine.* Early in 1972 reports from Australia stated that a positive correlation had been established between the taking of this antidepressant during the first third of pregnancy and the birth of infants with reduction deformities of the upper limb resembling those seen after thalidomide ingestion (McBride, 1972). Although press reports later indicated that these claims had been in part withdrawn, the fact that this and related tricyclic antidepressants had been found to show a low but variable level of teratogenicity in rabbits and rats (Robson and Sullivan, 1963; Aeppli, 1969) requires that the possibility of human teratogenicity be thoroughly investigated. A search through current literature by the present author yields 221 published cases in which one of these drugs was known or presumed to have been taken during the first trimester of human pregnancy (Barson, 1972; Crombie *et al.,* 1972; Kuennsberg and Knox, 1972; Scanlon, 1969; Sim, 1972; Report of the New Zealand Committee on Adverse Drug Reactions, 1971). A total of 6 children with various malformations was reported and, interestingly, none had limb defects such as were characteristic of McBride's cases. (These data do not represent a true incidence because the total number of pregnancies treated is not known and the search for malformations among offspring of reported cases was not exhaustive.) The Metropolitan Atlanta Congenital Malformations Report (Jan.–Feb., 1972) examined 120 cases involving reduction deformity of the limbs similar to those described by McBride and was unable to establish that any of the mothers had taken imipramine or related antidepressants. If these tricyclic antidepressant drugs have teratogenic potential in man, it is of low order when used at recommended therapeutic doses, and there is no new evidence to support the original view that reduction deformities of the limbs are typically produced by these drugs.

f. *Insulin.* This widely used drug has at times been the basis for some concern. Of 14 women subjected to insulin coma in psychiatric therapy during the first 14 weeks of gestation, 4 produced dead and 2 delivered malformed fetuses (Sobel, 1960), and 2 mentally defective children were associated with similar maternal therapy during the third month of pregnancy

(Wickes, 1954). The occasional malformed infant born to a diabetic woman maintained on insulin is probably coincidental (Pettersson *et al.*, 1970) or a reflection of the higher malformation rate associated with diabetes (see Section II, E,2).

4. *Drugs Involving Little or No Teratogenic Risk*

To state categorically that a drug or other environmental factor involves no risk to developing organisms, in view of accumulated experience in both animals and man, would be no less than foolhardy. In fact many teratologists accept the theoretical principle that all chemical agents could be shown, under the right conditions of dosage, developmental stage, and species selection, to have adverse effects on development (Karnofsky, 1965b; Wilson, 1964a), although the correlary must also be accepted that it is not always possible to demonstrate this principle. Nevertheless, it can be stated with some assurance that certain agents are unlikely to cause adverse effects within the limits of dosage ordinarily encountered. Drugs placed in this category have, for some reason at some time, been suspect but then found after further investigation to pose little risk in human therapeutic use, despite the fact that at higher dosage they may be detrimental to development in laboratory animals.

a. *Lysergic Acid Diethylamide.* There has been much controversy about claims of cytogenetic and teratogenic effects following use of lysergic acid diethylamide (LSD). A recent comprehensive review by Dishotsky *et al.* (1971) of more than 100 publications on the subject has done much to place the matter in perspective. In brief, the conclusions reached were that (1) when chromosomal damage has been found, it was among illicit drug users and therefore appears to be related to drug abuse generally; (2) pure LSD ingested in moderate dosage does not produce chromosomal damage that can be detected by current methods; (3) LSD may be a weak mutagen, but it is unlikely to be mutagenic in concentrations used by human beings; (4) early reports of teratogenic effects in rats and hamsters have for the most part not been confirmed and results in mice have been highly inconsistent; (5) the several instances of malformations among infants born to women having ingested illicit LSD during pregnancy may either be coincidental or related to the general drug-abuse problem; (6) there is no reported instance of a woman delivering a malformed child after taking pure LSD during pregnancy. Long (1972) reviewed 161 cases of children born to parents who took LSD before and/or during pregnancy and found 5 instances of limb malformation; but uncertainty about the number of other drugs taken, the time in pregnancy when taken, and other variables inherent in drug-abuse situations, together with the lack of a discernible pattern of defects, led the author to doubt that LSD was a causal factor. Dumars (1971) has as-

TABLE 3-6

EFFECTS OF LSD IN 100-DAY RHESUS MONKEY FETUSES[a]

Fetus No.	Treatment (oral)		Weight (gm)	Condition of fetus		
	Day(s) of gestation	Dose (μg) × repeated		External examination	Autopsy examination	Skeletal examination
♂22a	22	75	131	Normal	? Slight hydrocephaly	Normal
♂35a	25	75	154	Normal	Normal	No pubic ossification
♂2a	29	100	150	Normal	Normal	Bilateral cervical ribs
♀11b	27	200	145	Normal	Normal	Bilateral cervical ribs / Irregular thoracic ribs
♂16b	24,26,28	200 × 3	159	Normal	Normal	Normal
♀10b	22,24,26	200 × 3	95	Retarded	Normal	2 sternebrae / No pubic ossification
♀17d	20–46	200 × 12	151	Normal	Normal	Normal
♀51a	19–45	200 × 12	136	Normal	Normal	Normal
♀38a	22–45	200 × 12	131	Normal	Normal	Normal
♂58c	21–47	200 × 12	159	Normal	Normal	Normal
—53c	20–25	200 × 3			Aborted on day 25	
♀71a	23–49	200 × 12	141	Normal	Normal	Normal
♀39c	21–47	200 × 12	129	Normal	Normal	Normal
♂10g	20–46	200 × 12	159	Normal	Normal	Normal
15 untreated or vehicle			143±12	Normal	Normal	2 with extra ribs / 1 no pubic ossification / 1 with 2 sternebrae

[a] From dams given large doses early in pregnancy.

serted that parental use of illicit drugs does not cause differences in the incidence of chromosomal breaks or rearrangements from those seen in non-drug users.

Four pregnant rhesus monkeys were injected by Kato *et al.* (1970) with massive doses of LSD (0.125–1.0 mg/kg, approximately 90 times the human hallucinogenic dose), repeated several times during a period estimated to be in the third or fourth month of gestation. They observed 1 normal infant, 2 stillborn infants which "on gross inspection showed facial deformity," and 1 which died at 1 month postnatally. In the present author's laboratory 8 pregnant rhesus monkeys have been treated orally 3 times per week for 4 weeks between days 20 and 45 of gestation with doses of 200 μg (about 20 times the human hallucinogenic dose on per weight basis). One female aborted during treatment, but 7 were delivered of structurally normal fetuses at hysterotomy on day 100 of gestation (Table 3-6). Chromosomal abnormalities were not significantly increased in the 100-day fetuses or in the female monkeys during or after treatment. It appears that if rhesus monkeys show adverse effects on development it is at doses greatly in excess of the usual human dose.

b. *Sulfonamides.* These bacteriostatic drugs would theoretically seem to be likely teratogens by the nature of their biologic action, but such compounds have been found to have little effect on early human or other mammalian embryos. In recent retrospective surveys, one found no increase in malformations among women taking these drugs during pregnancy as compared with controls (Richards, 1969), whereas another reported a marginally significant increase in major malformations ($P = < 0.05$) in treated as compared with untreated pregnancies (Nelson and Forfar, 1971). Despite extensive use of these drugs for many years, there are no verified cases of association between taking sulfonamides during early pregnancy and subsequent delivery of a defective child. Although they have proved useful in studying teratogenic mechanisms in chicks (Landauer and Wakasugi, 1968), sulfonamides have usually been found to produce no or minimal effects in laboratory mammals (Giroud and Martinet, 1950; Paget and Thorpe, 1964). An exception has been the observation that those sulfonamides which are potent carbonic anhydrase inhibitors, acetazolamide in particular, are teratogenic in rodents (Wilson *et al.*, 1968), causing a uniquely localized malformation of the forelimbs (Fig. 3-5).

c. *Meclizine.* Meclizine and related antihistamines were thought to have had adverse effects on human development when taken during pregnancy, as reported in scattered instances soon after thalidomide was revealed to be teratogenic. Subsequently, however, several prospective studies involving large numbers of cases (Mellin, 1963; Smithells and Chinn, 1964; Yerushalmy and Milkovich, 1965) revealed that pregnant women taking these

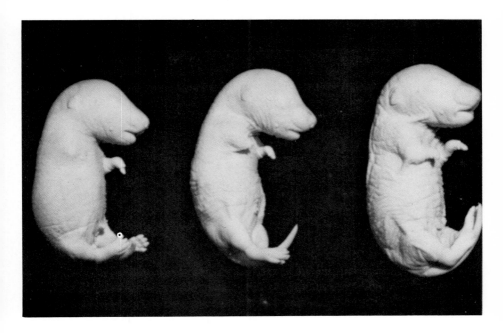

Fig. 3-5. Amelia, micromelia, and adactyly of the right forelimbs of 20-day rat fetuses from a maternal rat given the carbonic anhydrase-inhibiting sulfonamide, acetazolamide, on day 10 of gestation. The left forelimbs were also affected but usually to a lesser degree than the right ones. The hindlimbs and other external features of these fetuses were normal. (From Wilson *et al.*, 1968.)

drugs produced no more defective babies than other women. When 15 of the early studies were pooled by Lenz (1966), the 3333 infants from mothers given meclizine in the first trimester contained 12 with cleft palate or cleft lip or both, an incidence slightly higher than the expected number of such malformations in a group this size. Nevertheless, it must not be overlooked that the nutritional, fluid, and osmolyte imbalances associated with emesis gravidarum, for which meclizine was taken, might have contributed to the increased incidence of malformation found in the latter compilation. Recent studies continue to show no association between increased malformation rate and the taking of meclizine (Nelson and Forfar, 1971). By contrast, meclizine and several related antihistamines caused a high incidence of cleft palate in rats (King *et al.*, 1965), but the teratogenic dose in rats is much higher than the antiemetic dose in man.

d. *Cortisone.* As already noted (see Section II,F,1,b), cortisone is judged to have little or no teratogenic potential in man on the grounds that it has been widely used during human pregnancy and has not been shown, either in spontaneously reported cases or in epidemiologic surveys, to have been associated with the birth of defective children. The well-known teratogenicity of this compound in some rodent species undoubtedly has ensured that such associations have been looked for in man.

e. *Tranquilizers and Antiemetics.* Like cortisone, these assorted classes of drugs are assumed to have little or no teratogenic potential in man because they also have been extensively used without substantial reports of adverse effects on development. Both of these classes have, nevertheless, been held suspect, presumably because of their categoric association with thalidomide, a known teratogen, and meclizine, a drug at one time thought to be teratogenic.

5. *Overview of Drugs as Teratogens in Man*

Many drugs too numerous to name have never been mentioned in relation to teratogenesis. Prospective surveys have usually failed to indict any particular drug in association with developmental defects; furthermore, they have failed to show that the taking of drugs in general during pregnancy predisposes to a higher incidence of defects. For example, Mellin (1964) made special effort to ascertain the drugs actually taken by 3200 women during the first 13 weeks of their pregnancies. A total of 266 (8.3%) of these yielded structurally or functionally defective offspring. When these were compared with equal numbers of pregnancies yielding normal offspring born immediately before and immediately after those yielding abnormal infants, it was found that mothers producing abnormal children did not take more or significantly different drugs than the mothers in the two control groups (Table 3-7). Although these numbers were limited, the care with which this study was done strengthens the opinion that the mere taking of drugs during the first trimester does not predispose to abnormal development. In consideration of the findings in the foregoing review, one is inclined to agree with Mellin, who concluded that ". . . drugs in general are not an important factor in congenital malformations in general." Barring teratologic catastrophes such as thalidomide, the few drugs that have been identified as having some teratogenic potential in man represent only a very small fraction of either the drugs used or of the defects produced.

To avert any complacency that may result from the views stated above, however, it should be noted that two lingering questions remain unanswered: (1) Is it possible to devise tests and surveillance systems that will prevent another teratologic catastrophe such as thalidomide? (2) How are interactions between drugs and other environmental factors, or these and unstable genetic loci, to be identified, assuming that such interactions contribute significantly to the large "unknown" segment of causation in human teratology?

TABLE 3-7

Number of Mothers with Malformed Infants in Relation to the Number of Drugs Taken during the First Trimester of Pregnancy Compared with Two Groups of Control Pregnancies Yielding Normal Children[a]

No. drugs taken during first 13 weeks from last menstrual period	No. of mothers			Percentage of mothers		
	Congenital malformation	First control	Second control	Congenital malformation	First control	Second control
0	125	134	127	47.0	50.4	47.7
1	83	67	75	31.2	25.2	28.2
2	30	34	36	11.3	12.8	13.5
3	12	20	14	4.5	7.5	5.3
4	7	5	6	2.6	1.9	2.3
5	5	2	3	1.9	0.8	1.1
6	2	—	3	0.8	—	1.1
7	1	1	2	0.4	0.4	0.8
8	1	2	—	0.4	0.8	—
9	—	1	—	—	0.4	—
	266	266	266	100.0	100.0	100.0

[a] From Mellin (1964).

G. Environmental Chemicals

Concern is voiced with increasing frequency about the potential risks to reproduction and development of the large numbers of chemical substances being introduced into the environment. Actually the problem of detrimental effects on development from environmental chemicals such as lead is by no means a new one (Warkany, 1971), although recent recognition of some previously unsuspected types of exposure emphasize the need for close scrutiny of other seemingly unlikely situations involving pregnant women. For example, neuromuscular abnormalities and failure to grow in a child has been attributed to lead poisoning as a result of consumption by the pregnant mother of untaxed (moonshine) whiskey (Palmisano *et al.,* 1969); and a high abortion rate and the birth of a child with clubfeet, among pregnant women working in a media preparation laboratory, have been related to exposure to high selenium levels (Robertson, 1970). Other environmental chemicals that have been clearly implicated or recently brought under suspicion as being embryotoxic in man are discussed below.

1. *Methyl Mercury*

Mercury as well as lead has been regarded with some suspicion for a number of years (Butt and Simonsen, 1950). The demonstration that industrial effluents into Minamata Bay and other coastal waters of Japan were responsible for a congenital form of Minamata disease, however, was the first proved instance of organic mercury having accumulated as a teratogenic pollutant. Several newborn babies exhibited multiple neurologic symptoms resembling cerebral palsy. The mothers of these infants had eaten diets containing a large proportion of fish which, as a result of biologic magnification through the food chain, had accumulated high concentrations of methyl mercury (Harada, 1968; Matsumoto *et al.,* 1965). The fact that many of the mothers of affected babies did not themselves show symptoms of the adult form of the disease was further proof of the greater sensitivity of the fetus than of the mother to many chemical agents. The same type of congenital mercury poisoning occurred in the United States (Snyder, 1971) when a mercury-containing fungicide was applied to seed corn which was then fed to hogs, meat from which was subsequently eaten by a pregnant woman. The frank teratogenicity of organic mercury has now been confirmed in mice (Spyker and Smithberg, 1972) and in hamsters (Harris *et al.,* 1972).

2. *Industrial Solvents*

Several types of solvents have been shown to be teratogenic or otherwise embryotoxic in mammals, for example, acetamides and formamides in rats (Thiersch, 1962), dimethylsulfoxide in hamsters (Ferm, 1966), benzene in mice (Watanabe *et al.,* 1968), and several alkane sulfonates in rats (Helms-worth, 1968). Similar incidents in man are largely unknown, but the possi-bilities of industrial or household exposure to such substances during early pregnancy should be thoroughly examined. At least one report relates in-dustrial exposure of pregnant women to fat solvents such as zylene, trichlo-roethylene, methylchloroethylene, and acetone and the subsequent birth of children with sacral agenesis (Kučera, 1968). The same author points out that similar malformation can be induced in chicks by exposure of incubat-ing eggs to xylene.

3. *Pesticides*

Among the great variety of pesticides the defoliant 2,4,5-T has undoubt-edly been most often linked with teratogenesis. This compound has recently been the subject of exhaustive review of all of its effects on mammalian re-production (Report of the 2,4,5-T Advisory Committee, 1971), with partic-ular attention to possible teratogenic effects in man and laboratory animals. Claims have come from three areas of the world of embryotoxicity following alleged exposure during human pregnancy, namely, Vietnam (Cutting *et al.,* 1970; Meselson *et al.,* 1970); Globe, Arizona (Binns *et al.,* 1970); and Swedish Lappland (Rapport fram en expert grupp, 1971). When all available evidence from these localities was examined by qualified scientists, however, no basis could be found for regarding this herbicide as teratogenic in man. Data on its teratogenicity in six mammalian species were also evaluated. Mice showed moderate teratogenicity at the dose of 100 mg/kg/day throughout organogenesis, whereas rat and hamster embryos responded to doses that were nearer the maternal toxic level. Rabbits, sheep, and rhesus monkeys gave no indication of adverse effects at doses well in excess of any likely to be encountered in nature. None of the recent adequately controlled studies relating to this subject presents data indicating that this herbicide as present-ly marketed poses any risk to any aspect of human reproduction under like-ly conditions of exposure.

Positive embryotoxicity after application of some other pesticides during pregnancy in laboratory animals is known: organophosphorus cholinesterase inhibitors such as DFP, parathion, and methyl parathion caused intrauterine death and growth retardation but no anomalies in rats (Fish, 1966); captan caused malformations in rabbits (McLaughlin *et al.,* 1969); carbaryl pro-duced terata in very high doses in guinea pigs but not in hamsters and rats; and thiram was teratogenic in hamsters (Robens, 1969). Courtney *et al.* (1970) reported on a large-scale screening study in mice in which a number of pesticides were found to produce a statistically significant increase in the proportion of litters containing abnormal young, e.g., PCNB, captan, folpet,

2,4,5-T, 2,4-D isooctyl ester, 2,4-D butyl ester, 2,4-D isopropyl ester, carbaryl, and IPC. To obtain the adverse effects mentioned it was necessary to use large doses concentrated during the period of organogenesis. In contrast, exposure in nature would usually be in small doses over an extended period. There is no evidence that any of these compounds is embryotoxic in man.

It is noteworthy that DDT, the insecticide most often accused of adverse biologic effects, has not been reported to be teratogenic in any mammalian species (Khera and Clegg, 1969). It appears that relatively few of the numerous pesticides now in use have been found to be teratogenic, a somewhat surprising observation in view of the fact that these compounds were developed for the specific purpose of arresting growth in or killing living organisms. The failure of individual agents to be more widely embryotoxic in mammals may be attributable to one or more of the following: (1) They have not been adequately tested at high doses in pregnant mammals; (2) they possess a high degree of species specificity as regards their toxic effects; or (3) they possess a low ratio of maternal to embryonic toxicity. In the latter case pregnancy would be terminated or precluded before teratogenicity could be demonstrated.

4. *Cigarette Smoking*

Cigarette smoking during pregnancy has been reported (Fedrick *et al.,* 1971) to have possible teratogenic effects. Congenital heart disease was observed in 7.3 per 1000 births to women who smoked cigarettes (any amount) throughout pregnancy, whereas only 4.7 per 1000 such defects were seen among births to nonsmokers. The authors cautioned against accepting this 50% increase as proof of teratogenicity, in part because it was noted that the rate of smoking was higher among women of lower socioeconomic status. Other surveys have shown that cigarette smoking during pregnancy increased late fetal and neonatal mortality rates by 28% and reduced birth weight by an average of 170 gm (Butler *et al.,* 1972) and that the deficiency of weight and the excess of mortality among the offspring of smokers was not entirely dependent on race or socioeconomic factors (Rush and Kass, 1972). Thus, smoking by pregnant women increases the chances of perinatal death and decreases birth weight of their infants, but there is only suggestive evidence that it may increase the chance of malformation. Nicotine has been found to be teratogenic in chicks (Landauer, 1960) and mice (Nishimura and Nakai, 1958), but not in rats (Geller, 1959).

H. Perinatal Nutritional Deficiency

The teratogenic and embryolethal effects of specific dietary deficiencies during early pregnancy in animals has been reviewed earlier in this chapter

(Section I,C) and elsewhere (Asling, 1969; Giroud, 1971; Hurley, 1968b; Warkany, 1952–1953). Furthermore, some prenatal deficiencies have been shown to lead to irreversible functional deficits as well as structural abnormalities in the postnatal animal (Hurley, 1968a). It has often been stated that specific nutritional deficits such as interfere with development in animals are unlikely to occur in the human diet. General caloric restrictions and scarcity of several essential nutrients, however, exist today as they have at many times and places in human history. Whether such deficiencies during the developmental stages of man produce lasting deterimental effects has been much debated and still awaits final resolution.

For more than 30 years attempts have been made to evaluate the effects of inadequate diets on human reproduction and development. Miscarriage, stillbirths, premature birth, and postnatal morbidity were found to be considerably higher in Toronto among the offspring of mothers who ate a "poor diet" during pregnancy than among those of mothers whose diets were considered to be adequate (Ebbs *et al.,* 1941). A similar survey of pregnancies in Boston revealed that all stillbirths, all neonatal deaths except one, most congenitally defective infants, and all premature and functionally immature infants were born to mothers whose diets were judged to be "very inadequate" (Burke *et al.,* 1943). When the diet was "good to excellent" there was high probability that the infant would be in good physical condition. The wartime starvation imposed upon the inhabitants of several countries during World War II eventually resulted in infertility, but infants conceived before severe famine conditions prevailed were more often stillborn or were significantly below expected weight and length; however, prematurity and malformations were only slightly and not significantly increased (Antonov, 1947; Smith, 1947). These early studies indicated that extreme nutritional deprivation in man definitely could impair human reproduction and postnatal survival, and possibly contribute to an increase in the rate of malformations. In this connection it should be borne in mind that the socioeconomic factors often associated with malnutrition are also frequently correlated with genetic and other environmental factors that contribute to less than optimal development.

Much attention has been focused on the demonstration that severe malnutrition during infancy does produce biochemical and growth rate changes in the brain of children as well as animals (Zamenof *et al.,* 1971; Winick, 1969, 1971). Furthermore several investigators have related malnourishment in infancy to mental deficits in later life (Cravioto and Delicardie, 1970; Dobbing, 1970; Hertig *et al.,* 1972) and there is substantial evidence that kwashiorkor of such degree as to require hospitalization has a detrimental influence on intelligence during childhood (Birch *et al.,* 1971). There is little doubt but that permanent impairment of function can be induced in the brains of developmentally immature animals by agents causing relatively mild structural damage. For example, x-irradiation (Altman, 1971; Ostertag, 1969) or injection of drugs (Langman and Shimada, 1971; Langman *et al.*, 1972) in perinatal mice resulted in dose-dependent degrees of interference with the histogenesis of the brain, followed by associated motor disabilities.

That the brain of the human newborn is also vulnerable is illustrated in infants with phenylketonuria. When the congenital enzyme deficiency characteristic of this disease is recognized early enough to permit dietary restriction of phenylalanine, beginning soon after birth, most or all of the mental retardation associated with hyperphenylalaninemia can be avoided (O'Grady *et al.*, 1970). Thus, is seems to be established that the brain can have its final maturation diverted by adverse environmental influences during the early postnatal period, but the question of whether malnutrition alone is capable of causing permanent mental damage in human beings remains controversial at this time (Frisch, 1970; McKeown and Record, 1971).

CHAPTER 4

MECHANISMS OF TERATOGENESIS

The word mechanism has been used in many contexts in biology and medicine and consequently has come to have a less than precise meaning. It is perhaps most often used to indicate the means by which an effect is produced; for example, in teratology the means by which a malformation or other developmental defect comes into being. Such an unrestricted definition, however, can include everything or anything between the initiating cause and the final effect, without specifying how comprehensively or selectively the intervening events will be focused upon. It has already been noted that an ordered sequence of events occurs between the inception of abnormal development, when a causative agent first acts on a developing system, and its final manifestation as a structural or functional defect. Collectively these events can be properly referred to as the pathogenesis of abnormal development. There is, however, need to place special emphasis on the early events in pathogenesis because these are important, not only in initiating, but also in determining the direction of subsequent pathogenesis. Difficulty arises in identifying the first event, which probably often lies at the subcellular if not at the molecular level. Until the early events of pathogenesis are better known, therefore, it is proposed to apply the word mechanism to the earliest identifiable event thought to play a primary role in determining abnormal development.

Actually there is little precise information about how particular causes from the environment impinge on developing cells to produce the first recognizable reaction that is here called a mechanism. But by sifting through the literature of experimental teratology, it is possible to deduce that there are perhaps eight or ten general types of reactions by which developing cells might respond to outside influences in ways that would lead to abnormal embryogenesis. It can also be inferred that the different mechanisms are not

83

always triggered by the same type of cause. In other words, there is not necessarily a close specificity between a particular cause and a particular type of mechanism; possibly any one cause can activate any one or more mechanisms. Radiations, for example, seem able to produce several early effects in cells, such as point mutations, chromosome breaks, mitotic interference, and enzyme inhibitions. Similarly, dietary deficiency might result in substrate lack, altered energy sources, or osmolar imbalance. Thus, when the known causes are examined for probable initial effects in tissues, the mechanisms listed in Scheme 4-1 come to mind. It is probable that mechanisms not now suspected will be revealed by further research, just as some of those now listed are likely to be eliminated or consolidated with others as new data throw light on which effects are primary and which are secondary reactions. Existing data in support of those now listed are summarized as follows.

I. Mutation

This is the mechanism by which the nucleotide sequence in nuclear DNA strands is altered in such a way as to change the developmental potential of progeny cells. If the change occurs in a germinal cell, it is heritable and is called a germinal mutation; if in developing somatic cells, it is not heritable, is called a somatic mutation, and may cause a developmental defect or possibly a neoplasm, but only in that individual. Changes in nucleotide sequence take varied forms (Auerbach, 1967) (Fig. 4-1) depending on the numbers of nucleotides involved. The changes are mainly of three types: (1) interconversions within a single base pair, (2) deletions or insertions of

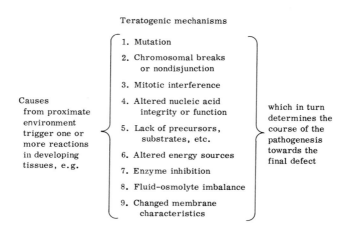

SCHEME 4-1. Diagram of the relationship of teratogenic mechanisms to prior causes and subsequent pathogenesis (see text for further explanation).

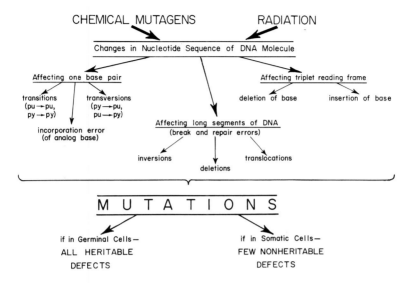

Fɪɢ. 4-1. The kinds of mutations as produced by two well-established types of causative agents, chemical mutagens and ionizing radiations. It is assumed that all mutations are induced by some environmental factor.

one or two bases so as to change the reading frame of the triplet codons, and (3) breaks with no or erroneous repair of longer DNA segments. Single base pairs may be modified by chemically converting one purine to another purine or a pyrimidine to another pyrimidine (transition), a purine to a pyrimidine or the reverse (transversion), or by the incorporation of an analog base which can lead to either of the foregoing (incorporation error). Since the nucleotides of a DNA strand are read in groups of three which code for individual amino acids, the deletion or insertion of a base changes the order of nucleotides within the triplet reading frame. As a consequence the message becomes garbled, as illustrated by the contrived triplet sentence that follows:

HER FAT CAT ATE HIS PET RAT

by deleting one letter but retaining the triplet reading frame becomes

HER FTC ATA TEH ISP ETR AT-.

When the molecule of DNA is disrupted, as in a chromosome break, one of the segments may be lost or erroneous repair may occur so that beyond the break the strand will be deficient or the sequence inverted, or made otherwise discontinuous by translocation of a segment from elsewhere. Ionizing radiations and a variety of chemical agents are able to cause chromosome breaks, both *in vivo* and *in vitro*. Such breaks are often repaired but restoration of the gross configurations of the chromosome does not preclude gene mutations. In addition to the obvious possibilities of inversions and translocations during repair, loss of only a few nucleotides at the site of the break, more or less than three, could result in changes in the triplet reading frame along the remainder of the strand.

Regardless of the nature of the change in nucleotide sequence, the result is a mutation (Fig. 4-1). Its future manifestations, however, depend on the type of developmental cell affected. If mutation affects a germinal cell, it will become heritable when the cell or its progeny participate in fertilization, except in the event there is a lethal effect on the germ cells initially affected. If mutation affects a somatic cell in an embryo, it will not become hereditary, but it may change the developmental potential of progeny cells sufficiently to produce a recognizable defect in that individual, either of a developmental or a neoplastic nature (Lederberg, 1970). The known environmental causes of mutation are ionizing radiations; a variety of chemical mutagens such as nitrous acid, alkylating agents, some carcinogens, etc. (Fishbein *et al.*, 1970); and such other factors as might lead to chromosomal breaks or crossovers (Jukes, 1966; Freese, 1971). Presumably mutations can occur at all times in the cell cycle. It is in the area of mutations that genetics and teratology overlap: Mutations produce the developmental defects that become hereditary.

II. Chromosomal Nondisjunction and Breaks

Chromosomal aberrations, including nondisjunction and loss or translocation of parts of chromatids, result in visible excess or deficiency of chromatin material in progeny cells. Nondisjunction is the failure of divided chromosomes to separate during cell division; it occurs most often during the meiotic divisions of germ cell maturation. Mosaic chromosomal abnormalities, however, in which there are two or more populations of cells with different chromosomal constitution in the same individual, take origin from mitotic errors in early cleavage stages of embryogenesis. Newly divided chromosomes fail to segregate one to each daughter cell, thereby tending to produce new strains of cells with trisomic and monosomic chromosomes, among the cells with normal ploidy. Nondisjunction occurs most often at the end of meiotic metaphase when chromatids fail to separate, although it may also occur during anaphase when one chromosome lags behind and is separated from its future cell mates and is lost. Parts of chromosomes broken during meiosis or mitosis are also lost during anaphase.

Regardless of when it occurs, the effect of chromosomal aberration is visible excess or deficiency in chromosomes or parts thereof, in surviving cells derived from affected germ cells or cleavage cells. Deficiency of chromosomal material is poorly tolerated, usually being lethal to the cell or the organism if involving more than one arm of an autosome, although absence of an entire X (or Y ?) chromosome is tolerated in Turner's syndrome with relatively minor adverse effects on development. Autosomal monosomic strains of cells probably occur in early stages of mosaic conditions but rarely do these survive long enough to be seen in postnatal individuals (Greenwood and Sommer, 1971).

Excess of chromosomes is only slightly less detrimental. Trisomy of some of the smaller autosomal pairs is compatible with survival beyond birth but results in severe developmental defects, as seen in Down's syndrome and in trisomies of the D and E types, but trisomy of larger autosomes is extremely rare (Caspersson *et al.,* 1972). Translocations of major parts of a particular chromosome to a chromosome of another pair (as in the transpositional type of Down's syndrome) can also lead to chromosomal excess that is tantamount to the more usual trisomy. On the other hand, excesses of either sex chromosome causes little or no phenotypic change in affected individuals.

The causes of chromosomal nondisjunction are not fully understood. Seasonal and socioeconomic factors have been suggested as contributory (Robinson *et al.,* 1969). There is substantial evidence that aged germ cells are more likely to exhibit nondisjunction than younger ones, both as regards germ cells from older parents (Lenz *et al.,* 1967; Robinson and Puck, 1967), and possibly also for germ cells that take part in fertilization after prolonged residence in the genital tract (German, 1968; Witschi, 1970). Considerable epidemiologic evidence indicates an association between viral infections and chromosomal abnormalities, particularly in Down's syndrome (Nichols, 1966; Stoller, 1968; Kučera, 1971b). An association has also been demonstrated between maternal irradiation and autosomal trisomy (Uchida and Curtis, 1961; Uchida *et al.,* 1968; Sigler *et al.,* 1965). Chromosomal breaks and other damage are known to have been induced in man by chemical agents (Shaw, 1970) and by a variety of agents in animals (see Saxén and Rapola, 1969, for review). A cause-and-effect relationship between induced chromosomal breaks and teratogenesis, however, remains to be proved (Bloom, 1972; Roux *et al.,* 1971).

III. Mitotic Interference

Changes in the rate of proliferation as a consequence of interference with mitosis have been known for many years to follow use of ionizing radiations (Hicks and D'Amato, 1966), some anesthetics (Andersen, 1966) and colchicine (Borisy and Taylor, 1967a, b), and more recently from podophyllin, vincristine, vinblastine, and griseofulvin (Malowista *et al.,* 1968). Among the probable ways that the mitotic cycle can be disturbed are (1) reduction of DNA synthesis, thereby preventing replication of chromosomes; (2) interference with formation or separation of chromatids such as the "stickiness" seen after irradiation; or (3) failure of formation or maintenance of the microtubules necessary for the mitotic spindle (e.g., colchicine effect). Agents that interfere with mitosis (stathmokinetic agents) have often been found to be teratogenic (Sinclair, 1950; Höglund, 1952; Nishimura, 1964), which is not surprising considering that the most characteristic feature of early embryonic development is rapid cellular proliferation. It is generally assumed that any interference with the mitotic process is likely to lead to death of affected cells, but there is now some evidence that the cell cycle may be slowed or even temporarily arrested by x-rays, without necessarily killing the cells (Tolmach *et al.,* 1971).

As mentioned above, the sites of action of these interfering agents undoubtedly vary widely, from production of peroxides and free radicals by x-rays passing in the vicinity of chromatin strands to dissolution of the microtubules making up the mitotic spindle by colchicine. These are not necessarily the primary effects; for example, the main effects of x-rays on mitosis may be secondary to the extensive chromosome breakage that is known to occur. In fact, this category probably represents more than one mechanism all of which share the common end point of interfering with mitosis. Even so, there is little doubt but that interference with the mechanics of mitosis, whatever its cause, will lead to abnormal embryogenesis if the end result is to exceed the capability of the organ or the organism later to restore the deficiency of cells.

IV. Altered Nucleic Acid Integrity or Function

The mechanisms by which many antibiotic and cancer chemotherapeutic drugs exert their initial effect on the cells of embryos, as well as on other rapidly proliferating systems, is by interference with the integrity, synthesis, or function of nucleic acids. Ultimately all of these agents cause faulty expression of the genetic information, albeit by diverse means (Table 4-1): (1) interference with the integrity or synthesis of DNA, as with cytosine arabinoside (Ritter *et al.,* 1971) or hydroxyurea (Scott *et al.,* 1971); (2) interference with RNA synthesis, as with actinomycin D (Jordan and Wilson, 1970; Waring, 1968); (3) incorporation of abnormal precursors, as with 5-fluorouracil (Schumacher *et al.,* 1969; Wilson *et al.,* 1969); and (4) interference with RNA translation during protein synthesis, as possibly with streptomycin (Filippi, 1967).

TABLE 4-1

TYPES OF INTERFERENCE WITH NUCLEIC ACID METABOLISM OR FUNCTION, DEMONSTRATED MAINLY IN CELL CULTURES OR MICROORGANISMS[a]

1. Interference with replication or integrity of DNA

Cytosine arabinoside[b]	Inhibits DNA polymerase
Hydroxyurea[b]	Blocks conversion of nucleotides to deoxynucleotides
Mitomycin C[b]	Cross-links complimentary strands of DNA
Streptonigrin[b]	Selectively binds DNA, inhibits incorporation of adenine

2. Interference with RNA synthesis (transcription)

Actinomycin D[b]	Binds guanosine residues of DNA
Nogalamycin	Binds adenosine and/or thymidine of DNA
Acridine orange	Binds euchromatin DNA, is mutagenic

3. Erroneous incorporation into DNA or RNA

6-Mercaptopurine[b]	Incorporated instead of normal purines
Tubercidin	Acts as analog of adenosine
8-Azoguanine[b]	Acts as analog of guanine
5-Bromouracil	Replaces thymine in synthesis, is mutagenic

4. Interference with RNA translation (protein synthesis)

Puromycin	Complexes with incipient protein
Cycloheximide	Interferes with transfer of tRNA to ribosome
Streptomycin	Binds with and causes misreading of mRNA
Lincomycin	Inhibits tRNA attachment to ribosome

[a] From numerous sources, but mainly from Balis (1968). In several instances the suggested mode of action is uncertain, although some evidence is available in support of the pathway cited.

[b] Known to be teratogenic in mammals.

This category thus encompasses several kinds of initial cellular responses which, until more information is available, are placed together because of the seemingly common feature that nucleic acid integrity or functions are affected. There is obviously some overlap between this category and mutations as described earlier in Section I, particularly as regards integrity of DNA molecules and the incorporation of analog precursors into DNA. Those types of compounds affecting DNA are not classified exclusively with mutagenic substances because some, such as acridine orange and 5-bromouracil, although they may alter nucleotide sequence in DNA and hence are mutagenic, may also act in other ways on nucleic acids (Table 4-1). Certainly all agents that affect nucleic acid synthesis or function are not mutagenic. Indeed, all have not been shown to be teratogenic, which raises the interesting question about the general relationship between mutagenic and teratogenic chemicals. This question has been examined in two studies (Kalter, 1971; Wilson, 1972c), which concurred in the view that there is only limited overlap between mutagenic and teratogenic chemicals, consisting mainly of such agents as those listed in Table 4-1 and the polyfunctional alkylating agents.

It is noteworthy that drugs and chemicals which interfere with RNA translation, that is, with protein synthesis (Table 4-1), are only slightly or not at all teratogenic in the sense of causing high rates of malformation, although they have been found to be embryolethal at high doses (unpublished data in author's laboratory). It is conjectured that protein synthesis is so essential and so ubiquitous to all embryonic cells that little interference can be tolerated without causing widespread cell death followed by organismic death.

V. Lack of Normal Precursors, Substrates, and Coenzymes for Biosynthesis

This is assumed to be the immediate effect of maternal nutritional deficiency, of placental transport failure, and of the presence of competitive antimetabolites. Furthermore, a breakdown at any point in the pathways of supply and distribution of essential nutrients and metabolites could also result in deficiencies in developing tissues. The latter would include failure of absorption of nutrients from the maternal digestive tract and inadequate transport of essential materials in maternal and embryonic or fetal bloodstreams, although little is known about these transport factors in relation to teratogenesis.

The necessity of an uninterrupted supply of nutrients to maintain normal growth and development in animals has been frequently discussed (Asling, 1969; Giroud, 1971; Hurley, 1967; Runner and Miller, 1956; Warkany, 1952–1953). Certain specific nutritional deficiencies such as a single vitamin are teratogenic in animals; but multiple deficiencies usually prevent pregnancy or lead to its early termination, suggesting that the rapidly growing embryo is unable to tolerate lack of more than one precursor, substrate, or coenzyme at any one time. Failure of reproductive function to continue under conditions of extreme undernutrition may serve a protective function, and probably explains why severe malnutrition in man is generally not associated with overt teratogenesis (see Chapter 3, Section II,H). Paradoxically, excesses of certain substances such as vitamins A and possibly D are also teratogenic (Cohlan, 1954; Friedman and Roberts, 1966). The reasons can only be guessed as having something to do with the production of metabolic imbalances.

In addition to maternal dietary deficiency, embryos and fetuses presumably could be deprived of essential anabolites as a result of inadequate maternal absorption or transport, inadequate placental transfer, or the presence of competitive analogs or antimetabolites. Instances of failure of maternal absorption and transport in relation to teratogenesis are not known, and the same may be said for transport by the chorioallantoic placenta, although nutritional lack as a consequence of occlusion of the yolk sac placenta of rodents and rabbits by diazo dyes (Beck *et al.,* 1967b) and certain antibodies (Brent, 1971a) may account for teratogenesis in these animals. A number of specific analogs and antagonists to nutrients or precursors such as antipurines, antipyrimidines, and antagonists to glutamine, adenine, leucine, folic acid, riboflavin, nicotinic acid, and others, are highly teratogenic in laboratory mammals (Cahen, 1966; Karnofsky, 1965a,b). The details of how shortages of essential metabolites disrupt developmental processes doubtless relate to the roles these substances play in normal development, but information on this subject is largely by inference from what is known of metabolic pathways in mature animals.

VI. Altered Energy Sources

In addition to the general need for anabolites from extrinsic sources noted above, biosynthesis and proliferation require an uninterrupted source of intrinsic energy generated in the developing tissues. Altered energy sources were implicated in mammalian teratogenesis several years ago when it was suggested (Runner, 1959) that a number of different teratogenic treatments produced similar results because they interfered with a series of common metabolic processes in the citric acid cycle. This view has since received some experimental support. Recent studies have revealed that the citric acid cycle was specifically impaired when defective embryos from riboflavin-deficient pregnant rats were found to have markedly reduced activity of the terminal electron transport system, as compared with control embryos or placental tissue from deficient females (Akzu *et al.,* 1968; Mackler, 1969).

It has not been possible to produce developmental defects in rats by direct application of agents capable of causing uncoupling of oxidative phosphorylation, e.g., with dinitrophenol (unpublished data from author's laboratory), although this procedure was used successfully to cause abnormality in early explanted chick embryos (Bowman, 1967). Landauer and Clark (1964) assumed that because the well-known teratogenic effects of insulin on developing chicks could be appreciably enhanced by simultaneous treatment with known uncouplers of oxidative phosphorylation, that insulin might also act as an uncoupling agent. Conversely, it has recently been shown that effects of other chick teratogens such as 3-acetylpyridine, 6-aminonicotinamide, and sulfanilamide were significantly moderated by concurrent treatment with high-energy intermediates such as succinate and ascorbate (Landauer and Sopher, 1970). Evidence relating interference with mitochondrial functions and other sources of cellular energy to abnormal development in mammalian embryos has also been advanced (Netzloff *et al.,* 1968; Verrusio and Watkins, 1969; Chepenik *et al.,* 1969).

As noted in Chapter 3, Section I, E, hypoxia is teratogenic under some conditions, but the effect is highly variable from species to species and at different times in the same species (Degenhardt, 1960). This variability undoubtedly is in part a reflection of the fact that the ratio of aerobic to anaerobic metabolism changes appreciably during early stages of organogenesis (Shepard *et al.,* 1970). Ten-day rat embryos in culture tolerated greatly reduced oxygen levels up to 30 minutes without appreciable effect on heart rate, but 11- and 12-day embryos showed significant drops in heart rate within 10 minutes after exposure to reduced oxygen, suggesting increasing reliance on aerobic metabolism with increasing gestational age.

VII. Enzyme Inhibition

The possibility that intraembryonic enzymes may be poisoned or inhibited in such a way as to be an initiating factor in teratogenesis has not been extensively investigated in mammals, but several experimental situations have provided suggestive evidence that such might be the case. For example, it is well known that folic acid antagonists are teratogenic in mammals (Nelson, 1963) and it is now generally accepted that these substances act by inhibiting the enzyme dihydrofolate reductase, thereby blocking the 1-carbon transfer system necessary for purine and pyrimidine biosynthesis and for certain amino acid conversions. Abnormal development of rat embryos has been shown to be associated with inhibition of thymidylate synthetase by the uracil analog 5-fluorouracil following treatment of the pregnant dam (Schumacher *et al.,* 1969). It is thought probably that the teratogenic action of hydroxyurea is related to the inhibition of ribonucleoside diphosphate reductase (Krakoff *et al.,* 1968; Scott *et al.,* 1971), and the possibility exists that the well-known teratogenicity of salicylates may be related to enzyme inhibition (Grisolia *et al.,* 1968). On the other hand, the teratogenic effects of the carbonic anhydrase inhibitor, acetazolamide, was shown to occur in rat embryos at a time earlier than this enzyme could be demonstrated by methods then available (Wilson *et al.,* 1968).

The foregoing examples assume that specific, usually single, enzymes have been interfered with. Widespread inhibition as with a general enzyme poison would probably be quickly lethal to the embryo or fetus, if not to the mother as well. Clearly much remains to be learned about the ontogeny of enzymes and how their *in vivo* susceptibility to inhibition may be related to teratogenesis.

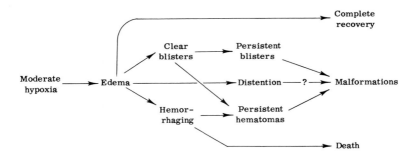

FIG. 4-2. The edema syndrome as visualized by Grabowski after exposure of developing chicks to hypoxia. A similar sequence of alternative pathways is thought to exist for other agents that produce fluid–osmolyte imbalance in embryos. (After Grabowski, 1964.)

VIII. Osmolar Imbalance

Convincing evidence now indicates that osmolar imbalance can act as a primary mechanism of teratogenesis by altering fluid pressures and viscosities in different compartments of an embryo, e.g., blood plasma versus extracapillary spaces, or intraembryonic versus extraembryonic fluid compartments. Such a mechanism has been postulated by Grabowski (1966) to explain abnormal fluid and blood accumulations in chick embryos subjected to hypoxia, trypan blue, hypertonic solutions, or adrenal cortical hormones. For example, a moderately teratogenic dose of hypoxia (10.5% for 5 hours) produced a sequence of osmotic changes called the "edema syndrome" which culminated in death, malformation, or recovery of the embryo (Fig. 4-2). The first symptom following exposure was a significant increase in all body fluids. Analyses of serum from hypoxic embryos revealed an increase in lactic acid, free amino acids, potassium, and carbon dioxide; a decrease in sodium, calcium, chloride, and glucose; and approximately normal levels of protein and inorganic phosphate.

Normally the osmolarity of chick serum and that of fluids surrounding the extraembryonic capillaries in allantois, in albumen, and in subgerminal space are markedly different. Grabowski assumed that the differences between serum and extraembryonic fluids was maintained by homeostatic devices which required energy expenditure. Oxygen deficiency and similarly acting teratogens were thought to interfere with such homeostasis, thereby tending to reduce the normal differences between serum and extraembryonic fluids by allowing an inrush of fluid into the embryo. The consequent excess of embryonic fluids resulted in internal and external hemorrhages and fluid-filled blebs and blisters. Most of the malformations later seen were attributed to the mechanical distortion caused by persistent hematomas and blisters adjacent to rapidly developing organs, rather than to direct cytotoxic effects in target organs. Slow injection of saline into normal embryos was shown to simulate the increase in blood pressure and to result in hemorrhages and blisters (Grabowski and Tsai, 1968), leading to the logical conclusion that mechanical factors were the immediate cause but that the underlying one was an imbalance of water and osmolytes. Of related interest is the fact that anomalies of the extremities and tail of mice have been produced by injecting pregnant females with hypertonic saline solution (Tanaka *et al.*, 1968). The subsequent defects were attributed to tissue damage as a result of the edema, blisters, and hemorrhages observable in embryos 4 to 6 hours after treatment.

Concern has been expressed about the possible adverse effects of hyperemesis gravidarum and its attendant fluid–osmolyte imbalance on the early embryonic development in man, but existing data do not seem to justify such concern (Farkas, 1969). On the other hand, the oral-facial malformations seen in the offspring of rats given benzhydrylpiperazine compounds during pregnancy has been attributed to the edema known to have occurred in the embryos after treatment (Posner, 1971). There no longer seems to be much doubt but that abnormal fluid accumulations can cause tissue distortions sufficient to lead to malformations; the critical question is whether osmotic disturbances are themselves primary reactions to environmental causes or are only secondary to some earlier change in developing tissues.

IX. Changed Membrane Characteristics

Instances wherein altered membrane characteristics in developing tissues have actually led to a teratogenic outcome are not known, but on logical grounds it is assumed that if such did occur the sequence of events would be similar to that described above for osmolar imbalance. The primary event, however, would be an alteration in permeability of a membrane rather than in the concentration of osmolytes in one or the other of the compartments separated by the membrane. The ease with which physiologic as well as foreign substances pass through epithelial, plasma, nuclear, mitochondrial, and other membranes is subject to change under certain conditions of stress; but whether this could be of such degree or duration as to affect the survival or subsequent developmental role of tissues and cells is a moot question. Ultimately the importance of membrane permeability as a teratogenic mechanism would depend on the degree to which particular cells and tissues were affected while others were spared, thus providing the necessary selectivity to achieve specific defects. For the present, altered membrane properties in an embryo can only be regarded theoretically to be a mechanism. To establish it as such will be difficult because of the need to distinguish it from osmotic imbalance which also involves the maintenance of osmotic differences on two sides of a membrane.

X. Other Possible Mechanisms

Other possible ways for initiating abnormal developmental sequences have been suggested, but when examined closely, little factual or logical support for such a role can be marshaled. For example, placental dysfunction has often been mentioned as a possible primary event in teratogenic action, but no instance is positively known in which impairment of placental function has led to abnormal development. On the contrary, Johnson *et al.* (1963) were unable to find evidence of damage in the placentae of rat embryos severely affected by a folic acid antagonist until after the embryo died. In fact, it is difficult to imagine placental impairment having the degree of specificity thought necessary for most teratogenesis. The most likely exception to the latter generalization is the inverted yolk sac placenta of rodents and related forms. This structure possibly serves essential transport and/or digestive function in the early stages of organogenesis; at least there is presumptive evidence that the impairment of such functions is responsible for the teratogenic properties of azo dyes (Lloyd and Beck, 1969) and certain antisera (Brent, 1971a). The manner in which physical presence of these substances in a transport membrane can produce localized effects in the embryo remains to be elucidated.

Destruction of microfilaments and microtubules within developing cells is known to occur *in vitro* following application of agents like colchicine and cytarbine (Spooner and Wessels, 1972). There is reason to believe that these cellular inclusions by contraction are instrumental in morphogenetic movements such as invagination and evagination of epithelial layers. Interference with these processes in an embryo would be expected to disrupt development, but it remains to be shown (1) that microtubules and microfilaments can be dissolved *in vivo* by chemicals that traverse the maternal body and the placenta, and (2) that in the absence of these cellular inclusions, morphogenetic movements do indeed fail to occur.

XI. Why Be Concerned with Mechanisms?

It is clear from the foregoing that precise information on teratogenic mechanisms is limited, but it may not be apparent why a knowledge of mechanisms is desirable. Some pragmatists would argue that a machinist is able to repair an engine without understanding the theory behind its operation. Be that as it may, teratology is concerned with more than repair. Surely one of the major objectives is to anticipate difficulty before it is at hand. The anticipation of teratologic risk in today's rapidly changing environment becomes an endless succession of screening tests of individual agents unless a knowledge of mechanisms can lead to extrapolations, generalization, and shortcuts that will simplify the task. Furthermore, the application of animal test data to the evaluation of human teratologic risk will become more than empirical to whatever degree the comparability of mechanisms between test animal and man is better understood. Finally, with a fuller knowledge of mechanisms, unrecognized causes may be anticipated and known causes in unfamiliar guise may be unmasked.

Correction and treatment of developmental defects should not be merely a search for palliatives at the symptomatic level. Correction of developmental errors at any point prior to their final manifestation, if not at the level of the initiating mechanism, at least at an intermediate point in the pathogenesis between the mechanism and the final manifestation, could be tantamount to prevention. For instance, there may be hope for correction of a deficient enzyme, avoidance of excessive accumulation of a substrate, or supplementation of an inadequate transport system before irreparable damage is done.

The prevention of "spontaneous" defects is thought to be a matter that lies largely in the future (Lederberg, 1970). This is not necessarily true when a defect lacking apparent single causation can be shown to be the result of interacting or multiple causes. There is no reason to suppose that multiple causes act through mechanisms other than the ones that are triggered by single causes. If so, a better understanding of mechanisms might simplify the difficult job of finding the multiple variables that combine to activate known mechanisms.

CHAPTER 5

MANIFESTATIONS OF ABNORMAL DEVELOPMENT

The manifestations of abnormal development can be characterized in two principal ways: (1) in the dynamic sense of tracing successive events that make up pathogenesis, between the initiating mechanism and the final defect; and (2) in the definitive sense of describing the qualitative or quantitative aspects of the final defect. Pathogenesis has been extensively studied only in its later stages when structures or functions are already recognizably abnormal and proceeding toward a predictable type of final defect. The earlier stages of pathogenesis, however, when the direction and pathways of abnormal embryogenesis are probably determined, remain largely obscure.

The quantitative aspects of the final defect, generally referred to as incidence, relate abnormal development to variables such as sex, race, geographical distribution, seasonal occurrence, and, of course, species. The qualitative aspects concern the nature of the final defect, that is, whether abnormal development culminates in death, malformation, growth retardation, or functional deficit. Each of these aspects of abnormal development is much too extensive for full discussion here. For example, a glossary of structural defects that are known to have developmental origin would include several hundred items, and the lists of known metabolic disorders that result from developmental error are increasing rapidly. Therefore these various manifestations of abnormal development can only be discussed in general and theoretical terms, with no attempt being made at comprehensive coverage.

I. Pathogenesis—Modes of Abnormal Embryogenesis

As indicated earlier, pathogenesis first becomes evident in the form of one or more modes of abnormal embryogenesis that are the result of one or

TABLE 5-1

MODES OF ABNORMAL EMBRYOGENESIS INVOLVED IN THE PATHOGENESIS OF
DEVELOPMENTAL DEFECTS

Modes of abnormal development	Probable effect in developing tissues	Example[a]
1. Excessive cell death	Too few cells to carry out morphogenesis or functional maturation	Ectrodactyly after necrosis in limb bud following x-rays or cytotoxic drugs
2. Changed rate of proliferation	Slowed differentiation schedule and/or growth	Probably cell deficiencies in localized tissues, e.g., small brain after irradiation
3. Failed cell interactions	Insufficient growth or activity of inductor tissue, or lack of competence of induced tissue	Agenesis of lens owing to failure of optic cup to contact ectoderm over forebrain region
4. Impeded morphogenetic movement	Obstruction of cell migration or interference with invagination, evagination, etc.	Lack of mesenchymal migration into cardiac region after folic acid deficiency
5. Reduced biosynthesis	Inhibition of nucleic acid, protein, or mucopolysaccharide synthesis	Growth retardation or embryo death following treatment with protein inhibitors such as puromycin
6. Mechanical disruption	Destruction of tissues or interference with growth by pressure, trauma, or vascular stasis	Limb, tail, and facial defects after hypoxia or other agents causing blebs, blisters, and hemorrhages

[a] See text for references.

more of the initiating mechanisms described in Chapter 4. These modes
have not all been widely studied in relation to teratogenesis, but their counterparts in normal embryogenesis are sufficiently well known to permit inferences as to their probable role in abnormal development. Those thought at
this time to be important pathways toward the final manifestation of abnormal development are listed in Table 5-1. Further study of this aspect of teratology is obviously needed.

A. EXCESSIVE CELL DEATH

This mode of abnormal embryogenesis has been studied in embryos exposed to teratogenic agents such as radiations (Hicks and D'Amato, 1966) and various chemical substances (Menkes *et al.,* 1970). In fact it has been suggested that all pathogenesis in teratology might involve excessive cell death, but this has not been proved and seems unlikely since highly effective teratogens like thalidomide appear not to cause necrosis in embryos receiving teratogenic doses (Battinich, 1971). On the other hand, extensive cell death is known to occur in the neural tube of rat embryos subjected *in utero* to hydroxyurea on day 12 of gestation but is not followed by overt malformation of the central nervous system in term fetuses (Scott *et al.,* 1971).

A distinction must be made between controlled or "programmed" cell death that is a part of normal embryogenesis in such tissues as the genital ducts (Forsberg, 1967) and the limb buds (Saunders, 1966; Saunders and Fallon, 1966) and the abnormal amounts of cell death that occur in response to cytotoxic agents. Although there may be some parallels between the types of tissues affected (Webster and Gross, 1970), it is generally true that the cell death associated with teratogenesis is both more widespread and more intense than is the controlled necrosis of normal embryogenesis. Furthermore, cell death in embryos exposed to cytotoxic agents is often accompanied by cytologic (Franz, 1971) as well as biochemical changes (Ritter *et al.,* 1971; Scott *et al.,* 1973) in surviving cells.

The intracellular events preceding induced cell death are usually not known. Several if not all of the mechanisms discussed in Chapter 4 would be expected to cause necrosis when present in sufficient dosage. The factors that determine the localization of cell death in certain tissues or organs so as to produce specific developmental defects, rather than death of the embryo as a whole, also are not always clear. Many studies, however, have reported that cell death induced by cytotoxic agents occurs most intensely in tissues undergoing rapid proliferation at the time of treatment. It is assumed but not firmly established that the killing of cells above some critical number exceeds the regenerative capacity of affected tissue, thereby leaving them with insufficient cells to proceed with normal developmental processes (Ritter *et al.,* 1973).

B. Reduced Proliferative Rate

Such teratogenic agents as hypervitaminosis A (Marin-Padilla, 1966), trypan blue (Stempak, 1964), and radiations (Franz, 1971) are known to reduce the rate of mitosis and consequently the proliferative rate in surviving cells, apart from the fact that other cells in the same tissue may be killed. Brent (1972b) reviewed the various effects of radiation on developing systems and concluded that growth retardation of the whole organism, as well as deficiency of cells in particular organs, can be induced by small to moderate doses at several stages of development. Growth retardation, however, cannot be attributed only to slowed rate of proliferation because deficiencies in numbers of cells obviously can result from cell death. Nevertheless, there is ample evidence that slowed mitotic rate can contribute significantly to growth retardation independently of cell necrosis (Franz, 1971; Wegner, 1966), although the relative contributions of each may be difficult to assess. The regulation of proliferative rates in normal tissues is poorly understood (Källén, 1956) and the manner in which this responds to conditions that produce teratogenesis is largely a matter of speculation.

C. Failed Cellular Interactions

It has long been accepted that cell interactions (induction) are an important part of normal embryogenesis, despite the fact that specific "inducer substances" have not been identified. Saxén (1972) has reviewed a variety of ways in which failure of normal interactions may lead to deviations in development, for example, lack of usual contact or proximity, as of optic vesicle with presumptive lens ectoderm; incompetence of target tissue to be activated in spite of usual relationship with activator tissue, as in certain mutant limb defects; and inappropriate timing of the interrelation, even though all parts are potentially competent. That the nature of cell-to-cell contacts and the manner of their adhesion are important determinants in both normal and abnormal development has been demonstrated by Abercrombie (1970). Insufficient or inappropriate cellular interactions usually result in arrested or deviant development in the tissue ordinarily induced or activated by the interaction.

D. Impeded Morphogenetic Movements

The movements of cells is an essential part of normal embryogenesis, with great variability displayed by different tissues, both as regards numbers of cells involved and the distances traversed. For instance, the short migration of spongioblasts in the neural tube from ependymal to mantle layers contrasts with the relatively longer distance traversed by the primordial germ cells from the endoderm of the cloaca to the mesenchyme of the future gonad. Adverse influences during development have in several experimental situations been shown to interfere with cell movements which resulted in permanent structural or functional damage. Limb defects in talpid mutant chicks have been attributed to decreased mobility of cells through abnormal aggregations of other cells in the limb buds (Ede and Agerbak, 1968). Heart abnormalities in chicks have been described after a chelating agent (EDTA) interfered with the migration of cells into the future cardiac region (De Haan, 1958), although cell migration and cardiogenesis were observed to be normal after simultaneous addition of Ca ions. Permanent structural changes in the central nervous system of rodents have resulted from interferences with cell migration by a variety of means (Bass, 1971; Langman and Shimada, 1970, 1971; Shimada and Langman, 1970).

Any extraneous influence that altered the viscosity or quantity of tissue ground substance or changed the quality of cell adhesions might be expected to interfere with the usual rate of cellular or tissue migrations. Such morphogenetic movements as invagination and evagination may depend on the contraction of intracellular microtubules and microfilaments (Burnside, 1971). Substances known to dissolve microfilaments and microtubules *in vitro,* e.g., Colcemid and vincristine, could be highly disruptive to embryogenesis if they reached epithelial layers *in vivo* while invagination or evagination were in process.

E. REDUCED BIOSYNTHESIS

Complete or partial inhibition of DNA synthesis has been shown to be associated with, but not necessarily responsible for, teratogenesis in the offspring of pregnant rats treated with cytosine arabinoside (Ritter *et al.,* 1971) and hydroxyurea (Scott *et al.,* 1971). The detrimental effects of interrupting RNA synthesis in developing organisms has been demonstrated in a variety of animals by using specific inhibitors such as actinomycin D (Flickinger *et al.,* 1967; Gross, 1967; Kafotos and Reich, 1968; Skalko and Morse, 1967). The necessity of the synthesis of specific proteins for cytodifferentiation as well as for other aspects of development can be taken for granted (Johnson, 1965; Rutter *et al.,* 1968) but it has not been possible to produce specific malformations in rats by using inhibitors of protein synthesis such as puromycin, lincomycin, and streptomycin (unpublished data from author's laboratory). The formation of other tissue components in the developing embryo has been less extensively studied but there is evidence that the synthesis of lipids (Miyamoto *et al.,* 1967; Noble and Moore, 1967) and of mucopolysaccharides (Gessner and Bostrom, 1965; Kochhar *et al.,* 1968) is also essential to normal embryogenesis.

F. MECHANICAL DISRUPTION

It was noted in Chapter 3, Section I,H that a variety of physical and mechanical factors in the environment could impinge on the embryos of submammalian forms to initiate abnormal development. Such extrinsic influences can be mediated through one of the mechanisms proposed in Chapter 4, but it is also possible that environmental factors can inflict mechanical injury directly on developing tissues. Examples would be physical trauma sufficient to displace or tear tissues or to interrupt their blood supply. Although these are less likely in mammals because of the shielding provided by the maternal body and by the hydrostatic cushions of fluids enclosed in the amnion and chorion, it is still possible for stab wounds and crushing injuries to involve the pregnant uterus. A number of experiments have shown, however, that chick embryos can survive surprising degrees of mechanical manipulation such as experimental clamping or displacement of major blood vessels (Gessner, 1970; Rychter, 1960), excision and transplantation of parts (Rosenquist, 1970) and various operative procedures involving the vitelline membranes (Silver, 1959); although malformation was a frequent consequence.

Conditions in embryos that favor the static accumulation of fluids, as in the hemorrhages, blebs, and blisters that follow osmolar imbalance (see Chapter 4, Section VIII), can result in local pressures and ischemia sufficient to cause necrosis and tissue breakdown. Damage of this type was associated with subsequent malformations in hypoxic chick embryos (Grabowski and associates, 1958, 1966, 1970), in mice after injection of hypertonic saline into pregnant females (Tanaka *et al.,* 1968), and in mice and rats after treatment of pregnant females with meclizine (Posner, 1971) or trypan blue (Kaplan and Grabowski, 1967; Waddington and Carter, 1952). Many years ago malformations in the extremities of certain mutant strains of mice were attributed to accumulation of blebs of leaked cerebrospinal fluid at the sites of later abnormality (Bonnevie, 1934); but there is no justification for assuming that the postulated "myelencephalic blebs" of the Bonnevie–Uhlrich syndrome in human teratology have a similar explanation (Warkany, 1971).

G. IS THERE A FINAL COMMON PATHWAY OF PATHOGENESIS?

The foregoing modes of abnormal embryogenesis without doubt often overlap or act concurrently to produce the abnormal organogenesis or the incomplete functional maturation that lead ultimately to the final defect. The possibility that all modes of abnormal embryogenesis converge in a common pathway, as suggested in Scheme 5-1, is an interesting subject for conjecture, but the details of pathogenesis of many more developmental defects than are now known must be analyzed to resolve this theoretical question. It is nevertheless true that a majority of developmental defects superficially seem to be attributable to too few cells or cell products to permit the completion of morphogenesis or of functional maturation.

The obvious exceptions to this hypothesis are malformations involving supernumerary parts, e.g., polydactyly, the duplications that occur in parts of the digestive and genitourinary tracts, and the localized overgrowth seen in hemihypertrophy and in gigantism of digits and extremities. Furthermore, situs inversus of the heart, aortic arch, respiratory tract, and digestive tract seem to involve neither excess nor deficiency of tissue but are mirror images

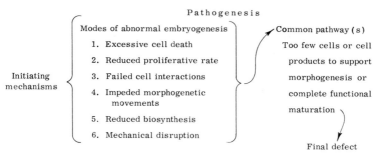

SCHEME 5-1. Diagram illustrating the hypothesis that the various modes of abnormal embryogenesis may all converge on one or a very few final common pathways. This view is supported by circumstantial evidence but it should not be regarded as proved (see text).

of the normal asymmetric pattern. Nevertheless, the structural defects that do not entail some deficiency of tissue are distinctly in the minority. As for the functional and biochemical defects referred to as inborn errors of metabolism, again most seem to result from a lack rather than an excess of a cellular product, frequently an enzyme. It must be borne in mind, however, that some functional defects including the various types of mental deficiency are not well enough understood to permit the judgment that the underlying disturbance involves deficiencies of cells or cell products. Thus, it appears that present knowledge of the pathogenesis of abnormal development is too limited to draw definitive conclusions about the existence of a final common pathway in teratogenesis.

II. Incidence of Developmental Defects in Man

A. RATE DEPENDS ON TYPE OF EXAMINATION

After reviewing the world literature covering 20 million births, Kennedy (1967) concluded that the frequency of individuals with some degree of congenital defect at birth almost certainly exceeded 2%. The prevalence of underreporting in unselected data of this type is demonstrated by the following breakdown: Data on 12 million births from official records, birth certificates, and retrospective questionnaires yielded a frequency of less than 1%; information on 7 million births from hospital and clinic records gave an incidence in most countries ranging between 1 and 2%; whereas in approximately a half million instances in which infants were subjected to intensive examination, the mean rate of defective individuals was 4.5%, with a range of less than 3 to more than 8%. Since all of these data were collected prior to 1965, it is safe to assume that even the more intensive examinations did not include as many chromosomal and metabolic tests as would be the case today.

B. IN STILLBORN AND NEONATAL INFANTS

Stillborn infants are known to have more malformations than liveborn infants. This fact has two important corollaries: (1) That severe malformations are responsible for many stillbirths, and (2) that autopsy reveals more malformations than any other type of examination. Among the data collected by Kennedy (1967) were 11,904 identifiable stillbirths in which the malformation rate was 12.7%. Other reports not included in the foregoing, in which higher proportions of cases were autopsied, yielded even higher rates of malformations. For example, Stevensen *et al.* (1950) found that 15.6% of 1100 stillbirths had defects that were regarded as incompatible with life. The frequency of developmental abnormality among neonatal deaths (infants dying within first month of postnatal life) has been found to be higher still, ranging from 19.7% (Hawkins and Meckel, 1950) to 26.0% (Ahvenainen, 1959) to 29.6% (McIntosh *et al.,* 1954).

C. IN ANTEPARTUM FETUSES AND EMBRYOS

Contrary to the view that gross malformations are more often associated with antepartum than with neonatal deaths, fetuses dying prior to term in two studies were found to have malformations in only 13 or 14% of cases (McIntosh *et al.,* 1954; Potter, 1962). Incidence figures based on the products of spontaneous abortion (less than 22 weeks of gestation) are not reliable because such material is often in some state of maceration when delivered. While examining a considerable quantity of such material the author found that the diagnosis of developmental abnormality was often questionable because of disortions of shape and proportion and actual resorption or maceration of anatomical parts.

Nishimura (1970) found that only 3.7 to 4.7% of 901 late embryos and early fetuses obtained from surgical abortions had externally visible malformations. Organogenesis had been largely completed in these well-preserved specimens and external malformations would not have been missed by the trained observers. Although internal malformations were not intensively studied, it is apparent from this and other studies that no large proportion of living embryos and fetuses is structurally abnormal. Certain malformations seen postnatally in the population are more frequent in the embryos and early fetuses (Lee, 1971; Nishimura, 1970), but there is little information on how and when types of defects rarely seen at term are selectively eliminated before birth. If selective elimination of defective individuals occurs *in utero*, it probably most often occurs early, as suggested by Hertig *et al.* (1956), who found that about 40% of human embryos between 2 and 17 days of age were abnormal.

D. PROBLEMS OF DEFINITION AND DIAGNOSIS OF DEVELOPMENTAL DEFECTS

Returning to the incidence of developmental defects at birth and subsequently, there are several factors that complicate the establishment of a realistic rate. One of the most troublesome problems is lack of agreement about what constitutes a developmental defect. There is an increasing acceptance of the view that all manifestations of abnormal development, i.e., death, malformation, growth retardation, and functional disorder, should be included within the scope of teratology. Nevertheless, considerable variability still exists among the investigators who compile incidence figures as to how far to depart from the traditional view that maldevelopment is synonymous with malformation. There remains a tendency to overemphasize structural defects above other types of developmental abnormality. The only logical justification for not including functional disorders of developmental origin in incidence rates for the perinatal period is the difficulty in diagnosing them. For instance, it is variously estimated that 1 to 3% of the population surviving beyond infancy is mentally deficient, but it is difficult to diagnose many types of this affliction until an age of 2 years or older is reached. Likewise some metabolic disorders of developmental origin do not show symptoms until months or years after birth.

Difficulties in early diagnosis, however, are not limited to functional defects. Thorough examinations directed specifically toward the detection of malformations in the neonatal period detected less than half of the malformations that were diagnosable at the end of 1 year (McIntosh *et al.,* 1954). An intensive study of congenital heart disease disclosed 3.8/1000 at birth, but at 6 months of age the rate was 10/1000 and after 3 years the cumulative rate had trebled to 11.5/1000 (Yerushalmy, 1970). Some developmental disorders of potential clinical significance may never be manifested as clinical disease, as is evidenced by the fact that Meckel's diverticulum, atrial spetal defect, incomplete rotation of the gut tract, to mention a few, are encountered with some regularity in the aged subjects of medical school dissecting laboratories.

The tendency to classify developmental errors as "major" and "minor," even when based on their potential to cause death or clinical disease, introduces subjective bias without affording much practical or theoretical benefit in epidemiologic terms. One study found that the overall rate of structural defects was 5.8% in Negroes, as compared with 2.7% in whites; but the higher rate in Negroes was largely accounted for by increased incidence of defects usually regarded as "minor," e.g., polydactyly, supernumerary nipples, and small branchial clefts (Berendes and Weiss, 1970). If the latter were ignored, the overall incidence by the author's definition became 2.5% for whites and 2.3% for Negroes. Although there may be medical justification for emphasizing life- and health-threatening defects, there is no close correlation between the magnitude of a developmental error and its potential to affect health. In the broader biologic sense small mutations probably influenced the course of evolution more than large ones because adjustment to the environment was less precarious after the former.

E. OTHER VARIABLES INFLUENCING INCIDENCE

Incidence rates are further complicated by differences in the frequency of malformations known to occur in different populations; for example, the same malformation may show surprisingly varied rates by countries, cities, or other geographic localities (Lilienfeld, 1970). Some of this can be attributed to racial differences and admixtures (Morton, 1970; Naggan and MacMahon, 1967) but other more subtle factors are probably also involved (Edwards, 1964; Leck, 1966; McKeown, 1961). It is well known that several malformations occur more often in one or the other sex (Hay, 1971). One study indicates that mothers younger than age 14 produce twice as many defective babies as older mothers (Coates, 1970). Thus the number of variables that seem capable of influencing rates of abnormal development (McKeown and Record, 1963), together with the variations imposed by the time and method of ascertainment and the interpretation of what is a teratic manifestation and what is not, collectively suggest that an overall incidence rate in man is almost impossible to determine.

Nevertheless, a reasonable approximation of the frequencies of develop-

TABLE 5-2

ESTIMATED INCIDENCE OF DEVELOPMENTAL DEFECTS AMONG LIVEBORN HUMAN INFANTS EXAMINED UNDER STATED CONDITIONS[a]

Condition	Estimated %
All live births over 500 gm, diagnosed at birth	3–5
Born alive, diagnosed by best available means during first 2 years postnatally	5–10
Born alive but dying during first postnatal year and autopsied	18–20
Born alive but dying during first postnatal month and autopsied	25–30

[a] Based on McIntosh et al., (1954) and several other sources.

mental defects of both structural and functional nature in liveborn infants under stated conditions of study is presented in Table 5-2. Regardless of the methods of ascertainment and the way in which defective development is defined, approximately twice as many defects are diagnosable a few months or years after birth than are diagnosable at birth (Neel, 1958). To this it should be added that several functional defects and a few cryptic structural ones (Meckel's diverticulum) may not be recognized until somewhat later. There is now general agreement that birth defects are associated with, if not responsible for, approximately 20% of deaths during the first year of life, more than any other single factor (Green, 1964; Stiekle, 1968).

III. Nature of the Final Defect

As emphasized in Chapter 2, Section V there are four types of final defects: intrauterine death, malformation, growth retardation, and functional deficit. It was also noted that these are not equally likely to occur after exposure to all adverse influences and that there are appreciable differences in their relative occurrence when exposure occurs at different times during the developmental span. It has not, however, been determined that all of the specific modes of abnormal embryogenesis discussed in Section I of this chapter can equally well lead to the various types of final defect. On logical grounds alone certain assumptions can be made (Table 5-1). Death of the organism or general growth retardation could result from different amounts of cell necrosis, but it is also likely that cell death in critical amounts in localized regions would lead to specific defects. On the other hand, mechanical disruption of tissues in a localized region would be expected to cause localized malformation or, if extensive enough, to kill the whole embryo; but such damage would probably not cause general growth retardation, and might affect specific functions only secondarily if at all. Reduced biosynthesis would seemingly be able to produce all four types of final defects and evidence has already been cited to indicate that inhibition of specific macromolecular synthesis, DNA and RNA, is associated with intrauterine death, localized structural defects, and general growth retardation. Little is to be gained, however, by such speculations. The prevention or reversal of certain abnormal developmental processes would seem theoretically possible by intervention during early stages of pathogenesis, but information is too meager at this time for a meaningful discussion.

A. STRUCTURAL DEFECTS—MALFORMATIONS

The descriptive aspects of human teratology have been extensively dealt with in terms of the anatomical and the clinical characterizations of developmental disease. Volumes have been written emphasizing various aspects: the bizarre and truly monstrous expressions (Gould and Pyle, 1896), the pathologic classifications (Ballantyne, 1902; Potter, 1953; Willis, 1958) and the clinical manifestations (Smith, 1970; Warkany, 1971). A vast accumulation of teratologic studies in animals have also dealt with the classification, causation, incidence, and anatomic descriptions of malformations. There is increasing interest in analytic approaches, however, as indicated repeatedly throughout this book. Further studies on the mechanisms and early pathogenesis of abnormal development are urgently needed.

B. Growth Retardation

Growth retardation has received much less attention than malformation, although it is now increasingly accepted as a manifestation of abnormal development in both man (Gruenwald, 1961) and in laboratory animals (Jensh and Brent, 1967; McLaren and Michie, 1963). Furthermore, in current research it is being related to such diverse factors as placental insufficiency (Myers *et al.,* 1971) and rate of DNA synthesis during the intrauterine period (Packard and Skalko, 1972; Roux, 1971). Intrauterine growth retardation in pigs has been shown not to be compensated for after birth and to be associated with reduced DNA and protein content between birth and maturity (Widdowson, 1972). Children with low birth weight have been found to have very few more "minor" congenital defects than controls (Crichton *et al.,* 1972). Other aspects of pre- and postnatal growth retardation will be discussed, particularly in relation to teratologic testing, in Chapter 9, Section II, A.

C. Intrauterine Death

Corner (1923) called attention to intrauterine death as a form of spontaneous pathology among the embryos of pigs some 50 years ago. It has been of interest to geneticists in connection with lethal mutations for many years, but death has only relatively recently been studied in animals as a manifestation of abnormal development in response to environmental factors (Adams, 1960; Beck and Lloyd, 1963; Larsson and Eriksson, 1966; Russell, 1965; Skalko and Packard, 1971). Prenatal death or "wastage," as it is sometimes called, has been sporadically studied in man (Nishimura *et al.,* 1968a; Robinson, 1921; Stiekle, 1968; Taylor, 1970), but only crude estimates of the cumulative mortality from conception are available. Warburton and Fraser (1964) concluded that at least 14.7% of known human conceptions are aborted, not including "habitual aborters," and that abortions were not correlated with a familial history of congenitally defective children, except that mothers of anencephalic infants had significantly more abortions than other women. Data on background rates of intrauterine death in domestic and laboratory animals are scarce; for example, it is estimated that rhesus monkeys have a rate of spontaneous abortion not exceeding 15% (Wilson, 1972b); but firm rates are not available for this or other species.

D. FUNCTIONAL DEFICITS

Functional disorders of developmental origin have not as a group been as well characterized as have structural defects, although certain types including mental retardation (Malamud, 1964) and the so-called inborn errors of metabolism (Holt and Coffey, 1968; Waisman, 1966) have been intensively studied in recent years. This class of developmental abnormality is often not recognized until some time after birth, owing in part to the fact that some functional parameters, particularly those of a mental and metabolic nature, do not reach maturity until months or years after birth. There is substantial evidence that many functional disorders may have their inception either prenatally (Chase *et al.,* 1971; Haddad *et al.,* 1969; Spyker *et al.,* 1972) or postnatally (Sechzer *et al.,* 1971) in animals and perhaps also in man. The mental deficiency associated with phenylketonuria is the consequence of high levels of postnatal phenylalaninemia, although the underlying enzyme deficiency is the result of a recessively inherited gene abnormality. Functional abnormalities of the central nervous system are sometimes associated with demonstrable structural defects and sometimes not: Malamud (1964) found at autopsy that 61% of 1410 mentally defective children had anatomic defects of the brain, whereas the remainder showed no structural variation outside of the normal range. As noted earlier, rubella virus causes, in addition to the familiar syndrome of anatomic defects, a number of functional disorders (Dudgeon, 1967; Menser *et al.,* 1967), some of which, e.g., mental deficiency, hearing defects, and jaundice, do not appear to be secondary to structural abnormality (Friedmann and Wright, 1966; Streissguth *et al.,* 1970).

CHAPTER 6

ACCESS OF ENVIRONMENTAL FACTORS TO DEVELOPING TISSUES

The nature of environmental agents determines whether or in what dosage they reach developing tissues. Germ cells as well as embryos are in large measure insulated by parental tissues from thermal and mechanical shock in the environment, although the male gonad may on occasion be exposed to unfavorable temperatures. Whether the latter increases the possibility of mutation is unknown. The exception to the general rule that parental tissues shield germ cells and intrauterine occupants from physical agents is ionizing radiations which are thought always to reach developing tissues in some fraction of the air dosage, the fractional dosage depending on the thickness and density of overlying parental tissues. The dosage of environmental chemicals reaching either the germ cells or the conceptus *in utero,* however, is always subject to modulation by the parental body and probably also by the placenta.

I. Parental Defenses against Chemical Agents

A. ABSORPTION

The route of entry of chemical agents, whether by absorption from the digestive tract, lungs, or skin, or introduced by some other route, is one of the determiners of concentration in parental plasma. Dosage, the area of absorptive surface, and the chemical nature and physical form of the agent also influence rates of absorption. These factors which collectively control the rate of entry of foreign chemicals into the blood of the parent are basic principles of pharmacology; but since they are not unique to teratology, the reader is referred to appropriate textbooks for further discussion (see Fingl and Woodbury, 1965).

Once foreign chemicals are present in the blood an active role in reducing their concentration is played by homeostatic functions of the parental organism. The critical question is whether homeostasis can prevent concentration from reaching detrimental effect levels. Little is known about the range of dosage over which germinal mutations may be induced, but it is thought to be broad for many chemical mutagens (Fishbein *et al.*, 1970), and it has been suggested that no threshold exists for the induction of mutagenesis. A threshold almost certainly exists, however, for other types of teratogenic effects, particularly those in which tissue repair and embryonic regulation can come into play (see Chapter 2, Section VI,A and Chapter 3, Section I,A). In any case, the probability of teratogenesis as a result either of mutations or of deviations in embryonic or fetal development depends on the concentration and duration of a potentially harmful chemical in the parental bloodstream. Both level and duration reflect the differential between the rate of absorption mentioned above and the rate of dispersal discussed below.

B. Dispersal of Chemical Agents from Plasma

Dispersal is used here as a collective term for the sum of all factors tending to reduce concentration of extrinsic chemicals in parental blood; therefore, it includes placental transfer as well as metabolism, excretion, storage, etc. This subject also is properly in the domain of pharmacology, but it is of such immediate importance to developing tissues that it must be emphasized in the present context. Presumably germinal tissues and the placenta are exposed to all chemicals in the parental blood, although the germ cells in both ovaries and testes are separated from direct contact with blood by at least an epithelial basement membrane and a capillary wall. Little is known about possible regulatory roles by such membranes, but it is probable that they are as freely permeable to foreign chemicals as to physiologic metabolites.

Chemical agents in parental blood are reduced in concentration by one or more of four homeostatic processes, namely, (1) excretion, (2) catabolism and other detoxication, (3) protein and tissue binding, and (4) storage. Excretion involves the removal from blood and the ejection from the body of the original chemical agent as well as any breakdown products that are formed. This occurs principally in the kidneys but skin, liver, lungs, and digestive tract may also participate. Catabolism is a more involved process by which the original compound is enzymatically degraded through oxidation, reduction, or hydrolysis to a simpler and often less toxic or more easily excreted form. Detoxication does not always involve chemical degradation; the extraneous compound may occasionally be complexed with a physiologic one in such a way as to reduce toxicity or facilitate transport. Both of these detoxifying processes occur mainly in the liver but other organs are sometimes involved. Binding of drugs or chemicals to proteins in plasma or in tissues can effectively reduce the concentration of the free forms, thereby lowering the effective dosage in contact with developing tissues at any one time. Storage is exemplified by those foreign chemicals (e.g., DDT) which by virtue of their ready solubility in fat or in other tissue components are more rapidly removed from blood than would otherwise be the case. Similarly, a dilution factor may operate in the case of compounds that quickly pass from plasma to other fluid compartments, such as into cerebrospinal fluid. Thus, these homeostatic processes tend constantly to reduce the concentration of foreign chemicals in the plasma, but at any given point in time plasma level is the differential between the rates of absorption and of dispersal of the compound.

II. Placental Defenses

The intrauterine occupant has another line of defense against foreign chemicals, one not available to the germ cells of postnatal individuals. This is, of course, the placenta. It provides added protection to the embryo and fetus by serving as a buffer able in many situations to reduce further the dosage reaching the conceptus. Present knowledge no longer justifies regarding the placenta as a "barrier" in the sense that it absolutely excludes any chemical substance. There is abundant evidence that a great variety of chemicals cross the placenta and are present in the conceptus in measurable amounts, both in laboratory animals (Panigel, 1971; Villee, 1965, 1971; Waddell, 1972) and in man (Adamsons, 1965; Apgar, 1966; Ginsburg, 1968, 1971; Lucey, 1965; Moya and Thorndike, 1963). Although much remains to be learned about the details of transfer of foreign as well as physiologic substances (Aladjem, 1970; Assali *et al.,* 1968; Boyd and Hamilton, 1970), information now available provides a working knowledge of normal placental transport. From the viewpoint of human teratology, however, many of the studies to date have two important limitations: (1) They were carried out during the latter third of pregnancy after the period of highest teratogenic susceptibility had passed, or (2) they were done in rodent or lagomorph species which may have atypical transport functions associated with the presence of the inverted yolk sac placenta (Payne and Deuchar, 1972).

It is established that the placenta of primates undergoes structural and ultrastructural changes as the conceptus passes from the period of early organogenesis, when teratogenic susceptibility is highest, to the near-term state when anatomical defects are less likely to be induced (Aladjem, 1970; Boyd and Hamilton, 1970; Panigel, 1971). The extent to which such structural changes are associated with changes in the physiology of transport is unknown. The following summary is based largely on studies on the mature placenta in the latter stages of gestation. Physiologic substances are thought to be transferred from maternal plasma to embryonic or fetal blood by one or another of five means. Nonphysiologic or foreign chemicals, however, are assumed to cross the placenta mainly by simple diffusion, except when they are analogs of natural metabolites, in which case the extraneous chemical is thought to cross by the same means as do the natural substances they resemble (Ginsburg, 1971).

A. Transfer of Physiologic Substances

1. *Simple Diffusion*

This is essentially a physicochemical process by which molecules of relatively small size and low charge are transferred according to the Fick diffusion equation:

$$\text{Rate of diffusion} = K \frac{A (C_m - C_e)}{X}$$

where K = a diffusion constant characterizing the placenta of the species concerned for the substance being diffused, A = the area over which diffusion occurs, C_m = concentration of unbound chemical in maternal plasma, C_e = concentration of unbound chemical in embryonic blood, and X = the thickness of the diffusion membrane. Both area (A) and thickness (X) of the placenta are known to vary markedly during development (Boyd and Hamilton, 1970; Panigel, 1971) and it is probable that the changing morphology also causes the diffusion constant (K) to change. Placental passage of some substances is known to change with increasing gestational age (Eliason and Posner, 1971), although the extent to which this may reflect such other factors as degree of plasma protein binding on either side of the placenta is not clear. Transfer always occurs down a concentration gradient and requires no metabolic energy. Oxygen and CO_2 are normally transferred in this manner, and it is thought that many drugs of small molecular size and low ionic charge also cross by diffusion. An important limiting factor for this mode of transfer would be rates of blood flow on maternal and embryonic sides of the membrane, a fact which could be instrumental in the teratogenicity attributed to serotonin and other vasoconstricting drugs in animals (Ward, 1968).

2. *Facilitated Diffusion*

This is the mode of transfer of substances that cross the placenta at a faster rate than would be compatible with their molecular size or charge or with their degree of lipid solubility. In other words, transfer is usually down a concentration gradient but faster than could be accounted for by simple diffusion. It appears to depend on a chemical receptor substance, "carrier," in the cell membrane which renders the molecule being transferred more soluble in the lipid component of the membrane. This differs from simple diffusion further in that a saturation phenomenon is apparent at high concentrations, thus there is competition for the transfer mechanism among chemically related substances, and the system may be impaired by inhibitors. Sugars, amino acids, and some salts are transferred by this means. Dancis *et al.* (1968) have shown that placentae of guinea pig and man maintain concentration gradients in favor of the fetuses for several amino acids, presumably by facilitated diffusion up the gradient. Certain analogs of amino acids, azaserine and DON, are teratogenic in rats at relatively small doses (Murphy, 1965), possibly owing to their accumulation on the embryonic side of the placenta by facilitated transport.

3. *Active Transport*

Many substances are known to be transferred across the placenta against a concentration gradient and in spite of the charge on the molecule. This requires the expenditure of metabolic energy, hence is called active transport. The details of this process are not clear, but it is thought to involve sequential enzymatic coupling and uncoupling of the transported molecule to an intracellular carrier molecule. Evidence for the existence of this mode of transport is seen in (1) transfer in the direction opposite from that of an electrochemical gradient, (2) presence of a gradient at equilibrium in the absence of other factors that would account for such, (3) decrease in transfer rate by the introduction of metabolic poisons, (4) competition for transfer by similar molecules, and (5) saturation of the transfer system. Some amino acids and divalent cations are transported by this means. No teratogens are known to be transported in this fashion, but some relatively large molecules that are teratogenic at minute dosage, e.g., actinomycin D (Jordan and Wilson, 1970), may be possible examples.

4. *Pinocytosis*

Trophoblastic cells have been shown in ultrastructural studies to form intracellular vacuoles by pinocytosis (Boyd and Hamilton, 1970; Panigel, 1971), that is, by engulfing a small quantity of maternal plasma, together with whatever solutes or particulate matter it might contain. The intracellular fate of such vacuoles and the materials they contain is not clear, but it is thought probable that large molecules such as intact proteins (e.g., antibodies) may be ejected on the opposite side of the membrane after having traversed the cells in a pinocytotic vacuole. Theoretically this mechanism would make possible the transplacental passage of almost any colloidal or particulate matter of subcellular size, perhaps including the viruses known to be capable of transplacental passage (Eichenwald, 1965).

5. *Leakage*

The presence of small rents or defects in the continuity of the membranes is known for the placentae of several species. These fortuitous openings are thought to provide the means by which blood cells cross the placenta from maternal to embryonic bloodstreams (Creger and Steele, 1957; Desai and Creger, 1963; Tuffrey *et al.,* 1969). The fetal red blood cells that serve as antigens in human erythroblastosis fetalis have for some time been assumed to gain access to the maternal bloodstream by this route. It is not believed that significant amounts of drugs or other chemical agents pass by this route (Ginsburg, 1971).

B. Possible Degradation of Chemicals by the Placenta

In addition to its transfer activities the placenta is known to serve several other functions. Of particular interest in connection with protection of the conceptus against possible adverse effects from extraneous chemicals is the possibility that the placenta itself may be able to take part in detoxication in a way similar to that in the liver. The subject of such biotransformation reactions in the placenta has recently been reviewed by Juchau (1972). It was concluded that present information is too meager for a final judgment. Although available data indicate that the placenta possesses the capability to transform drugs by each of the major processes, namely, reduction, oxidation, hydrolysis, and conjugation, there was reason to question the importance of such metabolic processes for the embryo or fetus. Certainly there is little evidence at this time to support the view that the placenta acts as a secondary liver able to protect the conceptus by catabolism of chemical agents present in maternal plasma. Nevertheless, the high metabolic activity of the trophoblast, particularly in the biosynthesis of RNA (Jordan and Wilson, 1970), would suggest that the possibility of biotransformation of some extraneous chemicals by the placenta should not be ruled out without further study.

C. The Embryo Dose

The dosage of an extraneous chemical that reaches the bloodstream of the embryo or fetus is the residue after the action of the biologic processes discussed above and diagramed in Fig. 6-1. As already indicated, the concentration of molecules in maternal plasma is by no means the only determinant of embryo dosage, and is itself only a secondary product of the original dosage to the maternal organism, the rate at which this is absorbed, and the

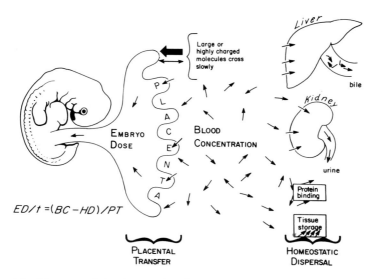

$$ED/t = (BC - HD)/PT$$

FIG. 6-1. Diagram of the factors that influence embryo dose of a foreign chemical present in the maternal bloodstream. The maternal blood concentration under usual conditions of exposure is subject to considerable change, representing as it does the differential between maternal absorption and the several routes for dispersal, including the maternal homeostatic processes of metabolism, excretion, protein binding, and tissue storage, as well as passage across the placenta to the embryo. These various biologic processes are all functions of time; therefore the embryo dose depends on the duration as well as the level of a chemical in maternal blood. Embryo dose is proportional to maternal blood concentration, however, only for substances that traverse the placenta by simple diffusion; otherwise the placenta imposes various rates of transfer depending on the nature of the substance being transferred. The formulation $ED/t = (BC - HD)/PT$ is in no sense a precise mathematical one, but does attempt to state the basic fact that embryo dose *(ED)* over a given period of time *(t)* depends on the maternal blood concentration *(BC)* which tends constantly to be reduced by homeostatic dispersal *(HD)* and by placental transfer *(PT)*.

rate at which it is being dispersed by maternal homeostasis. In simplest terms plasma concentration is the differential between input through absorption and dispersal by homeostatic processes. The aliquot of maternal plasma that passes over the surface of the trophoblast contains the concentration that will be a rate-determining factor in placental transfer. It is assumed that all chemicals in maternal plasma cross the placenta by one means or another at some rate; the critical question is at what rate.

Attempts to express in a precise equation all of the complex factors involved in placental transfer have not given practicable results, owing largely to difficulties in controlling the many variables (Assali *et al.*, 1968). For the present purpose it is sufficient to formulate a general statement which relates embryo dose (Fig. 6-1) to the fraction of maternal plasma concentration that is transported, as determined by the nature of the compound and the characteristics of the placenta in question. In addition to the latter factors which are relatively constant, rate of transport is to varying degrees influenced by a changing concentration gradient between embryonic and maternal circulations and by the minute-volume of embryonic circulation through the placenta which may also be variable but about which almost nothing is known. These variables make calculations of the level and duration of embryo dosage, even when the maternal plasma concentration is precisely known, little more than a rough approximation.

D. Role of Placental Failure in Teratogenesis

It is to be expected that partial detachment, infarcts, and other gross pathology that substantially reduce the effective transport surface of the placenta would lead to death or growth retardation of an embryo or fetus. On the other hand, reduced placental size and some types of overt pathology do not seem to influence adversely the welfare of the offspring (Longo, 1972). Little evidence exists to indicate that impairment of placental transport function is responsible for specific malformations or postnatal functional disorder in the offspring, although placental hemangiomata have been questionably associated with perinatal purpura and malformations in a few cases (Froelich and Fujikura, 1970).

The only exception to the general rule that the placenta is not often involved in teratogenesis appears to concern the inverted yolk sac placenta of rodents and rabbits. This double-layered membrane is thought to serve as the main means of transfer between maternal blood and the embryo during early organogenesis in these species. Substantial data indicate a transport function for this structure as regards macromolecules as well as some amino acids and other small metabolites (Deren *et al.*, 1966; Padykula *et al.*, 1966; Payne and Duchar, 1972). Pronounced teratogenic effects have been associated with the accumulation of tissue antisera (Brent *et al.*, 1971; Slotnick and Brent, 1966) and of trypan blue (Beck *et al.*, 1967) in the yolk sac placenta. In the latter instance the developmental defects were thought to be related to the breakdown of certain digestive functions as well as of transport activities usually attributed to this structure.

III. Do the Embryo and Fetus Have Their Own Defenses?

It is generally accepted that the fluids filling the amnion and chorion could serve as hydrostatic cushions for the intrauterine occupant in the event of mechanical trauma to the maternal abdomen. There is little evidence, however, that these fluid compartments serve as either a primary pathway of entry or as a repository for the accumulation of foreign chemicals, as has occasionally been suggested.

The possibility that the teratogenically susceptible embryo has intrinsic homeostatic devices that might moderate or eliminate potentially damaging chemical agents is a critical question that has been little investigated. Rane and Sjöquist (1972) have reviewed their own and other studies on livers removed from human fetuses at elective abortion, mainly during the second trimester of pregnancy, and have concluded that while the liver at this time contains drug-metabolizing enzyme components, it is not yet possible to generalize about the drug-metabolizing capacity of human fetal livers. According to these authors the several studies on drug metabolic functions in prenatal animals show that the capacity of animal fetuses to oxidize and conjugate drugs is negligible.

A number of studies on the autoradiographic localization of chemical agents in near-term animal fetuses and on the metabolism of drugs in isolated fetal tissues have been reviewed by Waddell (1972). It was concluded that the patterns of localization in such fetuses were essentially the same as in adults. Metabolism of drugs by the fetal liver at this time, however, was less than metabolism in adult livers, except for some steroids which were hydroxylated at as great or greater rate in early fetal life than during the perinatal or postnatal period. Autoradiography of pregnant mice at teratogenically susceptible stages of the embryo did not reveal any sites of localization in the conceptus that would suggest a mechanism for the known teratogenicity of cortisone and chlorcyclizine. Interestingly it was noted that the yolk sac placenta accumulates and excretes some drugs or their metabolites directly into the uterine lumen (Waddell, 1972). Whether this mechanism could be significant in reducing the effective dosage to the embryo is not known.

Certainly all drugs are not rapidly eliminated from the embryo or the fetus. Many experiments have shown that drugs can be incorporated into or bound to embryonic or fetal tissues (Cahen and Fave, 1970; Dagg *et al.,* 1966; Schumacher *et al.,* 1969). Hydroxyurea is known to have a half-life in the 12-day rat embryo that is approximately twice as long as that in the maternal plasma (Scott *et al.,* 1971) (Fig. 2-5), suggesting that this highly teratogenic compound was either bound or incorporated in the embryo. Nicotine given to pregnant rats maintains a high concentration gradient on the fetal side from 30 minutes through 20 hours after treatment on the nineteenth day of gestation (Mosier and Jansons, 1972). There are no data to indicate that the early mammalian embryo has inherent protective devices against extraneous chemicals during the period of high teratogenic suscepti-bility. The later fetus probably begins to develop some homeostatic mecha-nisms, e.g., excretion, but other protective devices, particularly metabolic degradation, seem to be much less effective than those of postnatal animals.

CHAPTER 7

NORMAL DEVELOPMENT AND SUSCEPTIBLE PERIODS

It has been emphasized that developing tissues and organisms, germ cells, embryos, fetuses, and immature postnatal individuals are more susceptible to environmental influences than are mature somatic tissues. It has also been pointed out that susceptibility to adverse stimuli varies widely during the developmental span; the types of response are likely to be qualitatively as well as quantitatively different in the successive epochs of development. Early predifferentiation embryos tend to die when the agent is applied in effective dosage, otherwise they survive more-or-less unscathed. Embryos undergoing organogenesis may also be killed by adverse conditions, but if not they are liable to sustain localized damage sufficient to lead to malformation. During the fetal period, histogenesis, growth, and functional maturation are the developmental processes most in evidence and, therefore, are the ones most vulnerable to abnormality under unfavorable conditions. After birth growth is the principal unfinished developmental process and accordingly is more likely to be impaired, but certain aspects of function, for example, higher mental activities, may still be susceptible to some types of stress such as severe nutritional deprivation. It is uncertain whether germ cells are more susceptible to mutagenesis at one time than another during their maturation.

I. Use and Abuse of the Concept of Critical Periods

Although susceptibility to various kinds of damage extends over much of the developmental span, undoubtedly it is greatest during organogenesis (see Chapter 2, Section II,C). It is thus appropriate to give particular attention to the timing of normal events during this period and to comment on the extent to which these may be changed by concurrent environmental influences. William Harvey in 1561 first pointed out that certain malformations seen after birth sometimes show considerable similarity in appearance to the primordia of the affected structures during organogenesis. For example, he noted that the facial features of newborn deer with cleft lip and palate were reminiscent of the undeveloped faces of deer embryos removed just prior to the time when the primordia united to complete the lip and jaw in normal embryogenesis. Thus arose the view that malformations represent an arrest of developmental processes at some point prior to their normal completion, still referred to today as the theory of developmental arrest. This notion has gained wide acceptance and has been extended to the unjustified assumption that a point-by-point correlation exists between the developmental conditions existing when a malformation was induced and the type of defect later observed. Accordingly, when Stockard (1921) produced similar malformations by exposing the embryos of sea minnows to either low temperature or reduced oxygen tension, he attributed the similarities of results to the fact that these different types of stresses were applied at comparable times in development. The occurrence of a variety of anomalies after subjecting embryos for a short time to a single agent was recognized as reflecting the fact that several organs were at critical stages in development when exposure occurred. These times of particular susceptibility in organogenesis were called "critical moments" by Stockard, a concept now usually referred to as critical periods.

It is often true that some correlation can be shown to exist between developmental conditions at the times an adverse influence is applied and the form of the structure later found to be malformed. In fact, schedules have been formulated to relate specific types of abnormal development with precise times for their inception, both in laboratory animals (Hicks, 1954) and in man (Lenz, 1964). The concept of critical periods may be misleading, however, if it is interpreted to mean that malformations can be induced only when primordia of affected organs are at a particular stage in organogenesis, or that organs at seemingly critical stages in organogenesis are necessarily always susceptible to induced maldevelopment. Numerous instances are known of malformations being induced at times when no recognizable primordia of the affected organ were present (see Chapter 2, Section II), or of the same malformation resulting from treatment applied at different stages in the organogenesis of the affected part (Russell and Russell, 1954; Shenefelt, 1972; Warkany and Schraffenberger, 1947). Thus attempts to localize precisely the time at which a teratogenic insult occurred by extrapolating backward to the time in organogenesis when an observed defect is assumed to have had a developmental counterpart or the affected organ to have failed to complete a critical morphogenetic event are not always trustworthy.

The concept of critical or susceptible periods is useful only in approximating the time of inception of abnormal development and should be used as a rule-of-thumb device rather than a scientific principle.

The following pages dealing with the chronology of specific events during human organogenesis are included to give the reader an overview of the sequences in which various structures appear, but are not intended to suggest that an adverse influence will necessarily affect any one or all events in progress at a particular stage.

SUMMARY OF HUMAN EMBRYOLOGY FROM FERTILIZATION THROUGH MAJOR ORGANOGENESIS

Figures 7-1 to 7-23 outline the main structural changes but make no attempt to deal with the complex developmental and biochemical interrelations also in progress during this period. The stated days of gestational age must be regarded as modal, not even as inclusive ranges, owing to the fact that human embryos, like those of other forms, develop at variable rates after fertilization. The timing of human gestation is further complicated by the unreliability of data on the menstrual cycle and the time of coition, and particularly by the lack of a reliable criterion for identifying the time of ovulation.

Staging follows that originally proposed by Streeter (1942, 1945, 1948, 1951) but his designation "horizons" has been dropped and the stages indicated by Roman numerals. Gestational ages have been revised in keeping with recent studies in which more reliable data as regards timing were available (Iffy *et al.,* 1967; Nishimura *et al.,* 1968a). Information from several sources has been used to expand the developmental events associated with each stage beyond the relatively few criteria used by Streeter. Figures 7-8 to 7-23 are retouched versions of photographs of actual embryos in the collection of the Carnegie Institution of Washington, which were originally published in the *Contributions to Embryology* as indicated.

II. Characteristics of the Human Fetus

It is customary to begin referring to the human conceptus as a fetus toward the end of the eighth week postconception, when major organogenesis is essentially completed. The most conspicuous developmental process during the fetal period is physical growth, but of equal or greater importance for postnatal life is functional maturation which begins at different times for different organs but is not complete in most instances until after birth. Preparatory to assumption of their functional roles, individual organs undergo further structural refinements to convert the relatively simple tissue groups

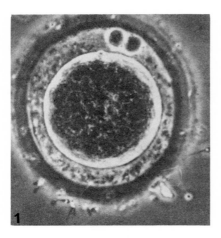

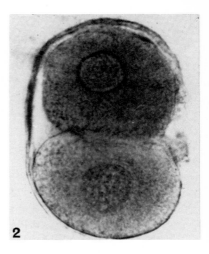

STAGE I

FIG. 7-1. *0–1.5 days postfertilization.*
One-celled zygote, second polar body
present, corona radiata dispersed, sperm
heads seen in zona pellucida and/or
perivitelline space, usually found in upper half of oviduct. (From Shettles,
1955.)

STAGE II

FIG. 7-2. *1.5–4 days.* Segmenting
blastomeres, 2-, 4-, 8-, 16-, and 32-cell
stages to morula, zona pellucida per-
sists, usually located in lower half of
oviduct (section of embryo No. 8698,
Hertig *et al.,* 1954).

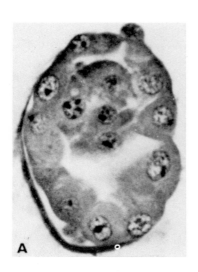

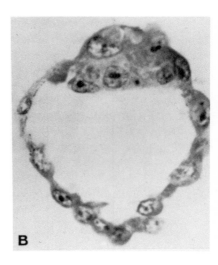

STAGE III A

FIG. 7-3A. *4–5 days.* Free blastocyst with segmentation cavity forming, zona pellucida dissolving, free-
floating in uterine cavity (section
of embryo No. 8794, Hertig *et al.,*
1954).

STAGE III B

FIG. 7-3B. *5–6 days.* Free blastocyst
with blastocele dilating, inner cell mass
clearly delimited, no germ layer formation apparent (section of embryo No.
8663, Hertig *et al.,* 1954).

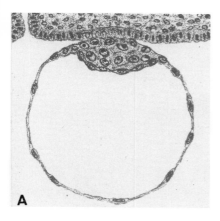

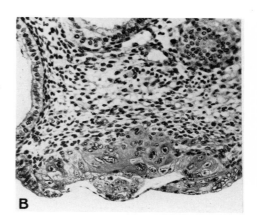

STAGE IV A

STAGE IV B

FIG. 7-4A. *6–7 days (?).* Attaching blastocyst with fully distended blastocele (composite drawing based on similar stages in animals—none yet recovered in man).

FIG. 7-4B. *7–8 days.* Implantation in progress, erosion of uterine wall, rapid proliferation of trophoblast, blastocele collapsed, amnion forms, bilaminar germ disc present, extraembryonic mesoderm begins (section of embryo No. 8020, Hertig and Rock, 1945).

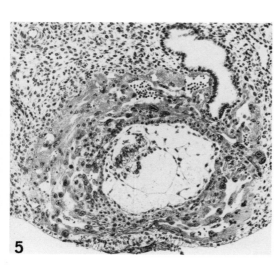

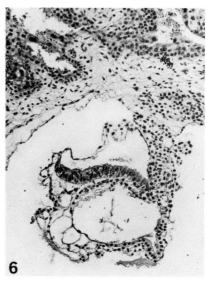

STAGE V

STAGE VI

FIG. 7-5. *9–12 days.* Embryo implanted, proliferation of trophoblast on all surfaces, no villi, amniotic cavity dilates, extraembryonic mesoderm proliferating (section of embryo No. 7699, Hertig and Rock, 1941).

FIG. 7-6. *13–14 days.* Primitive villi appear, yolk sac forms, body stalk indicated, extraembryonic coelom greatly expanded (section of Torpin embryo, Krafka, 1941).

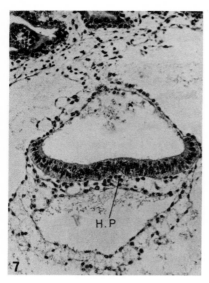

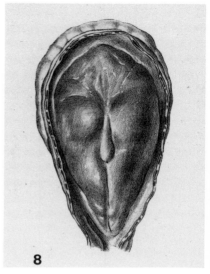

Stage VII

Fig. 7-7. *15–16 days.* True branched villi appear, axis of embryonic disc determined by head process (H.P), primitive node and streak indicated, few angioblasts in wall of yolk sac, allantois growing through body stalk (section of embryo No. 7802. Heuser *et al.,* 1945).

Stage VIII

Fig. 7-8. *17–19 days.* Embryonic disc elongates along future body axis, notochord begins, primitive node and streak well established, intraembryonic mesoderm forming, neural plate appears, angiogenesis in yolk sac wall (redrawn ectodermal surface of Heuser embryo, Heuser. 1932).

established during organogenesis to the more specialized ones associated with definitive function. This process is known as histogenesis. Despite its critical importance to functional normality in the postnatal individual, the study of histogenesis tends to be neglected, both in terms of normal morphology and of the pathogenesis of malformations. It is usually necessary to resort to the older editions of histology, embryology, and pathology texts to find accounts of histogenesis. The pathogenesis of metabolic diseases, many of which probably could be traced to abnormal histogenesis during the fetal period, would seem to offer many opportunities for investigation, particularly using the methods of cytochemistry and ultrastructure.

A. Normal Intrauterine Growth

This process appears to be under complex control, limited by the genetic characteristics of the species but capable of being modified by many envi-

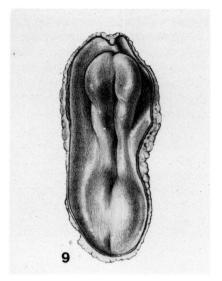

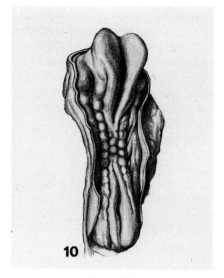

STAGE IX

STAGE X

FIG. 7-9. *20–21 days; 0–3 somites.* Head fold prominent, neural folds and groove form, notochord elongating, pericardium forms, heart primordia appear, intraembryonic blood islands initiate angiogenesis, foregut indicated, body stalk elongates (redrawn surface view of Ingalls embryo, Ingalls, 1920).

FIG. 7-10. *22–24 days; 1.5–3.5 mm; 4–12 somites.* Neural tube begins closure, optic sulcus present, otic placode forms, 1st branchial arch visible, 1st and 2nd aortic arches seen, bilateral cardiac primordia unite in single tube, first heart movement (?), pleural and peritoneal cavities begin, oral pit and pharynx indicated, hind gut begins, first pronephroi (redrawn surface view of Payne embryo, Payne, 1925).

ronmental factors. Availability of nutrients, both through the maternal dietary and as a consequence of transport across the placenta, is the major environmental determinant of the rate of intrauterine growth (Widdowson, 1968). Maternal physiologic state, particularly as regards endocrine function and the presence or absence of infections, is also a matter of considerable importance (Gruenwald, 1966a, b). The cause of intrauterine growth retardation in individual human cases, however, is often difficult to identify (Ounsted and Ounsted, 1968). Interspecies comparisons show that prenatal growth is dynamically very similar in a number of mammalian and avian species when final weights and the duration of the growth periods are adjusted to the same scale (Laird, 1966).

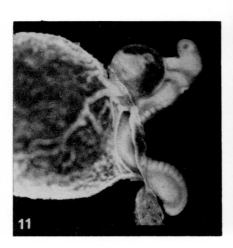 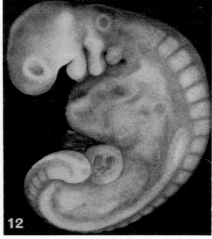

STAGE XI

STAGE XII

FIG. 7-11. *25–26 days; 2.0–4.5 mm; 13–20 somites.* Anterior neuropore closing, otic invagination, optic evagination, cranial nn. V, VII, VIII, IX, X, and XII seen, sinus venosus and cardinal vv. form, heart beats, heart tube convoluted, 2nd branchial arch appears, oral membrane ruptures, liver primordium evaginates, pharyngeal pouches form, yolk stalk beginning, cloaca formed, pronephros complete, septum transversum forms, body axis elongated and often dorsally curved (after embryo No. 6050, Streeter. 1942).

FIG. 7-12. *27–29 days; 3–5 mm; 21–29 somites.* Third branchial arch appears, 3rd aortic arch forms, arm bud appears, posterior neuropore closing, yolk stalk constricting, thyroid and laryngotracheal buds evaginate, dorsal pancreas appears, common bile duct and gall bladder form, mesonephric tubules and ducts begin, blood circulation begins, body axis C-shaped (after embryo No. 5923, Streeter, 1942).

1. Growth Retardation

As discussed more fully in Chapter 9, Section II,A, growth retardation is sometimes reversible, that is, it can be compensated for by a faster than normal rate at a later time, or it may result in permanent stunting or "runting." The factors responsible for reversible as opposed to irreversible growth retardation are not well understood. There is also uncertainty about the relative significance to be assigned to each; for example, should all prenatal growth retardation be considered a manifestation of developmental toxicity, or should only irreversible retardation be so regarded? The present author feels that statistically significant growth retardation, even if it is later reversible, should be considered as a sign of developmental toxicity, albeit of relatively benign nature.

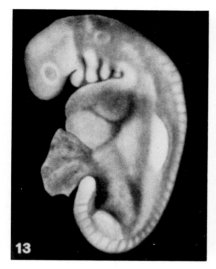

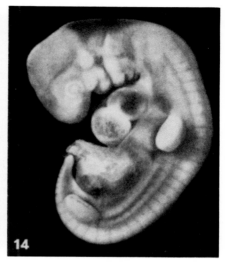

STAGE XIII

STAGE XIV

FIG. 7-13. *30–32 days; 4–6 mm; 30–40 somites;* Fourth branchial arch forms, optic vesicle contacts ectoderm, lens placode begins, otocyst closes, leg bud appears, amnion delimits umbilical cord, 4th aortic arch begins, heart chambers dilate, primary bronchi and lung buds separate, stomach indicated, mesonephric ducts reach cloaca, urorectal septum begins (after embryo No. 8066, Streeter, 1945).

FIG. 7-14. *33–35 days; 5–8 mm.* Olfactory placode forms, lens placode invaginates, cervical sinus begins, optic cup invaginates and stalk constricts, Rathke's pouch prominent, pharyngeal pouches differentiating, metanephric bud and blastema seen, zonation in spinal cord conspicuous (after embryo No. 6848, Streeter, 1945).

2. *Weekly Growth Increments during the Fetal Period*

Table 7-1 presents height and weight measurements of 704 human fetuses from the sixth through the thirty-eighth weeks of intrauterine development taken under uniform conditions at the Carnegie Institution of Embryology (Streeter, 1921). It is of interest to note that the human fetus increases in sitting height roughly at the rate of 1 cm/week after the sixth week, whereas the weekly increment in weight steadily increases from 1.6 to 255 gm.

B. NORMAL FUNCTIONAL MATURATION

The functional development of the human fetus and infant have been reviewed in a number of recent volumes (Assali, 1968; Barnes, 1968; Dawes, 1968) and is too extensive a subject for discussion here. Interference with

TABLE 7-1

HEIGHT AND WEIGHT OF HUMAN FETUSES FROM THE SIXTH TO THE THIRTY-EIGHTH WEEK[a,b]

Estimated ovulation age (weeks)	Sitting height at end of week (mm)	Increment in height		Formalin weight[c] (gm)	Increment in weight	
		(mm)	(%)		(gm)	(%)
6	23	—	—	1.1	—	—
7	31	8	26	2.7	1.6	59
8	40	9	23	4.6	1.9	41
9	50	10	20	7.9	3.3	42
10	61	11	18	14.2	6.3	44
11	74	13	18	26	11.8	45
12	87	13	15	45	19	42
13	101	14	14	72	27	38
14	116	15	13	108	36	33
15	130	14	11	150	42	28
16	142	12	8	198	48	24
17	153	11	7	253	55	21
18	164	11	7	316	63	20
19	175	11	6	385	69	18
20	186	11	6	460	75	16
21	197	11	6	542	82	15
22	208	11	5	630	88	14
23	218	10	5	723	93	13
24	228	10	4	823	100	12
25	238	10	4	930	107	12
26	247	9	4	1,045	115	11
27	256	9	4	1,174	129	11
28	265	9	3	1,323	149	11
29	274	9	3	1,492	169	11
30	283	9	3	1,680	188	11
31	293	10	3	1,876	196	10
32	302	9	3	2,074	198	10
33	311	9	3	2,274	200	9
34	321	10	3	2,478	204	8
35	331	10	3	2,690	212	8
36	341	10	3	2,914	224	8
37	352	11	3	3,150	236	8
38	362	10	3	3,405	255	8

[a] Based on 704 specimen in the Carnegie Collection, distributed as follows: white ♂ 252, white ♀ 241, Negro ♂ 66, Negro ♀ 60, others 15 ♂ 11 ♀, unidentified, 59.

[b] Adapted from Streeter (1921).

[c] Many of the specimens between the twenty-sixth and thirty-eighth weeks were embalmed, and in these cases the weight given is the fresh weight plus 5%.

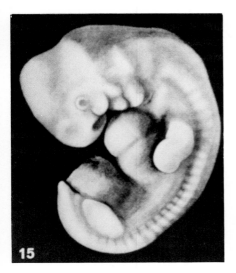

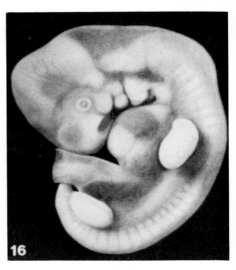

STAGE XV

STAGE XVI

FIG. 7-15. *36–37 days; 6–9 mm.* Lens vesicle closes, olfactory pits develop, cerebral evagination seen, aortopulmonary septal ridges forming, atrioventricular endocardial cushions forming, 6th aortic arch and pulmonary artery appear, secondary bronchi indicated, ventral pancreas seen, midgut loop projects ventrally, caecum dilates, musculoskeletal condensations in arm buds, hand plate evident (after embryo No. 3512, Streeter, 1948).

FIG. 7-16. *38–39 days; 8–11 mm.* Cervical sinus closes, pigment appears in retina choroid fissure closes, posterior hypophysis evaginates, auditory hillocks defined, all cardiac septa prominent but unclosed, A-V endocardial cushions fuse, midgut loop herniated into umbilical cord and begins rotation, mesentery attenuated, first division of ureteric bud, muscular and skeletal differentiation in upper limb, foot plate evident (after embryo No. 8098, Streeter, 1948).

normal maturation by environmental factors has also been discussed in these sources; for the present purpose it is sufficient to note that such factors as the taking of drugs, nutritional deprivation, and infections during the latter half of human pregnancy may lead to both low birth weight and poor functional state in the newborn infant. Such below-par infants rarely show structural malformations that could be attributed to adverse situations that prevailed during fetal life, even when the degree of functional deficits is severe. Thus the suggestion made in Chapter 2 to the effect that adverse conditions imposed during the fetal period would be expected to cause growth retardation and functional deficiencies but not gross malformation is in general borne out.

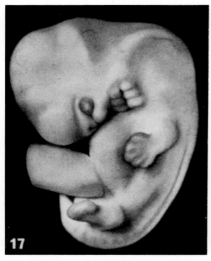 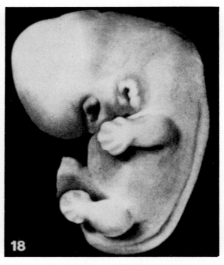

STAGE XVII   STAGE XVIII

Fig. 7-17. *40–41 days; 10–13 mm.* Upper jaw and nose forming, digital rays of hand appear, notable differentiation in diencephalon, tertiary bronchi formed, aortopulmonary septum nearing completion, cardiac semilunar valves appear, liver enlarges and shows biliary ducts, fusion of dorsal and ventral pancreas, stomach rotates, temporary occlusion in gut lumena by epithelial overgrowth, minor calyces of kidney form, chondrification of upper limb skeleton (after embryo No. 8101, Streeter, 1948).

Fig. 7-18. *42–43 days; 12–16 mm.* Facial primordia united, lids begin, auricular hillocks forming auricle, digital rays of foot appear, semicircular ducts forming, primary cardiac partitioning complete, Mullerian ducts begin, renal collecting ducts appear, active proliferation within gonads, urorectal septum complete, genital tubercle prominent, muscles identifiable in arm (after embryo No. 7707, Streeter, 1948).

III. Comparative Embryology

In the evaluation of potential teratogenic risks it is standard practice to apply the test substance to pregnant laboratory animals during the time of greatest susceptibility, namely, during the period of organogenesis. It is difficult to indicate precise times for the beginning and ending of organogenesis in particular species of animals, even in the more commonly used species such as the mouse, rat, and rabbit. This is due in part to the fact that different strains within these species show some differences in developmental schedule, but mainly it is because there is disagreement about the particular events that should be used to mark the beginning and ending of organogenesis.

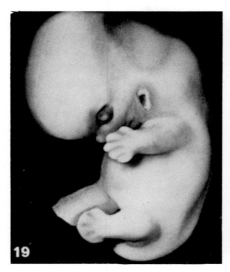

STAGE XIX · STAGE XX

FIG. 7-19. *44–45 days; 15–19 mm.* Cochlear ducts complete, tongue primordia unite, alveolar and dental laminae separate, salivary ducts evaginate, sexual differentiation of gonads occurs, earliest metanephric rudiments forming, suprarenal medulla invades cortex, muscular differentiation throughout body (after embryo No. 4501, Streeter, 1951).

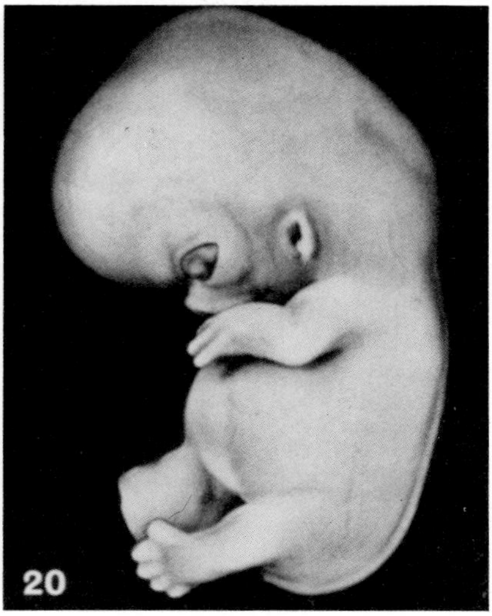

FIG. 7-20. *46–47 days; 17–22 mm.* Optic fibers reach brain, choroid plexus begins, tail regressing, palate folds present beside tongue, future ossification centers indicated by clearing of cartilage, anal membrane ruptures (after embryo No. 8157, Streeter, 1951).

Strictly speaking, organogenesis in the morphologic sense begins when the first organ rudiments are recognizable. In mammals the neural plate is the first such forerunner of true organ formation, although the cardiogenic plate is usually a very close second. These structural features are preceded by several hours to a few days by the establishment of the primitive node and streak which serve the critical functions of proliferating mesoderm, of indicating the future longitudinal axis of the embryo, and of inducing a number of important organs. Some embryologists equate the latter activities with what is called gastrulation in submammalian forms and would tend to regard these as the true beginnings of organogenesis. For the present purpose, however, the critical fact is not when recognizable organ formation begins, but when the embryo begins to show the high degree of teratogenic susceptibility typically seen during organogenesis. Information on the latter point is not precise, but experience has shown that little in the way of specific mal-

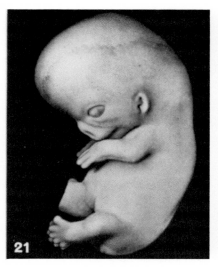

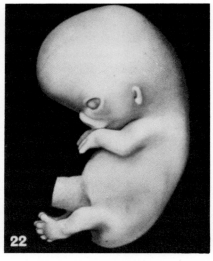

STAGE XXI

STAGE XXII

FIG. 7-21. *48–49 days; 20–24 mm.* Cornea formed, earliest nephrons unite with collecting ducts, first osteoblasts in humerus (after embryo No. 8553, Streeter, 1951).

FIG. 7-22. *50–51 days; 21–26 mm.* Calcification begins in humerus, few large glomeruli present, external genitalia undergo sexual differentiation (after embryo No. 8394, Streeter, 1951).

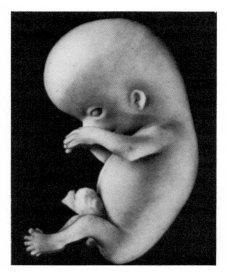

FIG. 7-23. *52–53 days; 24–30 mm.* Palatal closure begins, diaphragm forms, secretory tubules appear in kidney, ciliary body forming in eye, genital ducts undergoing sexual differentiation, midgut hernia may be withdrawn from umbilical cord, first marrow in humerus (after embryo No. 4570, Streeter, 1951).

STAGE XXIII

TABLE 7-2

Organogenesis and Related Events during Intrauterine Development of Several Mammals[a,b]

Species	Implantation begins	Primitive streak established	Organogenesis		Usual time of delivery
			Primordia beginning	Largely completed[c]	
Hamster	4.5–5	6	7	14	16–17
Mouse	4.5–5	7	7.5	16	20–21
Rat	5.5–6	8.5	9	17	21–22
Rabbit	7	6.5	7	20	30–32
Guinea pig	6	10	11	25	65–68
Pig	10–12	11	12	34	110–116
Sheep	10	13	14	35	145–152
Ferret	10–12	13	14	—[d]	40–43
Cat	12–13	—[d]	—[d]	30	60–65
Dog	13–14	13	14	30	60–65
Rhesus monkey	9	18	20	45	164–170
Baboon	9	19	22	47	172–178
Man	6.5–7	18	20	55	260–280

[a] From various sources.

[b] Timing is in estimated days after fertilization.

[c] For want of a more definite end point, closure of the palate was taken as the criterion of completed organogenesis, but it should be noted that such organs as the brain and the genitalia undergo appreciable structural change after this time.

[d] Little information available.

formations is likely to be induced by teratogenic treatment earlier than the time of appearance of the primitive streak (see Chapter 2, Section II,B). Overall embryotoxic susceptibility, particularly as manifested by malformations and embryolethality, increases rapidly after appearance of the primitive node and streak and often reaches a peak for many teratogenic agents soon after the time when organ primordia first appear. Thus, it seems appropriate to regard the appearance of the primitive node and streak as marking the beginning of organogenesis, and hence also of teratogenic susceptibility.

Table 7-2 presents data on important gestational events in several species that have been or are proposed (see Chapters 8 and 10) for use in teratologic investigations. It is obvious that the timing of particular events cannot be extrapolated from one species to another, except in a general way within closely related groups such as hamster, mouse, and rat among the rodents, or monkey, baboon, and man among the primates. The time of implantation is surprisingly variable and follows no ascending phylogenetic pattern. Some progression is seen, however, in the time of appearance of the primitive streak and in the beginning and end of organogenesis, from rodents to primates of the animals listed.

Since the order of organogenesis, that is, the sequences in which individual organs are formed, is basically similar in all mammals, some interspecies comparisons can be made on a sliding scale from the animals used in teratologic testing to man. For example, equivalent stages of mouse and human development were outlined by Otis and Brent (1954), of rat, chick, and human embryos by Monie (1965), and of mouse, rabbit, and man by Nishimura and Yamamura (1969). Several interspecies comparisons of organogenesis have also been made among mice, rats, and rabbits (Edwards, 1968; Ihara, 1970; Ogawa, 1967). Detailed comparisons of embryogenesis between animals species and between animals and man have not been made, but extensive timetables of developmental events are available for several species individually, e.g., hamster (Shenefelt, 1972), mouse (Rugh, 1968), rat (Witschi, 1962), pig (Kemp, 1962), rhesus monkey (Heuser and Streeter, 1941), baboon (Hendrickx, 1971), and man (*Biological Handbook on Growth*, 1962). An extensive bibliography on the embryology and pertinent aspects of reproduction of all animal species listed in Table 7-2 is presented in Appendix I of this book.

CHAPTER 8

THE ASSESSMENT OF TERATOLOGIC RISK

The rhetorical question, "Is a teratologic catastrophe such as was caused by thalidomide still possible?", would have to be answered in the affirmative today, 12 years after the fact. Although a recurrence today is much less likely than at the time of the original incident, the possibility may never be entirely eliminated. It must be accepted that absolute security from teratologic risk is unattainable because of the impossibility of predicting all biologic reactions to all variables and combinations of variables in the environment. Nevertheless, the probability of adverse effects on development from the environment has been lowered and there is reason for optimism that it can be further reduced. To do so, however, will require improved methodology in the two areas where teratologic risk can be best evaluated, namely, (1) early detection of unanticipated adverse effects in man, and (2) more reliable preclinical testing in animals.

I. Early Detection of Adverse Effects in Man

The statement is sometimes made that the most reliable test for teratologic risk in man is one carried out in man. This is probably true but even this, assuming widespread testing in pregnant women were practiced, would not preclude the possibility of adverse reactions. In general toxicology it is accepted that such things as unusual individual sensitivity, diseased states that reduce homeostatic functions of the liver, kidney, etc., and accidental overdosage, all can result in occasional unexpected effects, even after long use of a carefully tested agent. Thus, almost any new factor introduced into the environment is at risk sooner or later of being associated with adverse developmental effects in a small percentage of the population. If occasional adverse effects are in fact inevitable, then the unattainable goal of absolute safety should be abandoned in favor of intensified efforts toward early detection, followed by appropriate action to further reduce the demonstrated risk. Continued use of an agent found to be associated with any undesirable developmental effect would necessitate a decision as to what incidence level could be tolerated, balanced against the benefit expected from continued use. For example, should an insecticide or a herbicide that may carry a low risk of embryotoxicity for man be continued in use under controlled conditions when its use would significantly increase food production in areas of chronic food shortage?

Risk–benefit judgments are more easily discussed than acted upon because in practice they quickly involve subjective elements contingent on whose risk and whose benefit is at stake. Nevertheless, the growing complexity of man's relation to his environment will require that such judgments be made with increasing frequency. Decisions to restrict use of an agent found to cause detrimental effects raise two difficult questions: (1) Is the potential harm from continued use demonstrably greater than the anticipated benefit, and (2) can the agent be replaced by one that will yield equivalent benefit without introducing risks of its own? The latter is probably the more difficult of these questions because it implies the substitution of a new agent about which little is known under conditions of use for an older, better-known one the risks of which are to a degree already known.

A. RECOGNITION OF CAUSE-AND-EFFECT RELATIONSHIPS

When a change is introduced into the environment, whether a new drug, pesticide, radiation source, ultrasound, chemical pollutant, or a previously existing factor at an increased dosage level, how may adverse effects on development be associated with the cause? In mutagenesis this problem is frustrating in the extreme. In teratogenesis it is relatively less difficult because the clues needed to make the association may appear fairly promptly, e.g., (1) a catastrophe with obvious clustering of cases in space and time (as with rubella and thalidomide), (2) a gradual accumulation of spontaneously reported cases (as with androgenic hormones or folic acid antagonists), (3) the findings of an epidemiologic survey (no good examples to date), or (4) close surveillance of a population known to have been exposed (as with atomic radiations in Japan). Thus, assuming that sufficient numbers of adverse reactions were available to attract attention or to be revealed by statistical methods, the four criteria by which these reactions could be associated with their common cause are listed in Table 3-4.

The validity of these criteria was borne out in 1941 when within a few months the rubella virus was shown to be associated with a high incidence of congenital cataracts, deafness, and cardiovascular defects in Australia (Gregg, 1941). Again in 1961, within 2 years after its introduction and widespread use, thalidomide was associated with an abrupt increase in the incidence of previously rare forms of phocomelia and other limb defects in Germany (Lenz, 1961) and Australia (McBride, 1961). A somewhat longer time elapsed, approximately 1953 to 1960, before a connection was established in Japan between the ingestion by pregnant women of fish with high content of organic mercury and the birth of children with severe neurologic defects resembling cerebral palsy (Harada, 1968). The longer time needed to make the association between cause and effect in congenital mercury poisoning (Minamata disease) was in part owing to the smaller number of cases, 20 to 30 as compared with thousands in the rubella and the thalidomide episodes.

Is There Always Clustering of Characteristic Defects? The foregoing indicates that rapid association between teratologic cause and effect in man appears to depend on two conditions, namely, an appreciable number of cases clustered at one time and place, and an unusual if not unique defect or association of defects. These have not often been met, which suggests that some agents that are teratogenic in man are not always overtly so. Alternatively, other agents may have a low teratogenic potential that is only sporadically expressed or may not always produce a well-defined syndrome or recurring pattern of defect (see Chapter 3, Section II, F). In experimental teratology it is accepted that many agents produce characteristic patterns of defects, but these relatively uniform results are usually obtained with large doses given at known susceptible periods. Even under controlled experimental conditions, however, variability and overlap occur from pattern to pattern as regards individual malformations. For example, commonly occurring defects such as anophthalmia, hydrocephaly, or cleft palate may occur as components in the patterns of defects produced by a number of teratogenic agents, although the separate patterns usually can be distinguished by overall qualitative as well as quantitative differences. In fact, syndromes as sharply circumscribed as that caused by thalidomide in man are by no means regularly encountered in experimental teratology. The malformations produced by riboflavin deficiency in rats (Warkany and Schraffenberger, 1944) and acetazolamide in rats, mice, and hamsters (Layton and Hallsey, 1965; Wilson *et al.,* 1968) are among the more striking examples of circumscribed syndromes in animals. Thus it is likely that truly unique or highly characteristic syndromes are not always induced by environmental teratogens, either in the laboratory or in man. At least it would seem unwise to depend upon "sentinel" defects as an unfailing criterion in the recognition of induced teratogenesis. This tends to limit the quick recognition of adverse effects to a few special situations and requires that in human teratology more reliance be placed on such ancillary methods as the accumulation and evaluation of case reports, epidemiologic surveys, and close surveillance of high-exposure populations.

1. *Accumulation and Evaluation of Spontaneously Reported Cases*

a. *Adverse Effect of Drugs.* The spontaneous reporting of adverse effects of drugs, whether during pregnancy or otherwise, has been so incomplete and otherwise inadequate that the World Health Organization in 1968 convened a meeting for the express purpose of discussing means of improving this important aspect of safety evaluation (WHO Tech. Rep. No. 425). It was recognized that the quality of clinical observations, particularly those outside hospitals, is reduced by heavy work loads on individual physicians and by limited diagnostic facilities. The absence of immediate benefit to the physician together with a lack of feeling of responsibility to report were cited as reasons for widespread underreporting of adverse effects. The need for uniform and comprehensive monitoring of all adverse reactions to drugs with quick reporting to a central agency was stressed. It was recommended that such monitoring be hospital based, with qualified personnel assigned the responsibilities of diagnosis, documentation, and reporting. In subsequent meetings (National Academy of Sciences, 1971; World Health Organization Tech. Rep. No. 498, 1972) emphasis was placed on the formation of national centers for the collection and dissemination of information on all adverse reactions to drugs. The setting-up of such national centers, however, may be premature until some of the numerous problems of data collection and interpretation have been resolved in the smaller scale models that are now developing in some regional centers, some limited to inpatient (Jick *et al.*, 1970) and others on a broader base of inpatient and outpatient reporting (Friedman, 1972).

b. *Need for Better Reporting of All Adverse Effects on Development.* To date attention has been focused mainly on adverse reactions to drugs generally, but it is increasingly urgent that whatever monitoring programs are instituted will also include adverse reactions to other environmental agents (e.g., pesticides, industrial solvents, radiations, etc.). Particularly critical is the need for better reporting of developmental defects, as seen both at birth and in follow-up medical examinations in relation to drug treatment during pregnancy. Promising beginnings toward uniform hospital reporting of developmental defects have been made in Scandanavia (Källén and Winberg, 1968; Klemetti and Saxén, 1970) and in the United Kingdom (Stevenson, 1969). Hospital reporting combined with frequent analysis of results is being undertaken by the agencies participating in the

Metropolitan Atlanta Congenital Malformations Program (Flynt *et al.,* 1971), which issues a bimonthly compilation of defects diagnosed at birth in a number of associated hospitals. The latter program has already expanded beyond Atlanta to include Los Angeles and the Jacksonville area of northeast Florida, with 44 hospitals reporting 63,409 births during 1971 (several hospitals entered the program during the year). The express purpose is "to monitor the occurrence of malformations in a defined geographical area and to maintain a case registry for epidemiologic and genetic studies." With appropriate coordination to insure uniformity in diagnostic procedures, history-taking, and record-keeping, and with suitable data retrieval methods, this could become an extremely useful source of information.

A uniform interpretation of structural malformations, not to mention functional and biochemical defects of developmental origin, is an ever-present problem in monitoring birth defects. This problem, however, is amenable to solution through the preparation of suitable handbooks and glossaries, combined with periodic indoctrination conferences attended by responsible personnel in the regional hospitals. Follow-up studies 2 to 5 years after birth would be required to evaluate functional defects such as mental deficiency and inborn metabolic diseases, as well as structural abnormalities that become manifest only after the neonatal period, e.g., several gastrointestinal, cardiovascular, and genitourinary malformations. Follow-up studies on all births in a geographic area would be cumbersome and impracticable, but surveillance of randomized samples from the original population at suitable intervals could provide a valuable estimate of the totality of developmental abnormality. Realistic monitoring for increased mutation rates would involve many difficulties and considerable cost but the technical means to do so are probably now available (Neel, 1971). Such data are essential if the true impact of the rapidly changing environment on human development, including the genome, is to be evaluated.

c. *Case Reports in the Medical Literature.* Until systematized reporting of developmental defects is more effectively in operation, spontaneous reporting of one or a few cases at a time in the medical literature cannot be ignored. The inadequacy of the data obtained from such reports is well known to anyone who has attempted a literature survey in search of the causes of maldevelopment in man (see Chapter 3, Section II), but frustrating and cumbersome as this source may be, it has yielded useful information. It can provide suggestive evidence to serve as a stimulus to undertake both organized surveys in human populations as well as controlled animal studies directed at providing confirmation or elucidating mechanisms. Furthermore, it should not be overlooked that x-irradiation, androgenic hormones, and folic acid antagonists were gradually accepted as human teratogenic agents as a result of accumulated case reports in the medical literature. The greatest shortcoming of spontaneous reporting of cases is failure to report, and despite the lack of necessary facts to establish cause-and-effect relationships, medical journals should encourage the publication of case reports whenever reasonable presumption of causality can be shown between an environmental event during pregnancy and an adverse effect on development.

2. *Organized Epidemiologic Surveys*

These are of two principal types, prospective and retrospective. The former begins with a predefined population, for example, all diagnosed pregnancies within a given locality and time, and proceeds to record events thought to be pertinent to development, such as maternal medication, infection, trauma, etc., prior to delivery. After delivery the condition of the infants is correlated with information in the previously collected histories, or alternatively, infants from pregnancies known to have shared a common event, e.g., the taking of a particular drug, are closely scrutinized for similarities or for differences from the remainder of the survey population. Prospective studies to make meaningful correlations are dependent on the right observations being made during or soon after pregnancy. At best the chances of finding positive correlations are small because they are diluted within a largely negative sample, i.e., a high proportion of the pregnancies in any predefined sample will usually terminate normally.

The retrospective survey begins with a group of infants or children that exhibit a particular characteristic, such as being developmentally defective in a general or a specific way. Available records on the pregnancies producing the defective subjects are then examined in search of common events in the histories of similarly affected individuals. Even with very careful control and assuming that complete and accurate records are available, retrospective studies tend to have inherent biases that favor positive correlations and overlook negative ones. For example, they emphasize the instances in which the criterion defect is associated with a presumed causative factor, without ascertaining all of the instances in which the factor was present without being associated with the defect. To date neither retrospective (Nelson and Forfar, 1971; Richards, 1969) nor prospective surveys (Berendes and Weiss, 1970; Mellin, 1963, 1964) have clearly identified new human teratogenic agents. Furthermore, in one study in which the same group of pregnancies was subjected to both prospective and retrospective analyses, there was poor agreement as regards the association of the birth of dead or malformed infants with events during the pregnancies, owing largely to the unreliable memory of the mothers in the retrospective part of the survey (Klemetti and Saxén, 1967).

Difficulties in Recognizing Multiple Causation. The fact that epidemiologic surveys have generally failed to uncover new environmental causes of human maldevelopment is in itself significant. Emphasis in these surveys has often been focused on the identification of single causative factors, with less attention to the possibility of multiple causation or interacting factors, either multiple environmental agents or these interacting with genetic predispositions. The subject of interaction among two or more causative agents in teratogenesis was discussed in Chapter 3, Sections I, J and II, but in the present connection it is important to recall that although the phenomenon is well established in laboratory animals, well-documented examples in man are not known. To begin with a human developmental defect of unknown causation and work backward attempting to identify multiple causes from among the plethora of possibilities becomes a problem of considerable magnitude. With modern computer technology the necessary multifactorial analyses are possible (Fraser and Burnell, 1970; Smith, 1972), but great difficulty still exists in anticipating which data to collect and in deciding which to include in the analysis.

3. *Surveillance of High-Exposure Populations*

Some segments of human populations are exposed to higher doses of certain conditions that might be regarded as potentially harmful than is the population at large. When such conditions are recognized, particular effort should be made to examine the outcome of pregnancies in women known to have been so exposed. Much has been learned about the effects of high-energy radiations on human intrauterine development by intensive study of children born to women exposed during pregnancy to the atomic bomb explosions at Hiroshima and Nagasaki during World War II. The same can be said as regards the effects of extreme nutritional deprivation during pregnancy in the famine areas of Russia and the Low Countries during World War II. Although recent environmental changes may not have been as acutely stressful as those mentioned, it is likely that isolated situations could be found in which air or water pollution or industrial exposure to chemicals and certain radiations have approached potentially dangerous levels for human germ cells and embryos.

a. *Industrial Workers.* People who are routinely exposed by inhalation or direct contact to high concentrations of various chemical substances, and agricultural workers whose jobs entail intensive or long continued exposure to pesticides, are regarded as potential sources of information about general toxicologic effects of such substances. As women increasingly accept employment in industry, particular effort should be made, when pregnancy is diagnosed during such employment, to document exposure to chemicals and other agents that might have an adverse effect on intrauterine development. At present, however, there is little evidence that the course of human pregnancy has been influenced by industrial chemicals (Kučera, 1968). No acceptable data on human embryotoxicity following exposure to agricultural, household, or other use of pesticides is known (Khera and Clegg, 1969; Report of the 2,4,5-T Advisory Committee, 1971), but the nature of these compounds suggests that their continued use should be accompanied by careful surveillance of pregnancy outcome.

b. *Controlled Clinical Trial in Surgical Abortion.* The present system of testing new drugs under controlled conditions in selected human subjects, after completion of animal toxicity studies and before final marketing, has undoubtedly proved valuable as a means of reducing later untoward reactions in the general population. For drugs that are needed for use during the reproductive span of women, however, this method is not available because there is understandable reluctance to perform clinical trials in pregnant women, especially during early gestation when the human embryo is most sensitive to extrinsic teratogenic influences. Even if such tests were condoned during human pregnancy, they would lose much of their usefulness in ascertaining embryotoxic risk unless directed specifically at the embryo's most susceptible period, between the twentieth and thirtieth days postconception. Most physicians would not consent to conduct trials at this time except in the event that the pregnancy were already scheduled for surgical abortion, and some would also find this objectionable.

The use of therapeutic or volitional abortions for the purpose of testing the embryotoxic effects of drugs is said to have been explored in some parts of Europe and Asia, but only hearsay reports of the results are available at this writing. It is doubtful, however, that this type of clinical trial will be highly effective in screening for adverse effects on development, mainly because the situation itself imposes sharp limitations as to when and how such tests can be done. It is unlikely that recognizable effects could develop in the time elapsing between treatment and the early termination of pregnancy, which is in the best interest of the woman. Assuming that pregnancy is diagnosed within 4 weeks after conception, an infrequent occurrence under present circumstances, the decision to perform abortion and the making of necessary arrangements to carry out a controlled clinical test of a new drug would probably require an additional week or two. At best the embryo would be 30 to 40 days of gestational age before the test substance would be administered and, therefore, would have passed the period of greatest susceptibility. An even larger problem would then concern how soon to terminate pregnancy after the administration of the drug. The welfare of the pregnant woman would be best served by performing the abortion at an early date, but the likelihood of recognizing developmental deviation in the embryo would be enhanced by allowing intrauterine development to continue as long as possible after treatment. Aside from the ethical issues involved, legal considerations would prevent delaying induced abortion beyond the viable age of the fetus, i.e., 20 to 22 weeks of gestation. These circumstances now seem to mediate against meaningful use of induced abortions for the evaluation of teratologic risk of drugs. Nevertheless, human abortion material has been used to obtain valuable data on the transfer of drugs and vaccines from mother to fetus late in the first trimester (Bolognese *et al.*, 1972; Idämpään *et al.*, 1971; Wasz-Höchert *et al.*, 1970) and the possible use of such material for the evaluation of adverse drug effects on human intrauterine development is deserving of further consideration.

4. *Other Alternatives*

a. *Early Warning System.* Existing methods for anticipating teratologic risks in man are admittedly not satisfactory; but until more dependable ones are in the offing, the best alternative seems to be improvement in the reliability of present methods. There is no clear consensus as to how best to accomplish this, but it has been suggested (Brent, 1971b, 1972a; Ingalls and Klingberg, 1965) that strict clinical surveillance programs could be devised that would be capable of alerting regulatory agencies to adverse effects of drugs after only a very few cases were observed. In fact there is now in operation in Sweden a national registry, based on monthly reporting to a central agency, which is said to be sufficiently "sensitive" that had it been in operation in 1960 it would have detected thalidomide as teratogenic after the birth of only 7 affected infants (Källén and Winberg, 1968). In any event, the greatest need seems to be for prompt and accurate reporting to a central agency of all instances of developmental deviation that are, or are reasonably suspected of being, associated with an environmental factor such as the introduction of a new drug.

The inadequacy of voluntary reporting of adverse effects has recently been re-emphasized (Miller and Shapiro, 1972). Even a comprehensive system of hospital-based reporting, mentioned earlier in this chapter (Section I,A,1), to be fully effective would require mandatory reporting to a central agency of all developmental defects, whether diagnosed at birth or subsequently. Although compulstory reporting would be objectionable to some on ideological grounds, systems of this type are already in operation in Scandanavia (Klemetti and Saxén, 1970). The greater security achieved by mandatory reporting of all developmentally related defects would surely justify the expense and effort entailed. Thus, a truly effective early warning system would seem to require not merely governmental sanction but specific provisions under law for (1) mandatory reporting by hospitals or physicians of developmental defects and relevant history as soon as diagnosis is made to a central agency, and (2) establishment of agencies qualified to receive, evaluate, and act upon such reports as give significant indication of environmental causation.

Other approaches to monitoring for environmental effects on development and the germ cells have been the subjects of recent symposia (Hook *et al.,* 1971; Sutton and Harris, 1972) and of numerous publications emphasizing various aspects such as epidemiologic associations of defects (R. W. Miller, 1969), the use of vital statistics registries (J. R. Miller, 1969), and the prognostic meaning of major (Fraser, 1971) and minor (Smith, 1971) malformations. All considered, however, it is apparent that the foremost need is for comprehensive reporting, after which the sequential functions of collating, interpreting, and taking appropriate action regarding the accumulated data would be more meaningful than under the present haphazard arrangement.

b. *Continued Reliance on Animal Tests.* Although more effective methods for the early detection of adverse effects on development in man will doubtless be devised, there must be continued reliance on animal tests. Animals must be used for the initial screening for undesirable effects of all new environmental agents, and their use in preclinical testing of new drugs to minimize exposure of pregnant women to embryotoxic doses should be further refined. Methods for accomplishing the latter will be discussed in detail in Chapters 9 and 10. Nonhuman primates may be put to a further use that is appropriate to the foregoing discussion on surveillance in man. After new drugs, pesticides, etc., have been approved for regulated distribution and use by the public, there are likely to be sporadic claims of adverse effects. These cannot be ignored, but neither should they be the basis of ill-considered restrictive action on the part of regulatory agencies. Claims of unsuspected adverse effects are disquieting, but the often poorly substantiated nature of the claims, together with the benefits expected from continued use of the agent, should mollify too-hasty withdrawal of approval for use. Intensive studies in pregnant nonhuman primates given high doses of the substance in question may provide scientific data of value in resolving the issue of permitting continued human exposure during pregnancy. Such chemical agents as lysergic acid diethylamide, cyclamate, 2,4,5-T, some anticonvulsants, and a variety of antineoplastic drugs have been studied in this way in the author's laboratory, as noted elsewhere (Tables 3-5, 3-6; and Wilson, 1972b). Although this method has not been exhaustively applied, preliminary indications are that intensive spot-checking in pregnant primates has significant potential for the evaluation of sporadic claims of adverse effects on human development.

II. Evaluation of Human Teratologic Risk in Animals

It is now accepted that no animal test or battery of tests will provide complete assurance in the prediction of human teratologic risk. The best that can be achieved with animal tests is a statement that, under stipulated conditions of exposure, the probability of untoward effects in human populations will be low. Since the thalidomide incident progress has been made in devising test procedures that identify some potentially embryotoxic substances, but presently used procedures still do not provide all of the predictive value that is possible in view of present knowledge. Over the past 10 years a great many refinements of concept and procedure have been proposed by numerous investigators (Brent, 1964b; Cahen, 1964; Clegg, 1971; Dyban *et al.*, 1970; Fave, 1971; Ferm, 1965; Fraser, 1963; Frohberg and Oettel, 1966; Gibson *et al.*, 1966; Gottschewski, 1965, 1971; Nomura, 1969; Palmer, 1969a; Robson, 1970; Tuchmann-Duplessis, 1972; Zimmerman, 1964), and the World Health Organization has convened a Scientific Group to discuss methods for testing of drugs for teratogenicity (WHO Tech. Rep. No. 364, 1967). It is impractical to review these various sources, but information gleaned from them, together with the author's personal experience, form the basis of the following discussion. The remainder of this chapter is devoted to general considerations that should be taken into account when planning animal tests. Detailed discussions of protocol design and interpretation of results will be given in Chapters 9 and 10.

A. Dosage

1. *Route of Treatment*

The accepted practice of administering test substances to animals by the same route that will be used clinically is sound in most situations relating to teratologic testing. Problems may arise when the clinical route is to be percutaneous application (on the skin) because of the likelihood that animals will lick or scratch the site, rub it on the cage or on bedding materials, or otherwise alter the dosage or its rate of absorption. If the treatment area cannot be suitably protected, another route which produces similar blood levels should be sought. When the oral route is to be used, administration by stomach tube (gavage) or capsule is preferable to incorporating the dosage in the diet. By the latter route the amount of the test material actually consumed can only be estimated because of food wastage and possible chemical change owing to exposure to air, light, and other dietary ingredients. The possibility also exists that the taste or odor of the test material or its effect on appetite may alter the normal rate of food intake. Pair feeding of controls will equalize the problem of lowered food consumption but does not ensure intake of the desired dosage.

Subcutaneous treatment is advantageous if relatively slow absorption is desired in order to achieve prolonged, moderately constant plasma levels, but it entails the possibility of leakage unless the dosage is delivered with a long needle and small volumes are used. Intramuscular injection provides a moderate rate of absorption, but this varies somewhat with the physical state of the agent and the type of vehicle used. Intraperitoneal injection assures rapid absorption of most substances in quite large volumes, but acute discomfort and possibly peritonitis in the test animals may occur if care is not taken to avoid introducing irritating materials. There is always a chance that some or all of the dose introduced by this route may be unknowingly injected into the digestive tract. It must not be assumed that all materials administered by the intraperitoneal route immediately pass through the liver via the portal circulation. To be sure, absorption occurs mainly through the visceral peritoneum of digestive organs, blood from which passes immediately to the liver, but to a lesser extent it also occurs through the parietal peritoneum, the serosal surfaces of the urogenital organs, and certain areas of mesentery and other ligaments which are not drained by portal tributaries into the liver.

Highest plasma concentrations per unit of dosage are obtained immediately following intravenous injection. To maintain a moderately constant level of concentration, however, it is necessary to resort to repeated injection at frequent intervals or to continuous intravenous infusion. Large volumes, solutions with high acidic or basic reactions, or agents that might be thrombogenic should not be introduced by the intravenous route.

If more than one route is to be used clinically, the same ones should be used in testing unless it is known that the alternate routes produce comparable blood levels. The testing of food additives (preservatives, colorants, etc.) and contaminants (processing chemicals, pesticide residues, etc.) for teratogenicity must be done at a much higher level than the hopefully low dosage found in the marketed product. In these cases incorporation into the diet may reduce palatability and thereby limit food and dosage intake. It has been emphasized earlier that teratogenicity is an acute phenomenon; therefore, the justification for testing food additives and contaminants, which usually occur only in small amounts in food, is in anticipation of the possibility of accidental overdosage, or of overconsumption as in dietary idiosyncrasies.

2. Duration of Treatment

This is a subject about which there is diversity of opinion in teratogenicity testing. The earlier practice of treatment throughout gestation has now been largely abandoned in recognition of the fact that mammalian embryos are much more likely to show a teratologic response during the period of organogenesis than at earlier or later times. Accordingly, most protocols in use today specify treatment throughout the span of organogenesis (see Table 7-2) of the species used. This has the advantage that treatment covers the early formative stages of all organs, the time of maximal sensitivity for most organs, whether they develop early or late in the overall span of organogenesis. It also affords the convenience of an uncomplicated procedure. Nevertheless, continuous dosage throughout organogenesis may produce misleading results, a possibility less likely if the duration of treatment in at least some test animals is limited to no more than 3 or 4 days.

a. *Changing Plasma Concentrations versus Changing Embryonic Sensitivities.* The main objection to treatment throughout organogenesis is that it may activate maternal adaptative mechanisms or produce pathology, which could alter maternal plasma concentration, and hence cause fluctuations in embryo dosage during a test period. It is well known from experimental teratology that embryotoxic susceptibility normally varies during organogenesis (see Chapter 2, Section II), initially being low, then rising steeply to a peak, after which it declines slowly. Treatment started at the beginning of organogenesis and continued for several days allows ample time for maternal adaptative reactions such as the induction of catabolizing enzymes in the liver (Burns, 1970) to come into play, thereby possibly reducing plasma concentration before the peak of embryonic sensitivity is reached. For example, a number of teratogens are known to produce little or no embryotoxic effect when administered as a single dose on day 6 of rat gestation (Table 8-1), the time most often used for the first of ten daily treatments in tests employing this species, although the same agents may be highly teratogenic a few days later. If the compound being tested happens to be one that induces enzymes that speeds or slows the rate of its own metabolism (Table 8-2), plasma levels could be appreciably changed by 3 or 4 days of repeated daily dosage (Conney and Burns, 1972). In this way, the high teratogenic response that would be expected from a single treatment on days 9 or 10 of gestation could be significantly reduced below that shown in Table 8-1 by

TABLE 8-1

SOME RAT TERATOGENS THAT HAVE LITTLE EMBRYOTOXIC EFFECT ON THE SIXTH DAY OF GESTATION BUT ARE HIGHLY EFFECTIVE 3 OR 4 DAYS LATER

| | Treatment | | | 20-day fetuses | |
Agent	Dose (mg/kg)	Day	Total implants	% dead, resorbed	% survivors malformed
5-Fluorodeoxy-	20	6	114	6	1
uridine		9	209	10	38
Retinoic acid	20	6	95	5	0
		9	79	44	84
Actinomycin D	0.3	6	207	7	5
		10	88	48	65
Controls	(vehicle)		558	7	1

TABLE 8-2

Some Chemical Agents Known to Influence Rates of Metabolic Degradation of Themselves and/or Other Compounds after Repeated Dosage[a]

Increase metabolic degradation	Decrease metabolic degradation
Barbiturates	SKF 525-A
Thyroxine	Chlorthione
Some insecticides (DDT, chlordane, aldrin, dieldrin, heptachlor)	Iproniazid
	Metopirone
Some tranquilizers and antipsychotics (meprobamate, Librium, chlorpromazine)	Actinomycin D
	Puromycin
Some antihistamines (chlorcyclizine, diphenhydramine)	CCl_4
	Triparanol
Several hypoglycemic agents	Chloramphenicol
3,4-Benzpyrene	Any that competitively inhibit catabolic enzymes
3-Methylcholanthrene	
Steroid hormones	

[a] From various sources.

an enzyme inducing agent. Conversely, if the compound were one that slowed its own metabolism (Table 8-2), an exaggerated effect might be expected after repeated treatment. In either case maternal plasma level, and secondarily, embryo dose as well, would change during the course of protracted maternal treatment.

b. *Early Embryolethality May Mask Later Teratogenicity.* Embryos in early stages of organogenesis have sometimes been observed to be more subject to embryolethal than to teratogenic effects (Wilson, 1966). This was pointedly illustrated in recent rat experiments in which a single dose of cytosine arabinoside at 20 mg/kg of maternal weight on day 9 was sufficient to kill most of the embryos (unpublished data), whereas a single injection of this compound on day 12 at 100 mg/kg was found to cause 67% malformations but no increase in lethality above control level (Ritter *et al.,* 1971). Thus, continuous treatment with 20 mg/kg or more begun early in organogenesis would have led to the conclusion that this drug was only embryolethal, perhaps causing the high teratogenicity of treatment initiated at a later age to be overlooked. Continuous dosage at a level sufficiently low to have permitted survival to the teratogenically susceptible period on day 12 would have been too small to induce teratogenesis in the usual 6–15-day treatment protocol. Of related interest is the fact that some teratogens have been rendered less active by pretreatment of pregnant animals with related compounds that themselves were not, or were only slightly, teratogenic (Beaudoin, 1962; Posner *et al.,* 1967; Steffek *et al.,* 1968). Some of these instances are doubtless explainable in terms of enzyme induction, others possibly relate to saturation of reaction sites.

c. *Single Doses May Be More Effective than Multiple Doses.* Experimental demonstration of the way repeated treatment with a chemical agent may produce different embryotoxic results than a single treatment with the same compound was made by Robens (1969) using a number of pesticides. Groups of pregnant hamsters were treated on days 6 through 10 with the test compounds, while other groups were treated with smaller total amounts of the same compounds as a single dose on gestation day 7 or 8. Multiple treatments caused few developmental defects even at high doses but did cause some resorption and maternal death. The single treatments produced numerous defects in liveborn young. A similar phenomenon was observed by King *et al.* (1965), who gave chlorcyclizine to pregnant rats at 50 mg/kg/day from days 10 to 15 of gestation and produced a high incidence of cleft palate, but when other rats were given the same daily dosage from days 1 through 15 of gestation, malformations were greatly reduced. Again the probable explanation is that repeated treatments induced metabolizing enzymes which were able to lower maternal plasma levels of the test substance before the embryo's most sensitive period was reached. The foregoing experiments clearly show that teratogenicity could be missed when a potentially teratogenic compound is given in multiple doses.

d. *Repeated Doses May Cause Misleading Results in Several Ways.* The several ways in which long-duration dosage with drugs or other chemical agents may interfere with teratogenicity testing are summarized in Table 8-3. That implantation can be prevented by prior drug treatment has been shown or presumed to occur in a number of instances (Lucey and Behrman, 1963; Wilson, 1970). Thus a treatment regimen begun at a time prior to or coinciding with implantation (day 6 in rat, day 7 in rabbit) could preclude the birth of offspring, thereby obscuring teratogenicity, although the same or a lower dosage might be teratogenic if treatment were begun at later times. Even if implantation were not prevented, continuous treatment early in organogenesis could still obscure the teratogenic potential of a substance by causing early embryonic death. For example, irradiation of rat embryos with 100 R on day 8 of gestation caused moderate embryolethality and some growth retardation but no malformation, whereas the same dose on day 9 or 10 caused high rates of malformation (Wilson, 1954a). Furthermore, repeated doses are known to cause a broader spectrum of malformations than short-term treatments (see Chapter 2, Section II). The presence of many malformations in the embryo would probably favor intrauterine death, whereas the more discrete pattern of defects expected from short-term dosage would more likely permit survival to term.

TABLE 8-3

Ways in Which Repeated Treatment Prior to the Peak Susceptible Period of the Embryo May Produce Misleading Results[a]

Time of treatment	Primary effect	Secondary effect capable of altering test results
1. Before implantation	Interference with implantation	No issue
2. Early organogenesis	Early embryonic death	No issue
3. Before peak susceptibility	Induction of catabolizing enzymes	Reduced blood level during susceptible period
4. Before peak susceptibility	Inhibition of catabolizing enzymes	Increased blood level during susceptible period
5. Before peak susceptibility	Liver pathology or reduced function	Increased blood level during susceptible period
6. Before peak susceptibility	Kidney pathology or reduced function[b]	Increased blood level during susceptible period
7. Before peak susceptibility	Saturation of protein-binding sites[b]	Increased blood level during susceptible period

[a] See text for explanation.

[b] These effects have not been demonstrated in experimental teratology but their existence in other toxicologic situations makes likely their applicability to teratology.

Repeated treatments can produce aberrant results in teratogenicity testing in yet other ways (Table 8-3). Cumulative pathology in maternal rat liver was produced by repeated minute doses of actinomycin D given before organogenesis (Wilson, 1966); but this was sufficient to cause a four- to five-fold increase in the teratogenicity of a dose of this drug that was shown to be only mildly teratogenic when given to nonpretreated controls on day 9 of gestation. It was assumed that the liver damage induced by chronic treatment reduced the capacity of this organ to detoxify actinomycin D, thus causing a mildly teratogenic dose to produce a maternal blood level equivalent to that produced by a much larger dose. Similarly, pathology or reduced function of maternal kidneys might lead to slowed excretion and higher plasma concentration of a potentially teratogenic agent, such as might result from prior or concurrent treatment with a renotoxic agent or one that interferes with renal tubular secretion, e.g., probenecid. Experimental demonstration of an augmented teratogenic effect after reduced renal function, however, is not known to the author. Another theoretical possibility is that repeated dosage with a teratogenic chemical that is ordinarily bound by plasma proteins could saturate all available protein sites, thus eliminating the protection usually afforded by having part of each dose inactivated by protein binding. In either of these hypothetical situations a single or a few doses would be less likely to negate the normal homeostatic mechanism than would repeated treatments preceding susceptible periods in embryogenesis.

Thus, accumulating experimental evidence, as well as certain theoretical possibilities, indicates that long-continued dosage in teratologic testing can produce different results than a single or a few treatments at specific periods in organogenesis. In simplest terms chronic treatment may cause misleading results in three basically different ways: (1) by preventing implantation or causing early embryonic death, thereby precluding a teratogenic response, although both failed implantation and embryonic death should themselves be regarded as embryotoxic effects; (2) by inducing catabolizing enzymes that speed the degradation of the test substance, thereby reducing maternal blood levels; or (3) by inhibiting catabolizing enzymes, damaging liver tissue, reducing kidney function, or saturating protein-binding sites, all of which might tend to increase maternal blood levels (Table 8-3).

e. *These Potential Sources of Error Can Be Avoided.* The obvious alternative to treatment throughout organogenesis is treatment of different groups of animals for shorter periods that consecutively cover the span of organogenesis. Treatment of groups of animals on each single day of organogenesis is both impractical and unnecessary. A reasonable compromise is to divide the period of organogenesis of the test species into several 3- or 4-day time spans, with separate groups of animals tested at each of these shorter spans. For example, in an animal like the rat in which major organogenesis covers gestation days 8 or 9 through 16 or 17, the initial test could be conveniently carried out in three groups of pregnant animals, each treated for different 3-day spans for each dosage level tested. The use of three instead of the customary one treatment group at each dosage level would require more animals, but the additional cost would be more than balanced by the assurance that a period of special embryonic sensitivity had not been masked by changing maternal plasma levels, or one of the other possibilities mentioned above. When using a test animal with a long period of organogenesis, such as pig or rhesus monkey, a 4-day time span would probably accomplish the same purpose without significant loss of accuracy (see Chapter 10 for suggested protocols).

These shorter treatment spans undoubtedly provide more precise information about acute embryotoxic sensitivity than do longer spans. They do not, however, avert the possibility that longer treatment may itself lead to maternal toxicity in the form of cumulative effects, e.g., slowly developing pathology in liver or kidney, that could lead to increased plasma concentrations after a longer duration of treatment. To rule out this possibility, the highest dose that causes no embryotoxicity during the short-term treatment should be tested continuously throughout the period of organogenesis in one group of test animals. By thus using both short-term and long-term treatment groups, the predictive value of teratogenicity tests could be appreciably increased.

3. *Level of Dosage*

A teratogenicity test should not be regarded as complete until a dose is found that produces some embryotoxicity, that is, intrauterine death, teratogenicity, or growth retardation. Scientists conducting tests in the pharmaceutical and chemical industries may be reluctant to raise dosage to a level that produces unmistakable embryotoxicity because of concern that demonstrating an adverse effect with a newly developed compound will prejudice chances of approval by regulatory agencies. If this is the case, it is unfortunate because there is no scientific basis for assuming that any compound shown to be embryotoxic does not also have a no-effect range of dosage—in other words, a threshold below which safe tolerance levels could be set.

a. *The Threshold for Embryotoxic Effects.* As emphasized in Chapter 2, Section VI, there is ample experimental support for the belief that all teratogenic and embryolethal substances can be shown to have a threshold below which adverse effects are not found. Conversely, most if not all drugs and chemicals can be shown to produce some type of embryotoxicity if applied in sufficient dosage during an appropriate time in embryogenesis in one or more species of animal (Karnofsky, 1965b). The establishment of an embryotoxic level of dosage is important because this is the logical starting point from which to extrapolate downward in setting a safe tolerance level for chemicals and drugs that may be taken by or brought in contact with pregnant women. Technically the threshold of embryotoxicity could be defined as either the highest no-effect or the lowest effect level, but absolute precision in this regard is probably not necessary. A reasonable approximation would usually be sufficient in practice because the acceptable tolerance level for most substances would be set at a small fraction of a known effect level. In any event, if teratogenicity testing is to be put on a rational basis, the concepts of threshold and of safe tolerance levels below that level must be accepted.

Pregnancy involves two types of organisms, the maternal and the embryonic or fetal, and they often show wide divergence in the dosage required to produce toxic effects. This was illustrated in Table 2-4, in which a maternal effect as represented by LD_{50}, and an embryonic effect as represented by a typical embryotoxic dose, varied greatly for different types of compounds given to pregnant rats. Even though crude, such data demonstrate that maternal sensitivity is usually less than embryonic sensitivity, the only exceptions being two antibiotics in which maternal and embryonic sensitivities were approximately equal. Comparable data do not exist for man but the practical implication in teratogenicity testing of drugs is clear. When the therapeutic dose approaches the embryotoxic level, the benefit factor in the benefit versus risk ratio must be high, e.g., a drug that is health preserving if not life saving.

Although experience has shown that drugs generally are not embryotoxic at maternal therapeutic levels, the policy of drug abstinence during pregnancy except in cases of urgent need is still a prudent one. The unpredictable nature of pregnancy, however, makes it mandatory that any new drug likely to be used by a woman during any part of her reproductive span be rigorously tested for teratogenic potential. The dosage levels for such testing should begin at or above the highest anticipated therapeutic level and go upward until the threshold of embryotoxicity in appropriate test animals is found. As suggested above the establishment of a safe or, in some cases, an acceptable tolerance level below the threshold will vary with the therapeutic importance of the drug. Thus, as far as is consistent with the urgency for using the drug, the highest therapeutic level should be as far below the demonstrated embryotoxic threshold in test animals as possible to provide a maximal margin of safety against (1) species differences in sensitivity between the test animal and man, (2) occasional unusual sensitivity in man, and (3) overdosage.

b. *Safe Tolerance Levels.* A safe tolerance level is an empirically derived dosage set somewhere below the threshold level, depending on the nature of the compound and the purpose for which it will be used. It will vary greatly for different categories of chemicals such as drugs, pesticides, and food additives, and will vary within those groups according to the type of benefit expected from their use. Since drugs are often used at relatively high dosage to achieve the desired therapeutic effect, the ratio between threshold for embryotoxicity and acceptable tolerance levels for therapeutic use may be low, hopefully more than 1:1 but perhaps not exceeding 10:1. Antineoplastic and antibiotic drugs may be used therapeutically at levels above the threshold of embryotoxicity, but this is justified on the grounds of life-saving medication. On the other hand, an analgesic or tranquilizer could hardly be justified at an embryotoxicity to therapeutic ratio of 25:1 in women of reproductive age.

Usage levels for chemicals that are less directly involved with man's health and welfare than are drugs should be given much lower tolerance levels in reference to the embryotoxicity threshold in animals. Food preservatives, colorants, and other additives, as well as pesticides likely to occur as residues in food, are ordinarily ingested in only minute amounts in the daily diet and thus would usually not reach significant concentration in maternal blood. The possibility of unusual dietary habits or of excessive contamination, however, makes it advisable to set acceptable tolerance in the average daily diet at 100:1 or more below the embryotoxic threshold demonstrated in test animals. Pollutants in air, water, and food (e.g., organic mercury) should be tested for embryotoxicity when there is any reason to suspect appreciable exposure of pregnant women. The negative value of such substances in the environment would dictate extremely low tolerance levels. A ratio of 1000:1 of embryotoxic threshold level in test animals to mean daily human exposure might be taken as an upper limit of tolerance.

The foregoing comments on levels of dosage in testing can be summarized as follows. Test doses should be chosen with the intention of identifying an embryotoxic threshold which will then be used as a basis for extrapolating downward to an acceptable tolerance level. The setting of acceptable tolerance levels requires a value judgment of benefit vs risk. Benefit will vary from that associated with a life-saving drug, through the desirable use of some food preservatives, to the negative value of environmental pollutants. Under the best of conditions teratologic testing in animals provides only a rough estimate of the risk. Because of probable differences in the embryotoxic sensitivity of test animals and man, and the possibility of overexposure, human tolerance levels must be set as far below embryotoxic levels as is practicable in view of the need for the chemical or drug in question.

B. Choice of Test Animals

1. *General Criteria*

The first of many problems arising from the use of animals to assess teratologic risks in man is the choice of the most appropriate species for the tests. Rats, mice, and rabbits have been the most widely used species for the practical reasons that they are readily available, inexpensive, easy to maintain, and can be bred with relative ease in the laboratory. Unfortunately none of these reasons has much scientific bearing on the central problem of predictive value as regards environmental risks to human reproduction, although their relatively low cost does permit the use of larger numbers of these animals than is practicable with other test subjects.

Disregarding economic considerations, the ideal test animal would have the following characteristics: (1) absorb, metabolize, and eliminate the test substance in the same way as does man; (2) transmit the substance and its metabolite across the placenta at the same rate as in man; and (3) possess embryos and fetuses that have developmental schedules and metabolic pathways similar to those in the human conceptus. Existing comparative data are altogether too limited for a judgment as to which animal is most like man in any of these regards; but it is already apparent that no presently used species, including simian primates, is like man in all of these respects. Furthermore, it is evident that the degree of similarity to man exhibited by a given species varies from one test substance to another.

In view of the range of the criteria that should be considered in selecting test animals, it is not surprising that investigators in different disciplines rank the relative importance of these criteria differently. Pharmacologists tend to emphasize comparability of plasma levels of the test substance and its metabolites in man and the test animal, under the assumption that since this reflects rates of absorption, metabolism, and excretion of the test substance, it determines dosage to the embryo. The expert in placental physiology, however, would emphasize that rates of transport across the early placenta would be the limiting factor as far as embryo dosage is concerned. On the other hand, the developmental biologists with a biochemical bent would want to know where in the embryo the compound and its metabolites were localized and how they reacted in embryonic metabolism. Information on the latter subject is at present very meager, although in terms of mechanisms of embryotoxicity it could be the main determinant of whether the developing organism reacts adversely to environmental influences or is able to maintain a normal growth schedule in spite of them. Until experience proves otherwise, however, all of the above criteria should be considered, as far as available information permits, in the selection of test animals. The advantages and disadvantages of particular species of animals will be discussed later in this chapter.

2. Number of Species and Which Species

The current practice of performing teratogenicity tests in at least two species would seem laudable in view of the foregoing comments. Unfortunately, however, much of the benefit that might be expected from a diversity of test animals is lost because of the widespread tendency to select all test species from the closely related rodents (rat, mouse, and occasionally hamster or guinea pig) and lagamorphs (rabbits and hares). Although these animals have several dietary, reproductive, and metabolic similarities, probably of more significance is the fact that they all possess a highly specialized placental structure not present in higher mammals, namely, the inverted yolksac placenta. The embryos of these species may be dependent on this atypical structure for all interchange of essential materials with maternal blood during the critical first few days of organogenesis, the time when embryos generally are most susceptible to embryotoxic influences. Evidence has accumulated that the yolk-sac placenta is not only structurally, but very likely also functionally, different from the typical chorioallantoic placenta that serves other mammals (Beck *et al.,* 1967b; Brent, 1971a; Everett, 1935;

Padykula *et al.,* 1966). Furthermore, Brambell (1957) showed that molecules the size of immunoproteins were much more readily transported across the yolk-sac placenta than the chorioallantoic placenta.

Direct comparisons of the teratogenic susceptibility of rodents and rabbits, on the one hand, and of higher mammalian species, on the other, have seldom been attempted. In one study it was undertaken to compare the susceptibility of rat and rhesus monkey to several drugs known to be teratogenic in one or the other species (Wilson, 1971). Particular care was taken to administer the drugs at comparable stages in development. Rats were found to show embryotoxic effects after lower doses of most of the compounds tested than did monkeys. Thalidomide was a striking exception to this rule, however, and serves to deter a hasty generalization that rats are always teratologically more senstive than monkeys. Nevertheless, when the literature on experimental teratologic studies in nonhuman primates was reviewed (Wilson, 1972b), it became apparent that primates displayed little or no teratogenicity to many chemical agents that are highly teratogenic in rats, mice, and rabbits. When primate dosage was increased sufficiently to elicit some embryotoxic response, it was more often manifested as intrauterine death (abortion) or growth retardation than malformation. Further comparative studies of this type are needed, not so much to determine which of various test species has greater or lesser sensitivity to teratogenesis, but which reacts to given types of agents in ways most nearly comparable to those in man. As emphasized earlier in the choice of animals should be based on similarities to man in plasma concentrations, in placental transfer, and in reactions within the conceptus. Such data are not available for any compound today and a tremendous amount of research remains to be done if the choice of test animals is to be made on a less empirical and more truly scientific basis.

3. *Number of Animals per Test Group*

It has become customary to use 20 female rats or mice and 10 or more female rabbits at each dosage level when treatment is given throughout organogenesis. In general these numbers seem to have yielded sufficient numbers of offspring for statistical purposes. As suggested earlier in this chapter (Section II,A,2), however, a shorter duration of treatment (3 instead of 10 days) with smaller groups of animals (10 rats or mice instead of 20), treated at several consecutive time spans in organogenesis, would probably yield more meaningful results, and would not greatly increase the total number of test animals (see Chapter 10, Section II,A for protocol).

The tendency to use fewer rabbits than rats or mice reflects such factors as availability, cost, and ease of breeding. These considerations become even more compelling when primates or other large species are used. Nevertheless, members of the pharmaceutical and chemical industries are often willing to accept the significantly greater costs of primate tests. This is probably attributable both to the prevalent feeling that primate results are more direcly extrapolable to man than results from lower forms, and to the fact that primate tests are done only after a new compound has shown enough promise to warrant extra effort and expense in documenting its safety. It is generally agreed that there is no excuse for using fewer rodents or other smaller animals than are needed to satisfy statistical requirements. The desirability of full statistical numbers, notwithstanding, it may have to be compromised when the less available, less fecund, and more expensive animals, such as rhesus monkeys, dogs, sheep, or swine, are used. These larger animals probably would not be used unless rodents and/or rabbits had already indicated the general acceptability of a compound. Furthermore, there would hopefully be reasons, e.g., similarity in metabolism to man, for believing that the larger animals would yield results of greater biological significance, regardless of statistical numbers.

4. *Genetic Background of Test Animals*

A question is sometimes raised as to the desirability of using inbred or other highly homogeneous strains of animals in teratologic testing. Accumulated experience over many years of experimental teratology has shown that intrastrain variability in general, and spontaneous malformations in particular, are reduced when stocks of animals with some heterogeneity in genetic make-up are maintained by closed-colony but not brother–sister matings (Palmer, 1969b). Highly inbred animals as would result from brother–sister matings often show developmental defects unique to that strain but they also may be particularly resistant to teratogenesis by certain agents. Colony-bred stocks of a strain known to contain stabilized heterogeneity have generally been found to produce reproducible results. Palmer (1969b) summarized the advantages of random breeding over brother–sister mating as (1) alleviating the risk of mutation and overdominance, (2) preventing polygenic imbalance and inbreeding depression, and (3) retarding the development of subline divergence. In brief, random breeding tends to disperse the genetic variables throughout a colony. All colonies, however, whether inbred or random bred, will exhibit some spontaneous malformation, as well as varying degrees of lesser anatomic variations. The best safeguard against being misled by these is to use a stock for which extensive cumulative control data are available, in addition to the concurrent control run with each experiment. For example, when an unusual malformation occurs during a teratogenicity test, such background data can greatly facilitate interpretation by allowing the investigator to state that the defect has or has not occurred in a stated frequency among a large number of controls of the same stock examined in the same way over several years (see Chapter 9).

5. *Health and Parity of Test Animals*

It is superfluous to stress the need for cleanliness, adequate nutrition, constant temperature, and regular light-dark cycles to obtain reproducible results. Accordingly, when healthy animals are available and the best standards of animal care are ahered to, the use of specific pathogen-free animals is unnecessary and may add little except expense to teratogenicity testing. This is not to say that such animals do not have distinct advantages in chronic toxicity studies where longevity is important, but it will be recalled that teratogenicity is an acute phenomenon. The main concern is the maintenance of normal pregnancy, aside from the effects of the testing procedure.

Extraneous chemicals such as pesticides should not be used in the vicinity of test animals either during or for several weeks preceding a test, to avoid the possibility of the induction or inhibition of drug-metabolizing enzymes (Conney and Burns, 1972). The use of specific disease-control measures, such as daily dosage of primates with isoniazid as prophylaxis against tuberculosis, is preferable to the alternative; but its use during or immediately preceding the period of organogenesis in which a teratogenicity test is conducted is not advised. It is standard practice in the author's laboratory to discontinue isoniazid when a female rhesus monkey is bred and to resume its use only after pregnancy is terminated, by normal delivery, hysterotomy, abortion, or if the animal is determined not to be pregnant.

Questions are sometimes raised about the parity of test animals, but actually there are only a few situations wherein this is a matter of concern. If postnatal survival is to be used to evaluate functional normality of the offspring, it is advisable to use parous dams because some females, particularly rodents, are more likely to destroy or neglect the newborn of first litters than of subsequent ones. For general reproduction studies in which possible effects of the test substance on fertility are under scrutiny, all animals should be proven fertile before the test is begun. This still does not eliminate the possibility of spontaneous failure of fertilization or implantation, or of early resorption of conceptuses; but there are other means of recognizing these occurrences (see Chapter 9). Spontaneous abortions occur in 10–15% of macaque monkeys and baboons (Wilson, 1972b), and some of this rate is probably contributed by "habitual aborters." To eliminate such animals from testing procedures would require that all females used be multiparous, a luxury that is not easily afforded in small primate breeding colonies.

III. Advantages and Disadvantages of Specific Animals in Teratogenicity Testing

It has already been noted that no one animal species or group of related species is ideally suited for the evaluation of human teratologic risks. Accumulated experience, however, has shown that certain groups of animals may offer advantages for particular types of use, whereas others have been found generally inappropriate. In the inappropriate category must be placed all species or test systems that lack the all-important first line of defenses afforded by mammals to their developing tissues, whether these be germinal, embryonic, or fetal. This refers to the parental adaptative mechanisms by which mammals are usually able to reduce the dosage of most physical and chemical agents before they reach such developing tissues. A few nonmammalian species, mainly sharks and some snakes, like mammals do not expose their germ cells or their embryos to the outside environment; but for other reasons these animals are not recommended for teratologic testing.

The mammalian embryo and fetus benefit from a further and unique line of defense against chemical agents, namely, the selective transport functions of the placenta. As was emphasized in Chapter 6, most chemicals in the environment, specifically those in the maternal bloodstream, are subject to concentration gradients across the placenta, usually with the gradient favoring lower concentration in the conceptus than in maternal plasma. Although far from infallible, the placenta is so important as a dose-regulating device that its presence cannot be disregarded in realistic testing of the embryotoxic effects of environmental agents.

a. *Nonmammalian Forms.* For reasons just stated these are not considered suitable for use in the safety evaluation of human embryotoxic risks. Avian and other nonmammalian embryos have and doubtless will continue to contribute greatly to studies on embryologic and teratogenic mechanisms; but even the study of basic mechanisms of normal and abnormal development are not entirely comparable between birds and mammals. The relatively static nutritional and excretory functions in the incubating egg are in sharp contrast to the fluctuating interchange that occurs in both directions across the placenta. Foreign substances introduced into incubating eggs may remain in a slowly diminishing pool for a relatively long time, whereas most compounds as well as their metabolites have a short half-life in maternal and presumably also in embryonic bloodstreams of mammals.

b. *In Vitro Systems.* Whether involving whole embryo, organ, tissue, or cell cultures, these are all inappropriate for use in embryotoxicity evaluation. Among the many other obstacles to achieving and maintaining conditions that would even approximate the *in vivo* state, the problem of circulation of nutrients and metabolites surely ranks as a major one. These variables superimposed on and possibly interacting with whatever stress is introduced by the test substance would render results from *in vitro* cultures almost meaningless as compared with an embryo in dynamic balance with maternal homeostasis through the placenta. *In vitro* systems have been useful in basic studies on nutritional requirements for growth and differentiation over short spans of development, but to maintain normal growth and developmental schedules for longer than several hours or a few days has not been possible.

A. Rodents and Lagamorphs

The complications that may arise from dependence on the highly atypical yolk-sac placenta during early organogenesis in these animals has been discussed (Chapter 6 and elsewhere). Although this unique placental structure may not be wholly at fault, there is accumulating evidence that animals whose early embryos are dependent upon it for essential transport show embryotoxicity to lower doses of more chemical agents than do other mammals. On the other hand, the small size, short gestation period, large litter size, lack of seasonal breeding patterns, and ready availability of these animals add up to a strong inducement to continue their use in initial screening procedures. Not the least of the advantages is their modest cost which permits the use of ample numbers for statistical evaluation of results. These animals are already in such widespread use, that no specific references to teratologic testing with them are needed.

1. *Mouse*

Its small size can be a disadvantage, both in the examination of fetuses for defects as well as in studies on parental absorption, metabolism, and excretion of chemical agents, owing to the limited samples of tissues and body fluids. Breeding performance is sometimes erratic and several inbred strains are known to have high and occasionally variable rates of background malformations and intrauterine death (Kalter, 1968; Nomura, 1969), probably reflecting a greater degree of developmental instability than other rodents. Mice are known to respond readily to some substances that have limited teratogenicity in other animals, for example, cortisone and the herbicide 2,4,5-T, thereby earning a not altogether unjustified reputation for unusual sensitivity. The low cost of maintaining large colonies of mice may make this the preferred mammalian species for mutagenicity testing (Bateman and Epstein, 1971; Cattanach, 1971) and several inbred strains offer particular advantages in basic research, if not for teratologic testing (Smithberg, 1967). Its embryology is amply covered in monographs and research papers

(Appendix I, Section I). The genetics of the mouse is better known than that of any other mammalian species (Grüneberg, 1952, 1963).

2. *Rat*

The extensive use of this animal in both experimental studies and in routine teratologic testing attests to its several advantages, namely, (1) high fecundity, (2) low spontaneous malformation rate, (3) resistance to disease, and (4) convenient size for evaluation and analytical procedures. Surprisingly, there is no adequate single source of information on embryology, although most aspects of the subject are covered in numerous widely scattered research papers (Appendix I, Section III). Many stable, moderately heterogeneous stocks and strains are available throughout the scientific world, and intraspecies variation in routine teratologic tests seems to be lower than for any other wisely studied species (Palmer, 1969b). Rats are likely to be increasingly used in mutagenicity testing, particularly in the host-mediated test (Legator and Malling, 1971).

3. *Hamster*

This animal is gaining acceptance for use in teratology and other types of reproduction studies. It has many of the advantages and lacks some of the disadvantages of mice, particularly, it lacks the developmental instability displayed by many mouse strains. Owing to its short gestation period of 16 days, the hamster has virtually no fetal period. The somewhat abbreviated span of organogenesis may be advantageous or not depending on the type of study contemplated. Its general teratogenic sensitivity seems to parallel that of the rat. Many aspects of its embryology have been documented in the literature (Appendix I, Section II). Stable heterogeneous as well as closely inbred strains are now readily available from commercial suppliers.

4. *Guinea Pig*

This species offers particular advantage if there is need to test the influence of environmental factors on fetal development. It is like many higher mammalian forms and is unique among laboratory rodents in having an extended fetal period during which histogenesis and functional maturation are almost completed. After a 68-day gestation the offspring are born developmentally mature in most respects except physical growth. Guinea pigs are significantly less prolific than the foregoing rodent species because, in addition to the longer gestation period, the estrous cycle is 16 rather than 4 or 5 days in length. Furthermore, the litter size is 2 to 4 fetuses, instead of 8 to 16 commonly seen in the other rodents. Classic studies were done many years ago on its genetics and spontaneous malformations (Wright, 1934,

1960). Information on most aspects of embryology are available in the research literature (Appendix I, Section V).

5. *Rabbit*

The ease with which ovulation can be induced, permitting accurate timing of gestation, makes this animal particularly useful in studies where effects on implantation or on carefully timed events in organogenesis are of particular concern. The relatively large size of some breeds makes possible the collection of large volumes of body fluids and tissues for analysis, from both the maternal animal and the conceptus. Infectious diseases and parasites have proved to be obstacles to high reproductive performance in some laboratories, and good stocks of animals are not universally available. Extensive information on the genetics of anatomical variations (Sawin, 1955; Sawin and Crary, 1964) and on spontaneous malformations (Palmer, 1968, 1969a) has been published. Embryology is not fully documented but is adequate for most purposes (Appendix I, Section IV). This species has been credited with greater similarity in teratogenic sensitivity to man than is warranted because some strains were among the first animals to respond teratogenically to thalidomide (Somers, 1962). The malformations produced by thalidomide, however, are not typical of those seen in primates and there is no reason to regard rabbits as more valid test animals for evaluating human teratic risk than the closely related rodents.

B. CARNIVORES

The animals in this group have not been widely used in teratologic testing, but, in view of the urgent need for diversity in the choice of test animals, particularly for animals that do not possess the specialized placentation of the preceding group, available information is summarized here in the hope that investigators will be encouraged to explore further the use of these animals. Of the three species that can be maintained in the laboratory, namely, ferret, cat, and dog, all have the disadvantage of being seasonal breeders, usually having only one or two litters per year. On the other hand they are polytocous, with several young per litter, and the gestation period is relatively short so that test results are available within 2 months or less after treatment.

1. *Ferret*

Exploratory breeding and teratologic studies with this animal have been in progress in the laboratory of Prof. Felix Beck at the University of Leicester. In addition to the obvious advantage of its small size, it is readily bred, easily maintained in the laboratory, and seems to be responsive to most of the standard teratogens (Beck, personal communication). The greatest drawback to use of ferrets may be that the single yearly estrous period extends from April through July, ordinarily permitting only one pregnancy per year. There is a possibility that studies now in progress with artificial light schedules will improve this restricted breeding span. The female is induced to ovulate by coitus and consequently the timing of gestation can be precise. Unfortunately there is no background of pharmacologic or toxicologic information on this animal, and beyond the exploratory studies mentioned above, it has been infrequently used in teratologic studies (Rorke *et al.,* 1968; Steffek *et al.,* 1968; Steffek and Verrusio, 1972). A modest bibliography on reproduction and embryology is available (Appendix I, Section VIII).

2. Cat

Despite the extensive use of this animal in physiologic and pharmacologic studies, it has not been bred with much success in the laboratory. Several recent reports, however, have indicated that controlled breeding can be accomplished when the animals are allowed to range freely within a room rather than being confined to a cage. A disadvantage is lack of glucuronide-forming enzymes which eliminates an important drug-conjugating system in this species. Information on spontaneous malformations is sketchy (Bloom, 1965; Sheppard, 1951), but cats have been used in several experimental teratologic studies (Hoover and Grusemer, 1971; Malorney, 1969; Somers, 1962; Tuchmann-Duplessis and Lefebvres-Boisselot, 1957) and are deserving of further consideration. They offer the advantages of two or three litters per year and of accurate timing of gestation, owing to the fact that ovulation is induced by copulation. Average litter size is 4. The literature covers many but by no means all aspects of embryology (Appendix I, Section IX).

3. Dog

The smaller breeds of dog such as beagles are bred with relative ease under laboratory conditions and, like cats, have been extensively used in pharmacologic and toxicologic investigations. Published reports on the use of dogs in teratologic studies have appeared with increasing frequency in recent years (Delatour *et al.,* 1965; Earl *et al.,* in press; Friedman, 1957; Letavet and Kurlyandskaya, 1970; Miller, 1947; Phemister *et al.,* 1969; Savini *et al.,* 1968; Smalley *et al.,* 1968; Tapernoux and Delatour, 1967; Weidman *et al.,* 1963). Estrus occurs twice yearly and is easily recognized by the appearance of vaginal bleeding. Some information is available on the occurrence of spontaneous malformations in dogs (Calkins *et al.,* 1956; Fox,

1963; Gardner, 1959; Hamlin *et al.,* 1964; Mulvihill and Priester, 1971; Palmer, 1971), and most aspects of normal development have been adequately described (Appendix I, Section X). The main deterrent to more widespread use of the dog in teratologic testing is probably fiscal. The cost of buying dogs of known pedigree and of maintaining them under conditions favorable to breeding has been likened to that of rhesus monkeys. The larger litter size of dogs is a distinct advantage in terms of the total numbers of test offspring. Pedigreed beagles are widely used but they probably do not offer particular advantages over other small, nonpedigreed breeds that could be maintained as stable lines under closed-colony breeding conditions.

C. Ungulates

Among the smaller hooved mammals the pig and sheep, and possibly the goat, seem to be the most promising subjects for use in the evaluation of human teratic risk. The agricultural background of these animals assures a wealth of information on the breeding performance of various stocks. Although they have not been used as extensively in pharmacologic and toxicologic investigations as some of the preceeding species, a significant amount of information probably could be found. The larger size of these animals would require large samples of the test compound for dosing, but it is unlikely that sheep or pigs would be used in early stages of evaluation when only small samples of a new compound were available.

1. *Sheep*

Considerable information on the rates of spontaneous malformations and of intrauterine death is available in this species (Dennis and Leipold, 1972; Ercanbrack and Price, 1971; Evans *et al.,* 1966; Rosenfeld and Beath, 1947; Young, 1967) and most aspects of prenatal development are adequately described in the literature (Appendix I, Section VII). This animal has already been used in teratologic studies to a surprising extent (Dolnick *et al.,* 1970; James, 1972; James and Keeler, 1968; Keeler and Binns, 1968; Kerschbaum *et al.,* 1970; Knelson, 1971; Lapshin, 1968; Murphree and Graves, 1969; Suttle *et al.,* 1970). A disadvantage is its usual fecundity rate of only one or two lambs per year, but recent studies have shown that some breeds may regularly produce three or more lambs each year (Bradford, 1972).

2. *Pig*

The availability of the pig for teratologic research is well known because of its use in classic studies in nutritional deficiency during pregnancy (Hale, 1933; Palludan, 1966a, b); but a number of other types of agents have also been applied during pregnancy in this species (Barker, 1970, 1971; Davey and Stevenson, 1963; Earl *et al.,* 1964; Edmonds *et al.,* 1972; Emerson and Delez, 1965; Erickson and Murphee, 1964; Gerrits and Johnson, 1964; King, 1969; Menges *et al.,* 1970; Rosenkrantz *et al.,* 1970; Schnurrbusch and Möckel, 1969; Selby *et al.,* 1971; Ullery *et al.,* 1955; Young *et al.,* 1955). The organogenesis of the pig has been more thoroughly characterized than that of any mammal other than man (Patten, 1948 and Appendix I, Section VI), and several reports have described spontaneous malformations in this species (see Kalter 1968 for review; Cella, 1948; Freeden and Jarmoluk, 1963; Gustafsson and Gledhill, 1966; Selby *et al.,* 1971; Shaner, 1951; Warwick *et al.,* 1943). The average litter size is 10. With suitable animal husbandry facilities the cost of maintenance of the smaller breeds is probably less than that of dogs and macaque monkeys.

D. Nonhuman Primates

The advantages and disadvantages of using these animals have recently been reviewed in some detail (Wilson, 1972b) and the present discussion will be limited to generalities. To date only two genera, *Papio* (baboons) and *Macaca* (several species), have been demonstrated to be promising for use in the evaluation of human teratic risk. It was noted earlier in this Chapter that the cost is not much greater for maintaining breeding colonies of these primates than for pedigreed dogs and miniature pigs, but this may change because the future supply of primates is uncertain. Disregarding economic considerations, does the use of primates offer a greater degree of security in the evaluation of safety for man than does use of other forms?

The answer to this question is conditioned on the answers to two correlary questions. It is taken for granted that primates will not be used in mutagenicity testing or for preliminary teratogenicity screens, both of which uses require larger numbers than are practicable. The first and most basic question, then, concerns whether the agent to be tested is one that is needed for use during human pregnancy, for example, antiemetic, antidepressant, anticonvulsant, or oral hypoglycemic, for which an equally safe and effective counterpart does not already exist. (Life-saving procedures used against neoplasms or major infections are not questioned because their use would presuppose elective abortion when unexpected pregnancy is diagnosed.) Although not absolutely essential, these needed drugs when prudently used can alleviate much suffering and discomfort in pregnant women. Before use during human pregnancy, however, they must be subjected to the most rigorous animal test that can reasonably be devised.

The second question concerns the type of animal test or battery of tests that will have maximal predictive value for man. Actually, as will be more

fully explained in Chapter 9, a new concept is probably needed, one involving different levels of animal testing. Briefly, an initial level might consist of
a teratogenicity screen involving relatively large numbers of a readily available animal like the rat. A test substance causing no significant embryotoxicity would then advance to the next level in which a carnivore or an ungulate
would be used, depending on which showed greater similarity to man in the
metabolism of the compound in question, information that could be acquired during prior pharmacologic studies. The higher costs and lower fecundity of this second test animal, perhaps dogs or pigs, would dictate the
use of smaller numbers than were used in the initial screen, but the general
range of effective dosage would already have been defined.

The results of the second-level test would determine whether further animal investigations were necessary. If overt embryotoxicity occurred at levels
only moderately higher than the anticipated therapeutic level in man, the
compound would probably be disqualified for consideration for use in women
of reproductive age. On the other hand, if the compound caused no adverse effects at many times the expected human-use level, it might be considered ready for clinical trial without further animal test. If, however, there
were uncertainty about the margin of safety between the dose that caused
embryotoxicity in the second species and the therapeutic level in man, and if
the compound were still believed to fill a definite therapeutic need, then a
third level of animal tests in nonhuman primates would seem justified.

Thus, the use of nonhuman primates for embryotoxicity evaluation is recommended only for specific purposes, namely, (1) drugs clearly needed to
reduce severe discomfort or disease during pregnancy (e.g., anticonvulsants,
hypoglycemics) or (2) drugs that may be taken inadvertently during the
early part of undiagnosed pregnancy (e.g., contraceptives, anorexants). A
further use of primates might on occasion be justified as suggested earlier in
this chapter. Briefly, if, after a drug or an agricultural chemical had been
approved and been in use for some time, there were sporadic reports that
raised a question of low level embryotoxicity, intensive tests in pregnant primates using doses well above human-use levels or exposure might help to
resolve the question.

The foregoing has implied that embryotoxicity tests in nonhuman primates do indeed provide an added measure of security. This is probably true
when they are used in sequence with subprimate tests as proposed. It remains to be proved, however, that in absolute terms primates are more reliable predictors of human embryotoxic risk than are other mammals. Careful
scrutiny of available literature (Wilson, 1972b) reveals that man and other
primates may not have identical teratogenic sensitivity to more than a few
types of agents, namely, thalidomide, sex hormones, and probably ionizing
radiations. A degree of similarity in embryotoxic response could be found as

regards infections and some chemical agents, but it now seems very unlikely that a precise correlation in all aspects of teratogenic susceptibility can be expected. A preferential status for simian primates in preclinical tests can be fully justified only when such animals can be shown to be more like man than are other test species. The basis for comparison on which this judgment is made must take into account all of the following: (1) overall phylogenetic relatedness, (2) similarity of maternal metabolism of chemicals, (3) comparability of placental transfer functions, and (4) likeness in embryonic sensitivity to extrinsic agents generally.

1. *Phylogenetic Relatedness*

The phylogenetic closeness of the simian primates to man has been offered as ample justification for their use in safety evaluation, but this is based more on logic than scientific evidence, and in any case, must be examined closely. It would be surprising, however, if such relatedness did not impart a degree of similarity in embryotoxic sensitivity, in view of the close resemblance of simians to man in other reproductive parameters. It has been repeatedly emphasized that the rhesus monkey, for example, closely resembles man in the anatomic and temporal aspects of early embryogenesis; in placental structure and in known aspects of placental function; and in reproductive physiology generally (Wilson, 1972b). These recognized areas of correspondence common to all higher primates imply similarity as regards embryonic reactivity to chemical agents, as well as maternal capability to deal with such agents. There is little information on the former but acceptable data are now available on the latter point.

2. *Metabolic Relatedness*

The rhesus monkey has had widespread use as an animal model in the development and testing of human therapeutic agents such as antitubercular and antimalarial drugs. More to the point, Smith (1968, 1969) has reviewed the literature for the purpose of comparing the accuracy with which rhesus monkey and dog would predict drug metabolic pathways in man for 11 assorted drugs. It was concluded that monkey and dog each showed close similarity to man in five instances, but monkey showed fair similarity in four additional instances, as against two for dog, and dog showed no metabolic similarity in four cases, whereas monkey was totally unlike man in only one case. With 12 additional compounds dog was again found to metabolize like man in about half of the tests but "in man and rhesus monkey there was close correspondence between the metabolic patterns." When dog, monkey, and man were compared as to the presence of seven enzymatic pathways, dog was found to be strikingly different from the two primates, which were almost identical. Additional data are cited indicating that Old World monkeys and apes exhibit three metabolic reactions very much like man; New World monkeys showed less similarity; and prosimians were very little like man in these reactions. Peters (1971) also has compared different primate species with man as regards seven toxicologic and metabolic characteristics and has concluded that the rhesus monkey reacts more like man than does squirrel monkey in a ratio of 5:2. The latter is further indication that among simian primate groups, those closer to man (rhesus) metabolize more nearly as does man.

3. *Similarity of Placental Transfer*

Placental structure and circulation are highly analogous in man and rhesus monkey (Panigel, 1971; Ramsey and Harris, 1966) but little is known about the function of either type of placenta during the period of organogenesis when the respective embryos are teratogenically most vulnerable. Data on the dynamics of transport of the early human placenta, obtained by investigating the distribution of drugs to the conceptus of women scheduled for therapeutic or elective abortion, are becoming available in modest amount (Idänpään-Heikkilä *et al.,* 1971; Pitkin, *et al.,* 1970) but are still too limited to warrant generalizations. An innocuous dose of labeled or otherwise easily detectable drugs given at known times before the operation can provide useful information about rates of drug transport, as well as disposition in the embryo, but such studies are usually conducted after the period of high teratogenic susceptibility has passed. Parallel studies in pregnant laboratory primates and in women scheduled for abortion on the placental transfer and embryonic distribution of drugs would serve as a valuable indicator of the validity of extrapolating experimental data from monkey to man.

4. *Reaction within the Embryo*

The initial reaction produced in the embryo by an environmental factor, i.e., the mechanism of action, determines whether developmental deviation or regulation and repair will be the result. The extent to which these opposing reactions occur in different species has not been compared, although a few exploratory studies have demonstrated that some of the biochemical changes associated with the embryo's early reaction can be identified and measured in rats (Ritter *et al.,* 1971; Schumacher *et al.,* 1969; Scott *et al.,* 1971). These technical procedures can be adapted to drug distribution studies in the embryos of primates, including electively aborted human embryos as noted earlier, thereby providing access to the ultimate criterion in choosing the most appropriate test animal, namely, comparability of reactions within the embryos.

It was inferred above that general metabolic and toxicologic reactions are more like those of man the nearer an animal approaches man in the phylogenetic scale. If this is true for the maternal animal, it is not unreasonable to assume that it is also true for the embryo and the fetus. In fact, it is an accepted principle of comparative embryology that species differences in form and structure become less striking as earlier embryonic stages are examined; for example, rat, monkey, and human embryos are structurally quite similar in early somite stages and only later gradually develop the features characteristic of the respective species. It is an interesting but largely unstudied possibility that interspecies metabolic differences are also minimal in the embryo. In this eventuality, the well-known species differences in teratologic susceptibility would have to be attributed mainly to differences in placental transfer and in maternal metabolism, rather than to the embryo's reaction to the agent. This would simplify the problem of translating animal test data into human risk probability by eliminating one of the variables.

CHAPTER 9

COLLECTION AND INTERPRETATION OF RESULTS

Preceding chapters have dealt conceptually with various aspects of abnormal development in man and in animals without particular regard as to whether they were hereditary, spontaneous, or induced. The scope of the present chapter will be limited to manifestations of deviant development in laboratory animals, with emphasis laid on the means by which induced may be distinguished from spontaneously occurring abnormality. Discussions will be confined to the collection and interpretation of data obtained at the termination of pregnancies during which test or experimental procedures were applied. For a consideration of the transmissible defects that result from prior germinal mutations the reader is referred to Fishbein *et al.* (1970) and to Hollaender (1971).

I. Types of Observations to Be Made

In this chapter it is assumed that a pregnant mammal has been subjected to an environmental factor already known to cause developmental defects (experimental study) or to one being evaluated for such potential (teratogenicity test). Although the teratogenicity test and the experimental study in teratology have different objectives and may use different approaches (Palmer, 1969a), they share several problems relating to the interpretation of results. Since in both the collection and evaluation of data can be facilitated by the way in which the test or experiment is conducted, it may be helpful first to consider some of the problems met in evaluating data before proceeding to discuss the design of the protocols in Chapter 10. In any event and whatever the objective, the investigator should be aware that results or effects may be expected in one or more of four sectors when he applies a potentially stressful procedure to a pregnant animal, namely, effects on (1) the maternal animal, (2) the early embryo, (3) the perinatal offspring, and (4) the postnatal offspring.

A. Maternal Effects

Although it is not the primary aim of embryotoxicity tests to observe reactions of the maternal animal to the test procedure, any maternal toxicity that occurs should be included as part of the test result. In fact if significant maternal toxicity occurs in the range of dosage that causes teratogenicity, the latter is as a consequence less insidious because the agent is likely to be eliminated from further consideration unless it is an urgently needed drug the therapeutic value of which is expected to outweigh its toxic effects. The commonest maternal effect during embryotoxicity tests probably is failure to gain weight at the usual rate during pregnancy. This does not necessarily indicate interference with the growth of the conceptuses and may only reflect some transitory functional derangement in the mother such as loss of appetite, or loss of fluid, as a result of diuresis or diarrhea. At the other extreme, abrupt loss of weight or failure to gain any weight may signify termination of pregnancy. Whether this is to be attributed to maternal or embryonic reaction to the test procedure is not always apparent. If it can be determined that the endocrine or other conditions necessary to the maintenance of pregnancy have been interfered with, the problem may be assigned to maternal causes. If, on the other hand, the test procedure is of a nature that could cause early death of all embryos, then the dosage associated with failure of maternal weight gain should be regarded as primarily embryotoxic. Procedures causing death of all late embryos or fetuses, followed by resorption of the entire litter, may produce a secondary toxicity in the pregnant animal of such magnitude as to lead occasionally to maternal death. The examination of conceptuses at intervals after treatment should make it possible to recognize this situation. In any event, appreciable weight loss during a test treatment, or failure to gain after treatment is ended, while not necessarily indicating extensive embryolethality, is strongly suggestive of such, and the possibility should be ruled out.

Some authors have noted that certain chemicals and drugs have caused change in maternal liver weight (Courtney et al., 1970b), but unless this is shown to involve actual pathology of liver tissue, the meaning of such change is not clear. If treatment has been continued for several days, it is possible that fatty infiltration or the induction of liver microsomes might be responsible for increases in liver weight. Their main relevance to the interpretation of test results would seem to depend on the extent to which changes in liver can be shown or presumed to have affected plasma concentration of the test substance sufficiently to have altered embryonic dosage (see Chapter 8, Section II).

Maternal anemia may be observed during or after teratogenicity treatments, consequent to either suppression of hemapoiesis, hemolysis of erythrocytes, or hemorrhage at detached placental sites. These possibilities should, however, be distinguished from the lowering of hematocrit that normally occurs during pregnancy in many species. Maternal anemia per se is not teratogenic in rats, although it may be associated with intrauterine growth retardation of fetuses (Wilson, 1953).

B. Embryonic Effects

As emphasized elsewhere, the early embryo appears to be more susceptible to adverse influences than any other developmental stage. The effects on early embryos are usually not seen until near term when resorption sites or dead, malformed, or growth-retarded fetuses are found in routine examination. Some chemical agents, particularly if given before or during the time of implantation, however, are capable of interfering with the process or of killing the blastocyst while implanting. In either case the products of conception are lost or are implanted for so short a time as to leave no recognizable implantation site. The apparent result would be failure of maternal animals to produce any issue or to produce litters of the expected size.

The best means to evaluate early embryonic loss of this type is to count the corpora lutea of pregnancy in the ovaries and compare this number with the total of recognizable implantation sites, i.e., resorption sites plus placental attachments of surviving fetuses. In untreated mice, rats, hamsters, and rabbits this comparison rarely shows a discrepancy of more than one or two between numbers of corpora lutea and of implantation sites, probably because all embryos that become fully implanted leave an implantation scar (metrial gland), even though they may die and be resorbed soon thereafter. In the guinea pig, and possibly in other forms with long fetal periods, implantation sites associated with embryos that die early may fail to persist until term, thus leaving no evidence of embryolethality except an excess of corpora lutea.

In nonhuman primates the identification of early embryonic death requires special techniques. Species such as rhesus monkey regularly abort embryos that die early, but the resulting blood and tissue debris cannot be distinguished from the normal vaginal bleeding that occurs during the first 40 days of gestation. For this reason, all test procedures in such species should be preceded by a positive diagnosis of pregnancy, and the continuation of pregnancy should be ascertained by rectal palpation of the uterus at frequent intervals during and following treatment to detect arrest or regression of increase in uterine size (Wilson and Fradkin, 1969; Wilson et al., 1970).

C. EFFECTS IN FETAL OR PERINATAL OFFSPRING

The more familiar signs of embryotoxicity are observed in fetal or nearterm animals as resorption sites, dead and/or resorbing fetuses, and malformed or growth-retarded surviving offspring. To ensure that these manifestations are fully observed, it is necessary to interrupt pregnancy a few hours or days before expected term by either hysterotomy or necropsy of the maternal animal. Even animals not ordinarily carnivorous, including nonhuman primates, are nevertheless likely to eat dead and moribund offspring, as well as those with malformations that involve skin lesions allowing loss of body fluids or exposure of viscera. Early resorption sites in polytocous animals can be counted only by direct observation of the uterus before parturition begins. Dead fetuses that show any degree of maceration should not be weighed or included in the examination for malformation because of the frequent edema, distortions, and artifacts encountered in such specimens.

1. *External Examination of Fetuses*

Intact fetuses and newborns should first be determined to be living or dead by observing skin color and spontaneous or elicited movements. Recently dead and stillborn offspring may be either recorded as dead or included with those to be weighed and examined for malformations—but not both, to avoid duplication in accounting for the total of embryotoxic effects. It is probably logically more consistent to ignore the weight and malformations of dead fetuses, even if recently dead, and simply categorize them with other types of intrauterine death such as resorptions, abortions, etc.

Fetuses removed before term should be blotted to remove excess blood or amniotic fluid, the umbilical cord clamped or ligated in a uniform manner to prevent bleeding, and the specimens weighed individually. Growth retardation is better quantitated in terms of individuals affected than as mean weight per animal per litter because growth retardation, like malformation and death, may affect only certain fetuses in a litter. Sex ratio should always be recorded because it has recently been shown to vary with some types of chemical agents (Scott et al., 1972). Each fetus should then be thoroughly examined, using low magnification on small species, for variations in surface features, overall proportion, symmetry, intactness of skin, etc. This external examination is an important part of the search for malformations but it is never sufficient in itself if the object is the evaluation of all embryotoxicity.

TABLE 9-1
WEIGHTS AND MEASURES ON 15 CONTROL MONKEY FETUSES REMOVED BY HYSTEROTOMY ON GESTATION DAYS 99–101 FROM UNTREATED RHESUS FEMALES

Fetus	Body weight (gm)	Amniotic fluid (ml)	Weights of major viscera (gm)						
			Brain	Eyes	Lungs	Heart	Liver	Kidneys	Spleen
♀13d	133	70	20.6	1.10	2.4	0.80	6.3	1.29	0.18
♂16e	154	135	22.5	1.02	2.6	1.00	6.1	0.86	0.22
♂29d	149	150	23.4	0.96	2.6	1.10	5.2	1.25	0.33
♂41c	151	125	—	0.96	3.5	1.10	5.4	1.12	0.40
♂40e	148	130	21.1	1.16	2.8	1.00	5.3	1.06	0.34
♀47c	119	95	15.3	0.92	3.0	0.70	4.5	0.78	0.26
♀48c	142	84	25.4	0.96	2.7	1.08	5.8	0.90	0.24
♀60c	130	105	21.0	0.98	3.1	0.90	4.5	0.97	0.30
♂75b	125	85	18.0	0.90	2.5	1.33	4.8	0.91	0.25
♂39d[a]	143	85	23.1	1.06	2.7	1.10	—	0.96	0.20
♂70b	159	71	23.6	1.23	3.2	1.30	7.0	0.98	0.35
♂94a	146	93	22.2	1.08	3.0	1.26	6.1	0.97	0.35
♀98a	155	86	21.0	0.93	3.5	1.50	6.3	0.91	0.33
♂77c	154	84	21.1	1.11	2.9	1.09	5.5	0.80	0.33
♂58f	143	47	23.9	1.05	2.2	1.08	5.1	0.82	0.29
Mean	143	96	20.1	1.03	2.8	1.09	5.2	0.97	0.29
Standard deviation	12	28	2.9	0.10	0.4	0.20	0.8	0.15	0.06

[a] The mothers of this and the following 5 fetuses were given a vehicle, 15 ml of 0.3% tragacanth daily by stomach tube, days 20–45 of gestation.

It has been repeatedly shown that many teratogenic agents produce visceral and skeletal malformations that are not associated with external signs. Thus all fetuses should be fixed for further study of internal structure.

2. Detecting Internal Abnormality in Small Animals

Histologic serial sections are generally regarded as impractical in smaller species of test animals and impossible in animals as large as a rabbit. It is now common practice to divide the fetuses of smaller test species such as mouse, hamster, rat, and rabbit into two groups, according to a set proportion, half and half or one third and two thirds of each litter, for separate fixation to permit skeletal study in one group and visceral examination in the other. For skeletal visualization the best procedure for small animals is fixa-

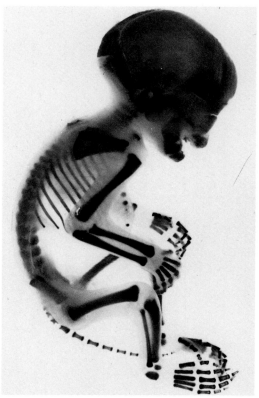

Fig. 9-1. Cleared, alizarin-stained monkey fetus removed by hysterotomy from an untreated rhesus female on day 100 of pregnancy. These specimens allow excellent visualization of the ossified skeleton but require 2 to 3 months for preparation. The sternum was displaced forward during postmortem examination of the thoracic viscera.

tion in 95% alcohol followed by clearing in 1 or 2% KOH, staining in alizarin red S, and preservation in glycerin (Schnell and Newbern, 1970). For visceral examination fixation in Bouin's fluid is advantageous because it is adaptable to various approaches, dissection, freehand sectioning, or histologic sectioning. Direct dissection of the cavities to expose and open major viscera (Monie *et al.*, 1965) is effective but time consuming and must be

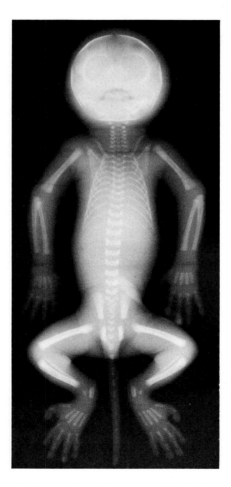

FIG. 9-2. Radiograph of a monkey fetus removed by hysterotomy from an untreated rhesus female on day 100 of pregnancy. Although the definition of skeletal structures is not as clear as that in Fig. 9-1, x-rays of this type have proved adequate for evaluation of the skeleton and they have the advantage of being made quickly and inexpensively.

done by a person with some knowledge of mammalian anatomy. The free-hand sectioning technique (Wilson, 1965b) is probably the fastest method for visualizing all major viscera and it has the advantage that relatively un-trained personnel can learn to recognize most malformations by the use of reference sections (see Appendix III). Accurate evaluation of skeletal and visceral preparations, whether dissections or freehand sections, will depend on the availability of professional personnel with training in mammalian pathology or anatomy to assist in making difficult diagnoses.

3. Detecting Internal Abnormality in Larger Animals

The skeletal and visceral examination of larger test animals presents no particular problems. Standard postmorten examination of the internal or-gans has been adapted for use in the 100-day monkey fetus (Wilson *et al.*, 1970) and should be equally suited to systematic study of fetuses and new-borns in other larger test animals. Tables of normal whole body and organ weights can be easily compiled (Table 9-1) and are useful in judging gener-al growth retardation as well as localized hypoplasia. Skeletal examination can be satisfactorily carried out on cleared-alizarin stained carcasses (Fig. 9-1) if care is taken during the postmortem exploration of cavities to mini-mize damage to or displacement of skeletal elements; but the preparation of larger fetuses by this method may require several weeks to a few months and is not inexpensive in the quantities of reagents required. x-ray visualization of the skeleton of larger fetuses is usually adequate as regards definition and detail (Fig. 9-2) and is much faster. It is also less expensive if radiologic equipment is already available.

D. POSTNATAL EFFECTS

These are usually of a functional nature and often are grossly manifested either in death during the early postnatal period or in failure to grow at the control rate thereafter. Specific tests for various functional parameters have been proposed, but unless there is reason to suspect particular functional deficits, survival and normal growth can usually be taken as ample indication of functional normality. At present a broad battery of specific physiologic tests seems impractical, except in the areas of behavioral changes, ataxia, and sensory losses; some tests are already available in the literature of experimental psychology and others may be modified from existing clinical tests. Postnatal growth is adequately measured by weekly weighing of offspring over a period of 2 or 3 months postnatally. Animals that die or fail to thrive during this period should be carefully examined for structural defects, and routine autopsy should be performed on all survivors at the end of the observation period.

Increasing concern is expressed about the effects on postnatal development of both prenatal and early postnatal exposure to adverse environmental influences (Nair and Dubois, 1968). Postnatal behavioral changes have for some time been known to follow such exposure (Furchtgott and Walker, 1969; Werboff and Havlena, 1962), but a number of other functional and some structural defects have been reported to follow perinatal treatments of experimental animals with radiations and other agents (Dekaban, 1969; Hazzard and Budd, 1969; Hicks *et al.*, 1969; Langman and Shimada, 1970, 1971; Langman *et al.*, 1972; Martin, 1969; Palludan, 1970; Windle, 1969).

II. Interpretation of Results

Variability seems to be inherent in all biologic systems and phenomena, and the average or mean condition may be more a statistical concept than an absolute state of being. This creates particular difficulties when, as after an embryotoxicity test, it is necessary to segregate a given sample of individuals into those to be considered normal and those to be labeled abnormal. Of the four manifestations of developmental deviation, only death of the conceptus is unequivocal. Growth retardation, malformation, and functional deficiency present varying degrees of difficulty in deciding where to draw the line between background variability and induced embryotoxicity. Clear-cut embryotoxicity of any of these types is readily recognized, but clear-cut cases are by no means the rule in embryotoxicity testing. Agents that are highly toxic would likely already have been eliminated from consideration before the stage of teratogenicity testing is reached. When a test reveals nothing that could be construed as embryotoxicity at any dose less than the maternal toxic level, there is still the lingering question of whether sufficient numbers of test animals were used to reveal a low level of embryotoxicity.

Thus, variability is implicit in the use of animals to evaluate human teratic risk. At best it will not provide more than a statement of probability as to the chances of adverse effects in man. One way to minimize the curse of variability in test animals used in embryotoxicity tests is to accumulate as much background data as possible on the spontaneous developmental variation in the stocks of animals used. Such accumulated control data on frequency of intrauterine death, malformation, and growth retardation, as well as of anatomic variations (see Section II,B) in untreated animals can sometimes be of greater value than the concurrent controls in interpreting an occasional deviation in a treatment group. For example, occurrence of anophthalmia during a teratogenicity test would be differently interpreted when it is known that this defect had previously been seen at the rate of 1 in 200 untreated offspring born in the colony than would an occurrence of spina bifida, a defect which had never occurred spontaneously in the colony.

A. WHAT IS GROWTH RETARDATION?

Many degrees of intrauterine growth retardation occur without known cause in man (Miller and Hassanein, 1971) and undoubtedly the same is true for other mammals. Aside from the known genetic, endocrine, and nutritional factors that influence growth, it must be accepted that many of the same agents capable of producing death and malformation can also cause growth retardation, depending on dosage and time of treatment. In fact malformed individuals are frequently smaller than their nonmalformed siblings. Quantitatively, growth-retarded individuals may be defined as those that are one or two standard deviations below the mean of control weight. When growth retardation is not proportionate throughout an affected individual, that is, if there is localized or regional retardation of particular parts, the affected part is hypoplastic and usually considered to be malformed, e.g., microcephaly, microphthalmia, or localized hypoplasia of any organ.

1. *Is Reversible Growth Retardation Abnormal?*

The question of the reversibility of growth retardation often arises. It is known that slowness of growth can be induced at almost any stage of development by nutritional deprivation, but normal weight increase may be resumed when adequate nutrition is restored. On the other hand, some environmental influences such as long-continued, low-level radiations cause permanent impairment of growth after which normal size is never attained (Jones, 1969). On logical grounds it is justifiable to question whether transitory growth retardation from which there is full recovery is in fact abnormal growth, rather than a transitory functional derangement. Failure to recover from growth retardation, on the other hand, is readily accepted as a developmental defect if the weight deficiency is different from the mean by a statistically meaningful amount. In the practical context of embryotoxicity testing, however, it is not feasible to determine whether the growth deficiency seen at brith, for example, in a rhesus monkey, is permanent or transitory when the animal reaches maturity 3 to 4 years later. In such situations an arbitrary criterion may have to be adopted, e.g., any animal more than two standard deviations from the mean weight of controls of the same age and sex is considered to be retarded.

B. WHAT IS A MALFORMATION?

An entirely satisfactory definition for a malformation does not exist. Developmental variations represent a continuum, from the infinite variety seen in the distribution of small blood vessels throughout the body to the infrequent deviations seen in large vessels such as the aorta. Pathologists and anatomists are well aware that structural variations of considerable magnitude are found in virtually every cadaver that is examined in detail. A majority of these were silent in that they produced little or no discomfort or functional limitation during the lifetime of the individual. Thus, neither frequency of occurrence nor magnitude of deviation from the mean provides an easily applied criterion for distinguishing anatomic variations from malformations.

1. *Detriment to the Affected Individual*

In medicine it is appropriate to define as a malformation any structural variant of developmental origin that actually or potentially causes disease, disability, or psychologic impairment. Even this definition does not eliminate uncertainty about what is detrimental and what is simply different from the usual. For example, the spleen is usually a single, moderately large organ attached to the mesentery of the stomach, but occasionally it consists of two or more separate organs situated in various locations. These accessory or supernumerary spleens are not known to be associated with any disease or other complication; according to the above definition they would not be malformations, even though they do represent an appreciable deviation in the usual anatomic pattern. This definition becomes less precise when applied to animals, but at least in principle it can be extended to all mammals. A more realistic wording, however, might be that in animals a malformation is a structural deviation of developmental origin that actually or potentially impairs the survival, health, or usual activity of the affected individual. Limiting the concept of malformations to only those variants with negative survival or health value, in animals even more than in man, puts at issue some rather conspicuous structural deviations such as polydactyly, ectrodactyly, agenesis of tail, and uncomplicated cleft lip. These generally do not impair survival or health, yet all are traditionally regarded as malformations, for no better reason than that they represent appreciable departures from the accepted view of normal morphogenesis. Clearly some latitude must be permitted if malformation is to be defined in terms of detriment to the affected animal.

2. *Infrequency of Occurrence*

It has been suggested that infrequency of occurrence of a particular defect in control animals might serve to distinguish spontaneous from treatment-induced malformations. In Chapter 2, Section I it was noted that the malformations seen in the offspring of treated pregnant animals sometimes seem to represent only an increased frequency of the malformations that occur at lower frequency spontaneously in that strain of animals (Andersen, 1949; Ingalls and Curley, 1957; Landauer, 1957; Runner, 1959; and many others). This is not always the case, however, for highly unusual malformations were induced in human beings by thalidomide and in experimental animals by vitamin A deficiency (Warkany *et al.*, 1948), acetazolamide (Wilson *et al.*, 1968), and other agents too numerous to mention. Thus, frequency or infrequency of occurrence in untreated animals does not provide a firm criterion, although it may be of some help in distinguishing spontaneous from induced malformations. A malformation that is unknown or occurs in less than 1/1000 in control offspring can reasonably be assumed to have been treatment related when it occurs in a test group, but one is never sure until it is shown to be increased in a dose-related fashion by treatment. An increase in the incidence of a malformation known to occur in untreated animals can be assumed to be treatment related if the increase is significant by the usual statistical methods, particularly if the increase is dose-dependent. A low incidence of a defect known to occur in controls, however, must always be regarded with suspicion.

3. *Variation versus Malformation*

A great deal of uncertainty in the interpretation of results has hinged about the spontaneous occurrence of minor anatomic variations, particularly of the skeleton. All mammalian species that have been adequately studied, including man, have been found to display anatomic variations in the segmental patterns of the axial skeleton, especially in the number and morphology of ribs, sternebrae, and lower thoracic and lumbar vertebrae (Fig. 9-3). These are so common in most strains of rabbits that they are accepted as normal occurrences by experienced investigators (Gibson *et al.*, 1966; Palmer, 1968; Sawin and Gow, 1967). They have been observed as the main developmental variant when pregnant animals were given massive doses of a drug that was generally not teratogenic in that species, e.g., thalidomide in rats (Dwornik and Moore, 1965; Globus and Gibson, 1968). They have been attributed to genotype and to assorted environmental influences in mice (Howe and Parsons, 1967; Ohmori, 1968). It is estimated that they occur in 5–15% or more of offspring from untreated pregnancies in mice, rats, rabbits, hamsters, guinea pigs, and rhesus monkeys.

Confusion arises from the fact that skeletal variations often increase above background level in the offspring of animals subjected during pregnancy to such mild stress as the injection of an inert vehicle, and when stressed more vigorously as in teratogenicity studies, the incidence may or may not show further increases. Table 9-2 presents data on skeletal variations seen in 20-day rat fetuses from Wistar females that were untreated or were given various control or teratogen treatments during pregnancy (Kimmel and Wilson, in press). Skeletal variations occurred with considerable frequency in the several control groups, but these were not clearly correlated with time or route of vehicle treatment. Among teratogen-treated groups skeletal variations tended to increase as malformations increased but the

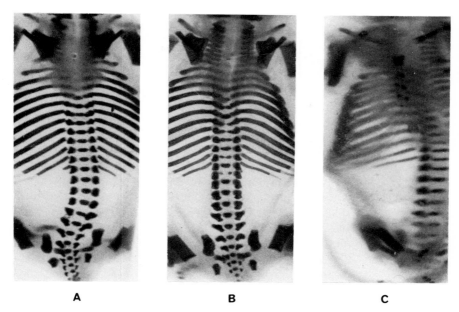

A	**B**	**C**

Fig. 9-3. Cleared, alizarin-stained rat fetuses removed on day 20 of gestation, showing the commoner skeletal variations in otherwise normal young. A. Rudimentary 14th rib on left side (less than half the length of 13th rib), and extra 14th rib on right side (greater than half the length of 13th rib). B. Cleft vertebral centra ranging from slightly constricted (T13), through "dumbbell"-shaped (T12) to completely divided (LI) conditions in the same animal. C. Cleft sternebrae in which the bilateral components have remained separate and are malaligned ("scrambled"). Intact, ossified sternebrae vary from 4 through 6 in number in normal 20-day rat fetuses.

correlation was not close. Some teratogenic agents such as aspirin produced greater degrees of variability than others; aspirin was particularly prone to cause supernumerary ribs and thoracic vertebrae.

The interpretation of anatomical variants, particularly supernumerary ribs, has been a matter of concern in the author's laboratory. It was noted a number of years ago that accessory riblike ossifications occurred either unilaterally or bilaterally at the level of the first lumbar vertebra in approximately 15% of newborn rats from untreated females of Wistar-derived stock. Originally it was assumed that the length of these varied as a continuum from barely visible nodules of bone to fully developed ribs almost as long as the preceding normal 13th rib. When a number were measured, however, they were found to represent a bimodal distribution, with a majority measuring 0.1 to 0.4 mm, but with another distinct peak between 1.2 and 1.7 mm (Kimmel and Wilson, in press). The practice was adopted of re-

TABLE 9-2
Skeletal Variations in 20-Day Rat Fetuses after Various Treatments during Pregnancy[a,b]

| Treatment | | | | | Percent survivors with specified skeletal variations | | | | |
Agent, route, and dose (mg/kg)	Day of gestation	Total implants	Percent dead or resorbed	Percent survivors malformed	Rud. 14th ribs	Extra 14th ribs	Various sternebral	Cleft vertebral centra 1 or more	5 or more
Control									
untreated	—	153	8	0	15	1	0	56	1
H₂O (ip, id)	7	65	12	2	21	0	0	26	0
	9	72	10	8	23	0	4	43	3
	11	67	22	0	14	0	2	56	2
H₂O (sc, bid)	9	62	0	0	24	5	0	84	12
	10	61	5	3	14	0	0	83	5
	11	72	3	9	14	1	1	94	7
CMC[c] (po, id)	11	69	9	3	11	0	0	21	0
Acetazolamide (sc, bid)									
500	9	65	6	3	18	5	2	90	23
	10	62	6	28	28	3	3	97	28
	11	68	1	3	13	0	0	79	7

Actinomycin D (ip, id)									
0.2	7	93	5	6	44	1	0	36	3
0.3	7	102	10	8	34	3	0	45	0
0.1	9	60	0	5	35	3	3	45	0
0.2	9	87	10	19	31	33	15	54	4
0.2	11	132	4	2	17	0	0	45	6
0.3	11	90	9	1	19	1	5	62	9
Aspirin[d] (po, id)									
250	9	60	3	3	33	33	0	6	0
500	9	89	34	62	—[e]	—[e]	24	71	0
500	10	127	18	64	—[e]	—[e]	16	88	84
500	11	118	9	20	25	0	6	81	44
750	11	169	21	66	53	0	15	78	53
1000	11	112	59	98	69	13	25	100	100

[a] Abbreviations: rud, rudimentary; ip, intraperitoneal; sc, subcutaneous; po, oral; id, once per day; bid, twice per day.
[b] From Kimmel and Wilson (in press).
[c] Carboxymethyl cellulose 0.2% at 5 ml/kg.
[d] Only approximately 1/3 of surviving fetuses in this group were cleared for skeletal study.
[e] Fourteenth ribs were greatly increased and 15th and even 16th ribs occurred as rudiments or as extra ribs in these treatment groups.

cording the shorter types of 14th ribs, those less than half the length of the normal 13th rib, as "rudimentary," and those greater than half the length of the normal 13th rib as "extra" (Fig. 9-3A). The occurrence of neither of these varieties of accessory rib structures is considered to be a malformation, but it is thought that an increase in their incidence during teratogenicity tests, if not already associated with increased malformations, indicates that the embryotoxic range of dosage is being approached.

Variations in the patterns of ossification of other skeletal elements—sternebrae, vertebral centra, and intramembranous bones of the skull—have also been observed with considerable regularity. Because of their frequent but inconstant occurrence it seems advisable not to consider any of these as malformations, although, as with accessory ribs, they may indicate that an embryotoxic effect is to be expected at higher dosage. Deficient or irregular patterns of ossification that are generalized throughout the skeleton may simply reflect growth retardation (Fritz and Hess, 1970). Thus, before classifying as abnormal such things as enlarged sutures and fontanelles in the skull and deficient numbers of sternebrae, metacarpals, metatarsals, and caudal vertebrae, the weight of affected animals should be compared with that of controls to determine whether the osseous deficiency is merely a reflection of general retardation. Beck and Smith (1972) found that three sublines of CBHA mice could be selected on the basis of susceptibility or resistance to trypan blue teratogenesis. These differed significantly in the frequencies of several skeletal characters and, interestingly, the subline most susceptible to trypan blue did not consistently show greater overall skeletal variations than the less susceptible lines.

C. What Is the Relationship between Malformation and Intrauterine Death?

This question was raised in Chapter 2, Sections E and F, but it needs to be considered in the present connection because of the varied interpretations that may be placed on these two manifestations during teratogenicity studies. As already emphasized, both types of abnormality often appear at comparable dose levels during organogenesis and they may tend to increase in roughly parallel fashion as dosage is increased, although when high embryotoxic doses are reached lethality increases at the expense of malformation. Embryolethality, then, is the ultimate expression of embryotoxicity in the sense that at a given stage of development higher doses produce only this manifestation of abnormality. A test dose that causes 100% embryolethality is clearly excessive and other embryotoxic effects must be sought at lesser doses if the study is to be in any degree comprehensive.

Although lethality and malformations are frequently associated in rodent litters after treatment during organogenesis, this is not necessarily true in other animals; in rhesus monkeys intrauterine death has been shown to be somewhat more prevalent than malformations at embryotoxic ranges of dosage (Wilson, 1971, 1972b). Little is gained by discussing which manifestation is the more sensitive or the more reliable in evaluating embryotoxicity because they have varied meanings in relation to times of treatment, as well as test species, levels of dosage, and types of agents used (Grauwiler, 1969; Chapter 2, Section E). In teratologic testing an increase in embryolethality or in malformations is equally indicative of adverse effect on development. In human teratology, however, intrauterine death would in most circumstances be regarded as preferable to the birth of a malformed or a functionally deficient infant.

D. NEED FOR POSITIVE CONTROL

The use of a positive control, that is, controls treated with a known teratogen, has from time to time been recommended to demonstrate the responsiveness of the particular stock of test animal being used. Under optimal conditions this should not be necessary because testing should be done in animals whose general sensitivity is already well-known to the investigator. Furthermore, there often is little carry-over of information about the responsiveness of an animal strain from one agent to another. For example, the lack of embryotoxic sensitivity of rats to thalidomide and cortisone would have no bearing on the sensitivity of this species to agents such as trypan blue, folate antagonists, 5-fluorouracil, or acetazolamide. Conversely, the susceptibility of one strain of rabbits or mice to thalidomide or cortisone does not signify that that strain will be more or less like man in embryotoxic responsiveness to a given test compound. Tests should be designed so that an embryotoxic level of dosage is found in more than one species preferably in two or more unrelated species (see Chapter 8, Section III, and Chapter 10). The present author believes that regardless of the strain or species used, the time, effort, and animals used in running positive controls would be better spent in subjecting more pregnant animals to the primary agent being tested.

E. THE "LITTER EFFECT"

It is often noted in embryotoxicity testing and in experimental studies that the litters of different females treated at the same dosage vary considerably in the degree and type of response (Jensh et al., 1970). A striking example was seen when pregnant rats treated with teratogenic doses of acetazolamide (Wilson et al., 1968) fell into two categories: those producing litters containing several pups with the typical reduction defect of the right forelimb, and those producing litters containing normal pups. A more usual expression of litter-to-litter variation involves quantitative and sometimes qualitative differences in rates of embryolethality, malformation, and growth retardation. Thus, the so-called "litter effect" is a toxicologic reflection of either genetic or environmental influences presumably acting through the maternal organism so as to make the offspring of one female react differently than those of another to the same dose. Nongenetic, maternal effects are well known in experimental teratology (Bornstein *et al.,* 1970; Davidson *et al.,* 1969; Kalter, 1969). The extent to which these can be related to differences in maternal metabolic parameters such as rates of absorption, catabolism, and excretion of a drug are usually not known, but these metabolic characteristics are in part themselves determined by heredity.

The question of how best to deal with this type of biologic variation, in which members of a litter may not vary independently but exhibit a tendency to react more like their littermates than like nonlittermates, is debatable. Statisticians seem generally to favor treating embryotoxicity data by litter units rather than by pooling all individuals from all litters comprising a treatment group. The propriety of the litter-unit approach may be justified on statistical grounds; but in actual practice there are few situations involving sufficient numbers of pregnant animals (10 or more per treatment group) that would be differently interpreted in terms of whole litters than of pooled offspring from all pregnancies in the dosage group. The pooling of all offspring simplifies the analysis as well as the presentation of data, and this advantage probably outweighs the small bias this method is said to introduce.

III. Sources of Error

Several factors already mentioned can be sources of error in the collection and interpretation of the results of embryotoxicity tests, namely, insufficient numbers of animals, inappropriate species, incomplete examination of test animals, etc. Other considerations are less obvious and for that reason perhaps they should be given particular emphasis. When equivocal or inconsistent results are encountered, the first recourse is to repeat or extend the previous studies. Repeating the study without careful consideration of possible sources of error in the original experiment, however, could be a futile gesture. The following are some attitudes and possibilities that may prove useful in recognizing and then either correcting or rationalizing the source of error.

A. REPRODUCIBILITY OF RESULTS

The fact must be accepted that teratology, as exemplified by embryotoxicity tests, is not in any real sense an exact science. The variability characteristic of all biologic systems is compounded in the maternal–embryonic relationship of mammalian pregnancy, involving as it does two individuals that are partly independent, partly dependent, and undoubtedly capable of interacting to varying degrees at different times in gestation. Investigators in the same laboratory are unable always to control the many variables in an embryotoxicity study, and the problem is magnified when results from two or more laboratories are compared. This was illustrated to a disturbing degree in a Collaborative Study by Sixteen Laboratories (1966), in which samples of three compounds were distributed to different laboratories in universities and pharmaceutical industries in Europe for embryotoxic evaluation in rats. Wide variations in results could in part be accounted for by the use of unlike stocks of animals maintained under different housing conditions, but probably of equal or greater importance was the fact that personnel of unstated experience and capabilities in the different laboratories treated the animals and collected and evaluated the results. It should be noted also that this test was done before methods in widespread use today had been generally adopted.

To determine the extent to which such variability could be minimized, repetitive experiments were carried out in the author's laboratory using the same personnel, the same stock of Wistar derived rats, the same sample of highly purified trypan blue, and the same dosage. First, a preliminary experiment was run to standardize and familiarize personnel with the procedures. The experiment was then repeated five times with all conditions such

TABLE 9-3

REPRODUCIBILITY OF TRYPAN BLUE TERATOGENICITY RESULTS IN RATS MAINTAINED AND TREATED UNDER STANDARDIZED CONDITIONS EXCEPT TIME OF TREATMENT[a]

Time of treatment	Total number implants	Percent dead or resorbed	Percent survivors malformed
Preliminary trial	103	37	24
August, 1969	119	35	33
November, 1969	111	52	34
February, 1970	115	57	51
May, 1970	143	55	58
August, 1970	128	37	31

[a] Given 50 mg/kg IP on day 8 of gestation. Pregnancy terminated day 20.

as temperature, humidity, light cycle, etc., remaining constant except the season of the year when treatment was given. The results in Table 9-3 indicae that even under these rigidly controlled conditions the results varied considerably from season to season, despite the fact that animals had no known cues as to the time of year. It was gratifying, however, to find that comparable rates of malformation could be produced during the same month on successive years (compare August, 1969, with August, 1970). Thus, although some variability is almost unavoidable, reassurance was derived from the finding that under closely controlled conditions a fair degree of reproducibility of results was obtained.

B. POSSIBLE INTERACTIONS

The possibility that one environmental factor may interfere with the accurate evaluation of the toxic effects of another needs no further discussion here. It is well to reemphasize, however, that the exquisite sensitivity of the embryo during early organogenesis is such that, what might under other circumstances be a negligible effect, could at this time lead to interference with or augmentation of the results of a test. Accordingly, variations in diet and the use of medications and extraneous chemicals such as pesticides must be avoided during embryotoxicity tests. When treatments are given orally by stomach tube or capsule it is well to fast all animals for a standard number of hours before treatment in order to minimize variations in rate of absorption, as well as the possibility of interaction that might result from food in the upper digestive tract. In situations where prophylactic medications are needed, such as isoniazid for prevention of tuberculosis in primates, such medication must be discontinued during and for several days prior to treatment with a test substance. The known fact that certain pesticides are able to induce catabolizing enzymes in liver, whereas others may cause inhibition of normal enzymes (see Table 8-2), contraindicates the use of such substances in the animal quarters during or for several days preceding a test.

C. OTHER POSSIBLE SOURCES OF ERROR

1. *Spontaneous Mutations*

Spontaneous mutations of either the germinal or somatic variety could occur as random events in such a way as conceivably to confuse embryotoxicity test results, although there is small probability of such an occurrence. If an unusual malformation occurs among the offspring of animals expected to show little or no effect, the occurrence of a new mutation might be invoked; but a practical way to deal with this situation would be to repeat that part of the test protocol to strengthen the probability that the effect was or was not related to treatment.

2. *Spontaneous or Infectious Abortion*

Abortion (either spontaneous or infectious) in domestic animals and non-human primates can simulate embryolethality during a test. Support for believing that abortion is or is not treatment-related requires that additional animals be treated, but examination of the past reproductive history of the aborting animal(s) may give a clue. Multiple abortions that do not appear to be dose-related would suggest that habitual abortion or infectious agents be considered.

3. *Inaccurate Timing of Fertilization*

Erroneous timing of fertilization can alter the embryotoxic sensitivity of test animals by causing treatment to be given at times other than that expected to coincide with organogenesis. This is more likely to occur in pregnant animals purchased from commercial breeders, or in domestic animals in which the time of ovulation with respect to insemination is difficult to estimate. The only practicable check on the possibility of erroneous timing is to extrapolate backward from the time of parturition, or from the weight of near-term controls, to estimate whether these factors can be reconciled with the presumed breeding date.

4. *Improper Administration of Dosage*

Improper administration of dosage was discussed in Chapter 8, Section II, A, but some points need further emphasis here. Intraperitoneal injection, even when done by experienced personnel, involves some risk that the dosage will be deposited in the gut tract and hence largely lost in the feces. Treatment by dietary incorporation is subject to possible wastage by the animal, decomposition by air and light, and the vagaries of the animal's appetite, all making dosage a matter of approximation. Subcutaneous injection can lead to leakage from the injection site, and percutaneous applications can be reduced by contact with other animals or cage and bedding materials. Dosage by means of stomach tube is sometimes lost by regurgitation in monkeys; repeated passage of the tube may cause esophageal inflammation or even perforation in rodents if not skillfully done.

Since these and other possible sources of error cannot be entirely eliminated, the investigator must be alerted to them. One of the best means of minimizing these problems is to use experienced and intelligent technical personnel who are also alerted to the possibilities for error. In fact it can be said, at the risk of saying the obvious, that the greatest possibility for error may lie in the quality of personnel with whom embryotoxicity testing is entrusted.

CHAPTER 10

SUGGESTED PROTOCOLS FOR EMBRYOTOXICITY TESTING

It is evident that there is no one animal species that can be considered ideal for evaluating human teratologic risk. Furthermore, there is uncertainty as to which of several criteria relative to man, e.g., phylogenetic relatedness, metabolic relatedness, similarity of placental transfer, or similarity of embryonic reaction, is most important in choosing animals to be used in testing. A great deal of research remains to be done before all of the information needed for making the wisest choice will be available (see Chapter 8). In the meantime testing must not only be continued but, in view of the rate of environmental change, it should be intensified and further refined.

Since soon after the identification of thalidomide as a human teratogen, there has been no want of recommended procedures to evaluate human teratologic risk using mammals generally (Cahen, 1964; Cook *et al.,* 1969; Palmer, 1969a,b; Report of WHO Scientific Group, 1967; Van Loosli and Theiss, 1964; Wilson, 1965b) or particular species of mammals (Brent 1964b; Ferm, 1965; Frohberg and Oettel, 1966; Gibson *et al.,* 1966; Giroux *et al.,* 1967; Tuchmann-Duplessis and Mercier-Parot, 1964b). A feeling of urgency about the need for better methods of testing still remains after the passage of ten years and in spite of a plethora of data and suggestions. Although much has been learned that reduces the probability of an occurrence like the thalidomide catastrophe, the introduction of new agents and higher levels of exposure to old ones tend to discount some of the progress that has been made.

Experience gained with one type of agent does not always provide a reliable guide in designing protocols for testing new agents. For example, thalidomide would be particularly unsuitable as a model of the embryotoxic

195

TABLE 10-1

A NEW CONCEPT IN TERATOGENICITY TESTING BASED ON MULTILEVEL TESTS IN DIFFERENT TYPES OF ANIMALS

Order of test[a]	Purpose	Suitable species	No. of pregnant animals
First level	Find embryotoxic dose range	Rat, mouse, hamster, or rabbit	130–150
Second level	Confirm or adjust above	A carnivore or an ungulate	40–60
Third level	Only if second level results are equivocal	Alternate to that used in second level	40–60
Fourth level	Only if use in human pregnancy needed or likely	Macaque monkey or baboon	40–50

[a] Tests would terminate at second or third levels in most instances.

properties of other drugs because (1) the disparity between maternal and embryonic toxicity is greater than for any other known teratogen; (2) it produces an atypically flat dose–response curve in simian primates, the most sensitive species; and (3) the range of effective dosage varies widely among susceptible species. The following suggestions for the design of protocols for embryotoxicity testing in laboratory animals are based on experience with a wide variety of chemical agents by a number of investigators.

I. A Multilevel Animal Test for Embryotoxicity

If better tests than are now in use are to be devised, it will probably call for a new concept involving the use of different levels of evaluation in different types of test animals (Table 10-1). The first level would logically consist of a teratogenicity screen employing large numbers of a readily available animal, such as rat or mouse, for the purpose of finding a general embryotoxic range of dosage. A test substance causing no significant embryotoxicity at appropriate multiples of the anticipated human dose would be advanced to the second level of testing, in which a carnivore (dog, cat, or ferret), or an ungulate (pig or sheep) would be used, depending on which showed greater similarity to man in the metabolism of the compound in question. Information on metabolism could be accumulated in the course of routine pharmacologic studies. The higher costs and lower fecundity of this second test animal, e.g., dogs or pigs, would dictate the use of smaller numbers than in the initial screen, but this would be acceptable because the general range of effective dosage would already have been defined. Thus, the second level test would be for the purpose of confirming or revising embryotoxic dosage found at the first level, in a species that hopefully would metabolize the test substance more like man than did the rodent-type animal; but, in any event, the second animal would not have the atypical yolk-sac placenta of the earlier animal.

The results of the second level test could determine whether further animal investigation were necessary. If the compound caused no embryotoxicity in either first or second level tests at for example, 10 times expected human-use level, and it was a drug not likely to be used during pregnancy, it might be considered ready for clinical trial without further animal tests. If, however, there were uncertainty about the margin of safety between the dose that causes embryotoxicity in either the first or second level tests and the expected therapeutic dose in man; or if the compound were of a type that might involve use by or exposure of pregnant women, a third level of subprimate tests should be considered (Table 10-1), using an alternate species to that used at the second level.

A fourth level involving nonhuman primates would be recommended only for either of two specific situations: (1) drugs clearly needed to control severe discomfort or disease during pregnancy (e.g., anticonvulsants, hypoglycemics) or (2) drugs that are almost certain to be taken inadvertently during the early part of undiagnosed pregnancies (e.g., contraceptives, antihistaminics, tranquilizers). An additional type of situation might on occasion also justify use of primates for embryotoxicity testing. If, after a drug or an agricultural or household chemical had been approved and been in use for a time, there were reports that raised some question of a low level of embryotoxicity, intensive tests in pregnant primates with doses elevated well above human exposure levels might help resolve the problem. Otherwise, in view of the time and cost involved in such tests and of the limited supply of animals, the use of primates for routine embryotoxicity tests is not recommended.

Until all of the requisite data needed for a better test system are available, e.g., on maternal metabolism, on placental transfer, and on embryonic reaction, the following multilevel animal tests are proposed. The suggested procedures have not been arbitrarily chosen, but are based on principles discussed in earlier chapters and on the practical experience of the author and other investigators. The underlying objectives are:

1. To introduce treatment groups involving short-duration dosage so that maternal adaptative systems will not be activated, thereby avoiding the possibility of changing embryo dosage during more prolonged treatment.

2. To diversify the tests by utilizing at least two species of animals that

are not phylogenetically closely related, thereby increasing the chance that one will metabolize the test compound like man and reducing the uncertainties that stem from atypical placentation.

3. To demonstrate a minimal embryotoxic or threshold level of dosage in at least one, preferably in both, of two unrelated species to serve as a basis for extrapolating downward to an acceptable tolerance or safety level for human use.

4. To reserve the use of simian primates for agents specifically needed or likely to be taken inadvertently during human pregnancy, and possibly for intensive testing of approved agents about which question of safety has been raised after being marketed.

5. To make some effort toward evaluation of postnatal function, the minimum of which would be survival and growth for a few weeks or months after birth, with some observations during this period on locomotion and other coordinated movements.

II. Sample Protocols

A. SUGGESTED PROTOCOL FOR RODENT-RABBIT SPECIES—USING RAT AS PROTOTYPE

1. *Animals*

Any standard, random-bred strain of rat the reproductive characteristics of which are well known to the investigators is acceptable. Young virgin females of 200–250 gm begin to run regular 4–5 day cycles within a few days after arrival from the supplier. Animals obtained from a reputable supplier usually require no conditioning or medication unless subjected to mishandling in transit, e.g., extremes of temperature.

2. *Breeding and Timing of Pregnancy*

Females are examined by vaginal lavage late in the afternoon for signs of proestrus (75–90% of nucleated epithelial cells). Females in proestrus are singly placed overnight with an experienced male residing in a solid-bottom cage containing litter or shavings. As early as practicable the following morning vaginal lavage is examined for sperm or the presence of a vaginal plug. The plug is not as reliable an indicator of successful copulation in rats as it is in mice. The mean time of fertilization in laboratory maintained rats is between 9:00 and 10:00 AM of the morning after mating (Blandau, 1955), and it is appropriate to regard this as time 0 in timing subsequent procedures.

TABLE 10-2

NUMBERS OF PREGNANT RATS TREATED AT CONSECUTIVE 3-DAY PERIODS

Dose level	Gestation days		
	9–11	12–14	15–17
X[a]	10	10	10
X/2	10	10	10
X/4	10	10	10

[a] X, highest tolerated dose over 10-day period, or half of adult LD_{50}, or other appropriate effect-level.

3. *Treatment of Pregnant Females*

The period of major organogenesis extends from days 9 through 17. A screen consisting of three short-term treatment periods at three dosage levels is suggested to cover the greater part of this period (Table 10-2). Concurrent controls may be run with the short-term treatment if desired, but a vehicle control should in any case be run concurrently with the long-term dosage. If the lowest of the three initial doses causes embryotoxicity at any of the 3-day periods, smaller fractions of X (highest tolerated dose) should be tested until one producing no effect is found. The highest dose producing no embryotoxicity during any of these short-term dosage periods is used for a long-term dosage throughout organogenesis. Accordingly, 20 pregnant rats are treated daily at this dose and an equal number treated with vehicle only, from days 9 through 17 of gestation. Ten treated and 10 control litters on the long-term dosage should be examined for intrauterine embryotoxicity on day 20 of gestation. The remaining 10 treated and control litters should be allowed to deliver and the pups permitted to survive for at least 1 month postnatally. The occurrence of embryotoxicity in the 10 litters subjected to long-term treatment and examined on day 20 would require that lower doses be tested until one is found that causes no prenatal embryotoxicity. Poor survival, slow growth, or impaired muscular coordination during the postnatal period would also require that dosage be lowered until no such toxicity is observed. The highest dose causing neither prenatal embryotoxicity nor postnatal functional disturbance as evidenced by normal survival, growth and motor coordination is taken as the threshold.

4. *Examination of Offspring*

All females treated for 3-day periods should be killed on day 20 by any means that does not traumatize the fetuses, and should be opened immediately to inspect the uterus *in situ*. A general plan for examination of fetuses was presented in Chapter 9, Section I, C. Half of the females treated for the long-term period should similarly be killed and their fetuses examined on day 20. The remaining long-term litters should be allowed to deliver normally and the number of living and dead fetuses determined as soon after delivery as is feasible. Living young should be reduced to no more than 8 pups per litter and allowed to survive, with weekly weighing, for at least 1 month. All dead or moribund young prior to this time should be autopsied, as should all survivors at the end of the observation period. Locomotion and other coordinated motor activities should be observed with some care a day or two before autopsy.

B. SUGGESTED PROTOCOL FOR CARNIVOROUS SPECIES—USING DOG AS PROTOTYPE

This species has not been used in the author's laboratory, and the following protocol is based in part on one developed at Huntingdon Research Centre, information about which was supplied through the courtesy of A. K. Palmer.

1. Animals

Pure-bred beagles, or other small breeds, are inoculated against distemper, canine hepatitis, and leptospirosis, treated with anthelminthic, and subjected to thorough veterinary examination on arrival in the laboratory, or prior to the spring or autumn estrous period.

2. Breeding and Timing of Pregnancy

Estrous females are placed with males of proved fertility and observed for successful coitus on two or three occasions during the first 5 days of "heat." The day of first successful coitus is considered day 0 of pregnancy because the time of actual ovulation is not easily determined in this species, although a recent study indicates that most bitches ovulate on the second or third day of estrus, following by 2 days a sharp peak in luteinizing hormone values (Phemister et al., 1972). The examination of vaginal lavage for motile sperm after observed mating may be helpful in placing the time of fruitful matings.

3. Treatment of Pregnant Females

The period of major organogenesis extends from days 14 through 30. A screen based on four successive 4-day short-term sequences of treatment would adequately cover this period. Because the approximate embryotoxicity threshold dose (X) in a rodent-rabbit species will already be known, this and one higher dose (2X) in a few animals at each short-term treatment

TABLE 10-3

Numbers of Pregnant Dogs Treated at Consecutive 4-Day Periods

Dose level	Gestation days			
	14–17	18–21	22–25	26–29
X[a]	3	3	3	3
2X	3	3	3	3

[a] X, approximate embryotoxic threshold dose (mg/kg) found in rodent-rabbit screen.

period may be adequate to locate the threshold level in the dog (Table 10-3). If embryotoxicity is observed at any time with the smaller dose (X), lesser doses are tested until a no-effect level is found. If not, this level or the next highest short-term treatment level that is nonembryotoxic is used as the dosage level to be given daily throughout organogenesis (days 14 through 30) to 10 pregnant dogs. A similar number of concurrent controls is treated with vehicle for the same period. Half of the test and half of the control females should be killed or hysterotomized before term for fetal examinations and the remainder of each group allowed to litter normally for observations on postnatal study. Embryotoxicity or postnatal function deficit would call for testing a lower long-term dose. The lowest dose producing no prenatal embryotoxicity or postnatal indication of functional impairment is taken as the threshold level for dogs. If this does not agree with the threshold level previously determined for a rodent-rabbit species, the value for the species that metabolizes more like man the compound being tested is taken as the embryotoxicity threshold to be used in extrapolating downward to an acceptable safety level for man.

4. *Examination of Offspring*

All animals on the short-term dosage and half on the long-term treatment are killed or hysterotomized on day 50 and the uteri examined *in situ* for total implantation sites, that is, resorption sites plus those with viable young attached. Living fetuses are weighed, sexed, and examined externally and internally by gross dissection of all cavity organs. Skeletal visualization by x-ray before dissection or by KOH clearing after dissection should be done on all fetuses.

Litters delivered at term should be weighed weekly and allowed to survive for at least 2 months for evaluation of survival, growth, muscular coordination, and sensory modalities. Pups that die or become moribund should be x-rayed and autopsied, as should all pups at the end of the postnatal survival period.

C. SUGGESTED PROTOCOL FOR UNGULATES—USING PIG AS PROTOTYPE

This species has not been used in the author's laboratory and the protocol outlined below is based in part on one used at the Huntingdon Research Centre, details of which were supplied through the courtesy of A. K. Palmer.

1. *Animals*

Several pedigreed breeds are readily available from suppliers of agricultural stocks. So-called miniature breeds require less of the test material but these animals have at times been scarce and they are said to be less docile than standard breeds. A period of at least 3 weeks is recommended for adjustment of the females to new surroundings.

2. *Breeding and Timing of Pregnancy*

Regular 3-weekly estrous periods occur throughout most of the year in nonlactating animals. The investigator has a choice between artificial insemination and natural breeding, said to be about equally effective. The former might have some advantage from the standpoint of timing of pregnancy, with day 0 being taken as the time of known insemination. Pregnancy cannot be readily diagnosed until 21 days later when the next expected estrous period is missed. In the interest of saving time it would be well to have several back-up pregnancies to substitute for females on treatment that prove not to be pregnant.

3. *Treatment of Pregnant Females*

The period of major organogenesis extends from days 12 through 34 and can be adequately covered by five consecutive treatment spans of 4 days each (Table 10-4). If embryotoxicity is observed in the lowest (X) treatment group, smaller doses are tested until a no-effect level is found. The

TABLE 10-4

NUMBERS OF PREGNANT PIGS TREATED AT CONSECUTIVE 4-DAY PERIODS

Dose level	Gestation days				
	13–16	17–20	21–24	25–28	29–30
X[a]	3	3	3	3	3
2X	3	3	3	3	3

[a] X, approximate embryotoxic threshold dose (mg/kg) found in rodent-rabbit screen.

highest no-effect level is then given daily throughout organogenesis to 10 pregnant pigs and a similar number of vehicle-treated controls is run concurrently. Half of the test and half of the control females are killed before term and the remainder of each group allowed to deliver for postnatal study of piglets. Threshold level is determined as in dogs. If the threshold level in pig does not agree with that previously determined for a rodent-rabbit species, the value for the species that metabolizes the test compound more like man is taken as the embryotoxicity threshold to be used in extrapolating downward to an acceptable safety level for man.

4. *Examination of Offspring*

This is the same as for the dog except that fetal examination is made on day 70 of gestation. Piglets delivered at term are weighed weekly and observed for muscular coordination and sensory modalities for at least 2 months postnatally before they are killed, x-rayed, and autopsied.

D. Suggested Protocol for Simian Primates—Using Rhesus Monkey as Prototype

1. *Animals*

Several species of macaque monkeys and baboons are presently thought suitable for embryotoxicity testing, but they should be reserved for the special purposes discussed earlier, for the following reasons: (1) limited supply of breeding animals; (2) need for specially trained personnel; (3) susceptibility to human pathogens, particularly tuberculosis; and (4) low fecundity. Newly arrived breeding stock must be maintained in quarantine for 2 or 3 months (Kaufmann, 1972) before being put on observation for reproductive cycles. Unless they are ready for breeding during the autumn or early winter (the natural breeding period) newly acquired animals are likely not to breed for several months, although after living under constant conditions in the laboratory for 1 or 2 years they tend to lose the seasonal breeding pattern and may run ovulatory cycles throughout the year.

2. *Breeding and Timing of Pregnancy*

No practicable means for determining the time of ovulation is yet available, perhaps excepting laparoscopic visualization of the ovaries, although acceptable results are had in rhesus monkeys by placing regularly cycling females with an experienced male from days 11 to 13 of the menstrual cycle. Vaginal lavage is examined on the morning of days 12 and 13, or after observed matings, and the day on which sperm are first observed is regarded as day 0 of pregnancy. Pregnancy is diagnosed occasionally as early as day

TABLE 10-5

Major Developmental Events at Each of the Five 4-Day Treatment Periods
Proposed for the Embryotoxicity Screen in Rhesus Monkeys

Four-day treatment period (gestation days)[a]	Developmental events
20–23	One to eleven pairs of somites, neural folds and early neural tube, heart primordia appear
24–27	Neural tube closes, brain vesicles form, branchial arches develop, heart chambers indicated, limb buds appear
28–31	Optic cup and lens forming, pharyngeal region differentiates, heart septation begins, midgut loop herniates
32–35	Face and sense organs form, heart septa completed, ureteric buds dividing, cartilaginous skeleton appears, digital rays present
42–45	Palate closing, skeletal ossification begins, renal glomeruli forming, external genitals developing

[a] Days 36 through 41 are not included in this preliminary screen because, although important histogenesis begins in several organs, no highly vulnerable organogenetic events are known to occur. This period is covered in the long-term dosage schedule (see text).

16 and regularly on day 18 or 19 (Wilson *et al.*, 1970) by chorionic gona-dotropin assay in mice, or by other proved methods. By the expediency of performing hysterotomy on day 100 of gestation, regularly cycling females may produce two pregnancies each year. Hysterotomy has been repeated as many as 7 times on some females in the author's breeding colony without untoward effect.

TABLE 10-6

Number of Pregnant Monkeys Treated at Consecutive 4-Day Periods

Dose level	Gestation days				
	20–23	24–27	28–31	32–35	42–45
HTD[a]	2	2	2	2	2
X[b]	2	2	2	2	2

[a] HTD, highest tolerated dose (25 days in nonpregnant monkey), in view of anticipated use during human pregnancy.

[b] X, embryotoxic threshold level (mg/kg) in subprimate species most like man in metabolism of test compound.

3. *Treatment of Pregnant Females*

The period of major organogenesis extends from days 20 through 45 of gestation. This can be dividied into five periods of 4 consecutive days each that will include most of the important organogenetic events (Table 10-5). A minimum of 2 pregnant females for each period at each of two dose levels is suggested (Table 10-6). These pregnancies are interrupted at 100 days and the fetuses removed by hysterotomy for fetal examination as described below, in Chapter 9, Section I,C, and elsewhere (Wilson *et al.,* 1970). If no embryotoxicity occurs at the highest tolerated dose (HTD) for any 4-day period, no smaller dose need be tested in short-term treatment and the HTD should be given daily throughout organogenesis to 10 pregnant monkeys, with a similar number of monkeys given concurrently the vehicle only for a similar period. If the HTD in short-term dosage produces embryotoxicity at any treatment period, the threshold value (X) in the subprimate species metabolizing the test compound most like man should be tested in monkeys indicated in Table 10-6. In case no embryotoxicity is observed at this level, it should be used in long-term dosage from days 20 through 45.

When embryotoxicity occurs in primates at the subprimate threshold dose, it is necessary to consider anticipated human use or exposure level, and whether the demonstrated embryotoxic level was sufficiently high above the former to permit an acceptable margin of safety. The existence of a large embryotoxic to human use ratio might warrant proceeding to find a nonembryotoxic, short-term level in primates that would then be used in the long-term and postnatal studies to find the highest no-effect level. No routine extrapolation to an acceptable use level is proposed here, however; all agents reaching this stage of testing, presumably all drugs urgently needed during human pregnancy, must be subjected to rigorous benefit-to-risk evaluation. In other words, scientific judgment and not laboratory data should be the basis for the final decision.

4. *Examination of Offspring*

All pregnancies on short-term treatment and half of the test and half of the control pregnancies on long-term treatment are to be interrupted on day 100 of gestation and the fetuses examined grossly, autopsied, and x-rayed or cleared for skeletal study. The remaining pregnancies are allowed to go to normal delivery and the young weighed weekly and observed for behavior, muscular coordination, and sensory modalities for at least 3 months postnatally. At the end of this observation period surviving young should be x-rayed and autopsied.

SELECTED REFERENCES ON EMBRYOLOGY AND REPRODUCTION OF LABORATORY ANIMALS

I. Mouse

Allen, E. (1922). Estrous cycle of the mouse. *Amer. J. Anat.* **30**, 297–371.

Allen, E., and MacDowell, E. C. (1940). Variations in mouse embryos of eight days gestation. *Anat. Rec.* **77**, 165–173.

Balinsky, B. I. (1950). On the prenatal growth of the mammary gland rudiment in the mouse. *J. Anat.* **84**, 227–235.

Bonnevie, K. (1950). New facts on mesoderm formation and proamnion derivatives in the normal mouse embryo. *J. Morphol.* **86**, 495–545.

Chen, J. M. (1952). Studies on the morphogenesis of the mouse sternum. I. Normal embryonic development. *J. Anat.* **86**, 373–386.

Dagg, C. P. (1966). Teratogenesis. *In* "Biology of the Laboratory Mouse" (E. L. Green, ed.), 2nd ed., Chapter 14, pp. 309–328. McGraw-Hill, New York.

Dickson, A. D. (1966). The form of the mouse blastocyst. *J. Anat.* **100**, 335–348.

Farbmann, A. I. (1968). Electron microscope study of palate fusion in mouse embryos. *Develop. Biol.* **18**, 93–116.

Forsthoefel, P. F. (1963). Observations on the sequence of blastemal condensations in the limbs of the mouse embryo. *Anat. Rec.* **147**, 129–130.

Frommer, J. (1964). Prenatal development of the mandibular joint in mice. *Anat. Rec.* **150**, 449–461.

Grüneberg, H. (1943). The development of some external features in mouse embryos. *J. Heredity* **34**, 88–92.

Grüneberg, H. (1963). "The Pathology of Development." Wiley, New York.

Healy, M. J. R., McLaren, A., and Mitchie, D. (1961). Fetal growth in the mouse. *Proc. Roy. Soc. Ser. B* **153**, 367.

Hoshino, K. (1967). Comparative study on the skeletal development in the fetus of rat and mouse. *Congen. Anomalies (Japan)* **7**, 32–38.

Johnson, M. L. (1933). The time and order of appearance of ossification centers in the albino mouse. *Amer. J. Anat.* **52**, 241–271.

MacDowell, E. C., Allen, E., and MacDowell, C. G. (1927). The prenatal growth of the mouse. *J. Gen. Physiol.* **11**, 57–70.

McLaren, A., and Michie, D. (1960). Control of prenatal growth in mammals. *Nature (London)* **187**, 363–365.

Mintz, B. (1960). Embryological phases of mammalian gametogenesis. *J. Cell. Comp. Physiol. Suppl. 1,* **56**, 31–47.

Ogawa, T. (1967). Comparative study on development in the stage of organogenesis in the mouse and rat. *Congen. Anomalies (Japan)* **7**, 27–31.

Otis, E. M., and Brent, R. (1954). Equivalent ages in mouse and human embryos. *Anat. Rec.* **120**, 33–63.

Rugh, R. (1964). "Vertebrate Embryology; The Dynamics of Development." Harcourt, Brace, New York.

Rugh, R. (1968). "The Mouse, Its Reproduction and Development." Burgess, Minneapolis, Minnesota.

Sano, M., and Sasaki, F. (1969). Embryonic development of the mouse anterior pituitary studied by light and electron microscopy. *Z. Anat. Entwickl.-Gesch.* **129**, 195–222.

Smiley, G. R. (1967). A profile cephalometric appraisal of normal growth parameters in embryonic mice. *Anat. Rec.* **157**, 323.

Snell, G. D., and Stevens, L. C. (1966). Early embryology. In "Biology of the Laboratory Mouse" (E. L. Green, ed.), Chapter 12, 2nd ed., pp. 205–245. McGraw-Hill, New York.

Turner, C. W., and Gomez, E. T. (1933). The normal development of the mammary gland of the male and female albino mouse. I. Intrauterine II. Extrauterine. *Res. Bull. Mo. Agric. Exp. Sta. No. 182.*

Walker, B. E., and Fraser, F. C. (1956). Closure of the secondary palate in three strains of mice. *J. Embryol. Exp. Morphol.* **4**, 176–189.

Wessells, N. K., and Cohen, J. H. (1967). Early pancreas organogenesis: morphogenesis, tissue interactions, and mass effects. *Develop. Biol.* **15**, 237–270.

Wirtschafter, Z. T. (1960). The genesis of the mouse skeleton. "A Laboratory Atlas." Thomas, Springfield, Illinois.

II. Hamster

Adams, F. W., and Hillemann, H. H. (1950). Morphogenesis of the vitelline and allantoic placentae of the golden hamster *(Cricetus auratus)*. *Anat. Rec.* **108**, 363–383.

Boyer, C. C. (1948). Development of the golden hamster, *Cricetus auratus,* with special references to the major circulatory channels. *J. Morphol.* **83**, 1–38.

Boyer, C. C. (1953). Chronology of development for the golden hamster. *J. Morphol.* **92**, 1.

Einerth, Y., and Forsberg, J. G. (1959). On the development and regression of the Müllerian ducts in the male hamster. *Acta Morphol. Neer. Scand.* **2**, 379–385.

Foote, C. L., Norman, W. P., and Foote, F. M. (1954). Formation of the extra-embryonic cavities of the hamster. *Amer. J. Anat.* **95**, 291–307.

Forsberg, J-G. (1960). On the development of the hamster vagina, *Acta Anat.* **41**, 16–37.

Graves, A. P. (1945). Development of the golden hamster, *Cricetus auratus waterhouse,* during the first nine days. *Amer. J. Anat.* **77**, 219–251.

Lavelle, F. W. (1951). A study of hormonal factors in the early sex development of the golden hamster. *Carnegie Contrib. Embryol.* **34**, 19–53.

Oritz, E. (1945). The embryological development of the Wolffian and Müllerian ducts and the accessory reproductive organs of the golden hamster *(Cricetus auratus). Anat. Rec.* **92**, 371–387.

Oritz, E. (1947). The postnatal development of the reproductive system of the golden hamster *(Cricetus auratus)* and its reactivity to hormones. *Physiol. Zool.* **20**, 45–67.

Purdy, D. M., and Hillemann, H. H. (1950). Volume changes in the amniotic fluid of the golden hamster *(Cricetus auratus). Anat. Rec.* **106**, 571.

Purdy, D. M., and Hillemann, H. H. (1950). Prenatal growth in the golden hamster *(Cricetus auretus). Anat. Rec.* **106**, 591.

Ramm, G. M., and Swartz, G. E. (1955). The development of the hamster metanephros correlated with general body growth and compared with the metanephroi of other species. *Anat. Rec.* **123**, 259–277.

III. Rat

Addison, W. H. F., and How, H. W. (1921). The development of the eyelids of the albino rat, until completion of disjunction. *Amer. J. Anat.* **29**, 1–31.

Adelmann, H. B. (1925). The development of the neural folds and cranial ganglia of the rat. *J. Comp. Neurol.* **39**, 19–171.

Alden, R. H. (1948). Implantation of the rat egg. III. Origin and development of primary trophoblast giant cells. *Amer. J. Anat.* **83**, 143–181.

Angulo, A. W. (1932). The prenatal growth of the albino rat. *Anat. Rec.* **52**, 117–138.

Barr, M., Jr., Jensh, R. P., and Brent, R. L. (1970). Prenatal growth in the albino rat: Effects of number, intrauterine position and resorptions. *Amer. J. Anat.* **128**, 413–428.

Bartelmez, G. W. (1962). The proliferation of neural crest from forebrain levels in the rat. *Contrib. Embryol. Carnegie Inst. Wash.* **37**, 1–12.

Bhaskar, S. N. (1953). Growth patterns of the rat mandible from 13 days insemination age to 30 days after birth. *Amer. J. Anat.* **92**, 1–53.

Booneville, M. A. (1968). Observation on epidermal differentiation in the fetal rat. *Amer. J. Anat.* **123**, 147–164.

Brock, N., and von Kreybig, T. (1964). Teratogenese als pharmakologisch-toxikologisches Problem. I. Allgemeine Grundlagen: Normale Embryonalentwicklung von Ratte and Meerschweinchen. *Arzneimittelforsch.* **14**, 655–664.

Burlingame, P. L., and Long, J. A. (1939). The development of the heart in the rat. *Univ. Calif. Publ. Zool.* **43**, 249–320.

Christie, G. A. (1964). Developmental stages in somite and post-somite rat embryos, based on external appearance, and including some features of macroscopic development of the oral cavity. *J. Morphol.* **114**, 263–286.

Coleman, R. D. (1965). Development of the rat palate. *Anat. Rec.* **151**, 107–118.

Edwards, J. A. (1968). The external development of the rabbit and rat embryo. *Advan. Teratol.* **3**, 239–263.

Forsberg, J-G. (1961). On the development of the cloaca and perineum and the formation of the urethral plate in female rat embryos. *J. Anat.* **95**, 423–436.

Hafez, E. S. E. (1970). "Reproduction and Breeding Techniques for Laboratory Animals." Lea and Febiger, Philadelphia, Pennsylvania.

Henneberg, B. (1926). Beitrag zur ontogenetischen Entwicklung des Scrotums und der Labia majora. *Z. Anat. Entwickl.-Gesch.* **81**, 198–219.

Henneberg, B. (1937). Normaltafel zur Entwicklungsgeschichte der Wanderratte *(Rattus norvegicus* Erxleben). "Normaltafeln zur Entwicklungsgeschichte der Wirbeltiere." (F. Keibel, ed.), Vol. 15. Gustav Fischer Verlag, Jena.

Huber, G. C. (1915). The development of the albino rat, *Mus norvegicus albinus. J. Morphol.* **26**, 247–358.

Keibel, F. (1937). "Normentafeln zur Entwicklungsgeschichte der Wanderratte." Gustav Fischer Verlag, Jena.

Lejour-Jeanty, M. (1965). The morphologic and cytochemical study of the development of the primary palate in the rat. *Arch. Biol.* **76**, 9–168.

Long, J. A., and Burlingame, P. L. (1938). The development of the external form of the rat with observations on the origin of the extraembryonic coelom and fetal membranes. *Univ. Calif. Publ. Zool.* **43**, 148–184.

Moffat, D. B. (1959). Developmental changes in the aortic arch system of the rat. *Amer. J. Anat.* **105**, 1–35.

Myers, J. A. (1917). Studies on the mammary gland. II. The fetal development of the mammary gland in the female albino rat. *Amer. J. Anat.* **22**, 195–223.

Odor, D. L., and Blandau, R. J. (1951). Observations on fertilization and the first segmentation division in rat ova. *Amer. J. Anat.* **89**, 29–61.

Price, D. (1936). Normal development of the prostate and seminal vesicles of the rat with a study of experimental postnatal modifications. *Amer. J. Anat.* **60**, 79–128.

Puchkov, N. F. (1957). Equivalent embryonic ages of chick, rat and man. *Dokl. Akad. Nauk S.S.S.R. Biol. Sci. Sect. Transl.* **125**, 221–224.

Rogers, W. M. (1929). The development of the pharynx and the pharyngeal derivatives in the white rat *(Mus norvegicus albinus). Amer. J. Anat.* **44**, 283–329.

Schmidt, W., and von Kreybig, T. (1965). Die vorgeburtliche Entwicklung der Gonaden der Ratte. *Z. Anat. Entwickl.-Gesch.* **124**, 588–600.

Schwind, J. L. (1928). The development of the hypophysis cerebri of the albino rat. *Amer. J. Anat.* **41**, 295–319.

Shearer, E. M. (1933). The development of the arteries in the anterior limb of the albino rat. *Amer. J. Anat.* **53**, 427–467.

Shepard, T. H., Lemire, R. J., Aksu, O., and Mackler, B. (1968). Studies of the development of congenital anomalies in embryos of riboflavin-deficient, galactoflavin fed rats. I. Growth and embryologic pathology. *Teratology* **1**, 75–92.

Shepard, T. H., Tanimura, T., and Robkin, M. A. (1970). Energy metabolism in early mammalian embryos. *Develop. Biol. Suppl.* **4**, 42–58.

Spark, C., and Dawson, A. B. (1928). The order and time of appearance of centers of ossification in the fore and hind limbs of the albino rat, with special reference to the possible influence of the sex factor. *Amer. J. Anat.* **41**, 411–445.

Stotsenberg, J. M. (1915). The growth of the fetus of the albino rat from the thirteenth to the twenty-second day of gestation. *Anat. Rec.* **9**, 667–682.

Strong, R. M. (1925). The order, time and rate of ossification of the albino rat *(Mus norvegicus albinus)* skeleton. *Amer. J. Anat.* **36**, 313–355.

Torrey, T. W. (1943). The development of the urogenital system of the albino rat. I. The kidney and its ducts. *Amer. J. Anat.* **72**, 113–144.

Torrey, T. W. (1945). The development of the urogenital system of the albino rat. II. The gonads. *Amer. J. Anat.* **76**, 375–397.

Torrey, T. W. (1947). The development of the urogenital system of the albino rat. III. The urogenital union. *Amer. J. Anat.* **81**, 139–153.

Wilson, J. G., and Warkany, J. (1948). Malformations in the genito-urinary tract induced by maternal vitamin A deficiency in the rat. *Amer. J. Anat.* **83**, 357–407.

Wilson, J. G., and Warkany, J. (1949). Aortic-arch and cardiac anomalies in the offspring of vitamin A deficient rats. *Amer. J. Anat.* **85**, 113–155.

Witschi, E. (1962). *Development:* Rat. *In* "Growth, Including Reproduction and Morphological Development" (P. L. Altman and D. S. Dittmer, eds.), pp. 304–314. Fed. of Amer. Soc. for Exp. Biol., Washington, D.C.

Wright, H. V., Asling, C. W., Dougherty, H. L., Nelson, M. M., and Evans, H. M. (1958). Prenatal development of the skeleton in Long-Evans rats. *Anat. Rec.* **130**, 659–672.

IV. Rabbit

Assar, Y. H. (1931). The history of the prochordal plate in the rabbit. *J. Anat.* **66**, pt. 1, 14–45.

Assheton, R. (1894). A reinvestigation in the early stages of the development of the rabbit. *Quart. J. Microsc. Sci.* **37**, 113–164.

Atwell, W. J. (1918). The development of the hypophysis cerebri of the rabbit *(Lepus cuniculus L.)*. *Amer. J. Anat.* **24**, 271–337.

Baden, W. (1927). Zur Entwicklung der äusseren Genitalien des Kaninchens. II. Über die Entwicklung der Klitoris beim Kaninchen. *Z. Anat. Entwickl.-Gesch.* **84**, 334–413.

Berke, J. P. (1965). The development of the rostral neuraxis and neural crest in the rabbit embryo up to 16 somites. *Bol. Inst. Estud. Med. Biol. Univ. Nac. Mex.* **23**, 185–212.

Bruce, J. A. (1941). Time and order of appearance of ossification centers and their development in the skull of the rabbit. *Amer. J. Anat.* **68**, 41–67.

Chaine, J. (1911). "Tableaux synoptiques du développement du lapin." L'Homme, Paris.

Crary, D. D. (1964). Development of the external ear in the Dachs rabbit. *Anat. Rec.* **150**, 441–448.

Crary, D. D., and Sawin, P. B. (1957). Morphogenetic studies of the rabbit. XVIII. Growth of ossification centers of the vertebral centra during the 21st day. *Anat. Rec.* **127**, 131–150.

Davies, J., and Routh, J. I. (1957). Composition of the foetal fluids of the rabbit. *J. Embryol. Exp. Morphol.* **5**, 32–39.

Elchlepp, J. G. (1952). The urogenital organs of the cotton tail rabbits *(Sylvilagus floridanus)*. *J. Morphol.* **91**, 169–198.

Fuchs, H. (1905). Zur Entwicklungsgeschichte des Wirbeltierauges. I. Über die Entwicklung der Augengefässe des Kaninchens. *Anat. Hefte* **28**, 1–251.

Gottschewski, G. H. M. (1967). Embryonal development of the rabbit. *Zeiss* **14**, 128–131.

Gottschewski, G. H. M. (1970). Analyse der Säugertierembryonalentwicklung. *Naturwissenehaften. Rdsch.* 23 Jahrg. Heft 4, pp. 132–143.

Gregory, P. W. (1930). Development of the rabbit embryo. *Carnegie Contrib. Embryol.* **21**, 141–168.

Günther, G. (1927). Zur Entwicklung der äusseren Genitalien des Kaninchens. I. Über die Entwicklung des Penis beim Kaninchen. *Z. Anat. Entwickl.-Gesch.* **84**, 275–333.

Hunter, R. M. (1935). The development of the anterior post-otic somites in the rabbit. *J. Morphol.* **57**, 501–532.
 Arch. Anat. Microsc. Morph. Exp. **36**, 151–200, 242–270, 271–315.
Jost, A. (1947). Recherches sur la différentiation sexuelle de l'embryon de lapin.
Leeson, T. S., and Baxter, J. S. (1957). The correlation of structure and function in the mesonephros and metanephros of the rabbit. *J. Anat.* **91**, 383–390.
Leeson, T. S., and Leeson, C. R. (1958). Observations on the histochemistry and fine structure of the notochord in rabbit embryos. *J. Anat.* **92**, 278–285.
Minot, C. S., and Taylor, E. (1905). Normal plates of the development of the rabbit *(Lepus cuniculus L.).* "Normaltafeln zur Entwicklungsgeschichte der Wirbeltiere," Vol. 5. Fischer, Jena.
Rosahn, P. D., and Greene, H. S. N. (1936). The influence of intrauterine factors on the fetal weight of rabbits. *J. Exp. Med.* **63**, 901–921.
Sawin, P. B., and Crary, D. D. (1956). Morphogenetic studies of the rabbit. XVI. Quantitative racial differences in ossification pattern of the vertebrae of embryos as an approach to basic principles of mammalian growth. *Amer. J. Phys. Anthropol.* **14**, 625–648.
Togari, C., Sugiyama, S., and Sawasaki, Y. (1952). On the prenatal histogenesis of the thyroid gland of the rabbit with special emphasis on its histometrical measurements. *Anat. Rec.* **114**, 213–229.
Waterman, A. J. (1943). Studies of normal development of the New Zealand white strain of rabbit. I. Oogenesis. II. External morphology of the embryo. *Amer. J. Anat.* **72**, 473–515.
Zimmerman, W. (1964). Methoden für experimentelle Untersuchungen am Kaninchen während der Frühen Embryonalentwicklung. *Zbl. Bakt.* **194**, 255–266.

V. Guinea Pig

Amoroso, E. C. (1959). The attachment cone of the guinea pig blastocyst as observed under time lapse phase-contrast cinematography. In: Implantation of ova. *Mem. Soc. Endocrinol.* **6**, 50–53.
Blandau, R. J. (1949). Observations on implantation of the guinea pig ovum. *Anat. Rec.* **103**, 19–47.
Blandau, R. J. (1949). Embryo-endometrial interrelationship in the rat and guinea pig. *Anat. Rec.* **104**, 331–360.
Bookhout, C. G. (1945). The development of the guinea pig ovary from sexual differentiation to maturity. *J. Morphol.* **77**, 233.
Brock, N., von Kreybig, T. (1964). Teratogenese als pharmakologischtoxikologisches Problem. I. Allgemeine Grundlagen: Normale Embryonalentwicklung von Ratte und Meerschweinchen. *Arzneimittelforsch.* **14**, 655–664.
Broman, I. (1949). Über die Embryonalentwicklung der Blinddärme bei *Procavia. Acta. Anat.* **7**, 86–126.
Draper, R. L. (1920). The prenatal growth of the guinea pig. *Anat. Rec.* **18**, 369–392.
Eaton, O. N. (1932). Correlation of hereditary and other factors affecting growth of guinea pigs. *U. S. Dept. Agr. Bull.* **279**, 1–35.
Gruber, C. (1906). Bau und Entwicklung der äusseren Genitalien bei *Cavia cobaya. Gegenb. Morphol. Jb.* **36**, 3–26.

Harman, M. T., and Derbyshire, R. C. (1932). The development of the suprarenal glands in the guinea-pig *(Cavia cobaya)*. *Amer. J. Anat.* **49**, 335–349.

Harman, M. T., and Prickett, M. (1932). The development of the external form of the guinea pig *(Cavia cobaya)* between the ages of eleven days and twenty days of gestation. *Amer. J. Anat.* **49**, 351–378.

Harman, M. T., and Dobrovolny, M. P. (1933). The development of the external form of the guinea pig *(Cavia cobayas)* between the ages of twenty one days and thirty five days of gestation. *J. Morphol.* **54**, 439–519.

Harman, M. T., and Saffrey, O. B. (1934). The skeletal development of the anterior limb of the guinea pig, *Cavia cobaya*, from the 25-day embryo to the 161-day post natal guinea pig. *Amer. J. Anat.* **54**, 315–331.

Harman, M. T., and Smith, A. (1936). Some observations on the development of the teeth of *Cavia cobaya*. *Anat. Rec.* **66**, 97–111.

Hill, J. P., and Sansom, G. S. (1929). Observations on the structure and mode of implantation of the blastocyst of *Cavia*. *J. Anat.* **64**, 113–115.

Hunter, R. H. F., Hunt, D. M., and Chang, M. C. (1969). Temporal and cytological aspects of fertilization and early development in the guinea pig, *Cavia porcellus*. *Anat. Rec.* **165**, 411–429.

Ibsen, H. L. (1928). Prenatal growth in guinea pigs with special reference to environmental factors affecting weight at birth. *J. Exp. Zool.* **51**, 51–91.

Kennedy, J. A., and Clark, S. L. (1941). Observations on the ductus arteriosus of the guinea pig in relation to its method of closure. *Anat. Rec.* **79**, 349–371.

Klapper, C. E. (1946a). The development of the pharynx of the guinea pig with special emphasis on the morphogenesis of the thymus. *Amer. J. Anat.* **78**, 139–180.

Klapper, C. E. (1946b). The development of the pharynx of the guinea pig with special emphasis on the fate of the ultimo-bronchial body. *Amer. J. Anat.* **79**, 361–398.

Lohle, B. (1913). Die Bildung des Gaumens bei *Cavia cobaya*. *Gegenb. Morphol. Jb.* **46**, 595–654.

Maclaren, N. (1926). Development of *Cavia:* Implantation. *Trans. Roy. Soc. Edinburgh* **55**, 115–123.

Moog, F., and Ortiz, E. (1960). The functional differentiation of the small intestine. VII. The duodenum of the fetal guinea pig, with a note on the growth of the adrenals. *J. Embryol. Exp. Morphol.* **8**, 182–194.

Payne, P. R., and Wheeler, E. F. (1967). Growth of the foetus. *Nature (London)* **215**, 849–850.

Rabl, H. (1927). Die Entwicklung der form der Zunge und des Kihlkopfeinganges beim Meerschweinchen. *Z. Anat. Entwickl.-Gesch.* **83**, 1–44.

Rajtova, V. (1967). The development of the skeleton in the guinea pig: II. The morphogenesis of the carpus in the guinea pig *(Cavia porcellus)*. *Folia Morphol.* **15**, 132–139.

Rajtova, V. (1967). The skeletogeny of the guinea pig: III. Prenatal and postnatal ossification of the skeleton of the pelvic limb. *Folia Morphol.* **15**, 258–267.

Rajtova, V. (1968). Development of the skeleton in the guinea pig: IV. Morphogenesis of the tarsus in the guinea pig *(Cavia porcellus)*. *Folia Morph.* **16**, 162–170.

Rajtova, V. (1968). The development of the skeleton in the guinea pig: V. Prenatal and postnatal ossification of the axial skeleton in the *Cavia porcellus*. *Folia Morph.* **16**, 233–243.

Rajtova, V. (1969). The development of the skeleton of the guinea pig: VI. Prenatal and postnatal ossification of the bones of the neurocranium in the guinea pig *(Cavia porcellus L.)*. Folia Morphol. **17**, 48–55. VII. Prenatal and postnatal ossification of bones of the splanchnocranium in the guinea pig *(Cavia porcellus L.)*. *Folia Morphol.* **17**, 56–65.

Sansom, G. S., and Hill, J. P. (1931). Observations on the structure and mode of implantation of the blastocyst of cavia. *Trans. Soc. Zool.* **21**, 295–354.

Scott, J. P. (1937). The embryology of the guinea pig. I. A table of normal development. *Amer. J. Anat.* **60**, 397–432.

Squier, R. R. (1932). The living egg and early stages of its development in the ginea

Squier, R. R. (1932). The living egg and early stages of its development in the guinea pig. *Carnegie Contrib. Embryol.* **23**, 225–250.

Turner, C. W., and Gomez, E. T. (1933). The normal development of the mammary gland of the male and female guinea pig. Res. Bull. Mo. Agr. Exp. Sta. No. 194.

Yoshinaga, T. (1921). A contribution to the early development of the heart in mammalia, with special reference to the guinea pig. *Anat. Rec.* **21**, 239–308.

VI. Pig

Baker, L. N., Chapman, A. B., Grummer, R. H., and Casida, L. E. (1958). Some factors affecting litter size and fetal weight in purebred and reciprocal cross matings of Chester White and Poland China swine. *J. Anim. Sci.* **17**, 612–621.

Berton, J. P. (1965). Anatomie vasculaire du mésonéphros chez certains mammifères. I. Le mésonéphros de l'embryon de porc. *C. R Ass. Anat.* **124**, 272–290.

Broman, I. (1946). Über die Entstehung und sekundäre Verschiebung der äusseren Geschlechtsteile beim Schwein. *Acta Anat.* **1**, 418–440.

Done, J. T., and Hebert, C. N. (1968). The growth of the cerebellum in the foetal pig. *Res. Vet. Sci.* **9**, 143–148.

Durbeck, W. (1907). Die äusseren Genitalien des Schweines. *Gegenb. Morphol. Jb.* **36**, 517–543.

Glenister, T. W. (1956). The development of the penile urethra in the pig. *J. Anat.* **90**, 461–477.

Jost, A. (1947). Recherches sur la differentiation sexuelle de l'embryon de lapin. *ton Contrib. Embryol.* **21**, 141–168.

Green, W. W., and Winters, L. M. (1946). Cleavage and attachment stages of the pig. *J. Morphol.* **78**, 305–316.

Hafez, E. S. E. (1958). Reproduction, placentation and prenatal development in swine as affected by nutritional environment. *J. Anim. Sci.* **17**, 1212.

Hafez, E. S. E., Ed. (1968). "Reproduction in Farm Animals," 2nd ed. Lea and Febiger, Philadelphia, Pennsylvania.

Henneberg, B. (1922). Anatomie und Entwicklung der äusseren Genitalorgane des Schweines und vergleichend-anatomische Bemerkungen. I. Weibliches Schwein. *Z. Anat. Entwickl.-Gesch.* **63**, 431–494.

Henneberg, B. (1925). Anatomie und Entwicklung der äusseren Genitalorgane des Schweines und vergleichend-anatomische Bemerkungen. II. Männliches Schwein. *Z. Anat. Entwickl.-Gesch.* **75**, 265–318.

Heuser, C. H. (1923). The branchial vessels and their derivatives in the pig. *Carnegie Contrib. Embryol.* **15**, 121–139.

Heuser, C. H. (1927). A study of the implantation of the ovum of the pig from the stage of the bilaminar blastocyst to the completion of the fetal membranes. *Carnegie Contrib. Embryol.* **19**, 229–243.

Heuser, C. H., and Streeter, G. L. (1929). Early stages in the development of pig embryos, from the period of initial cleavage to the time of the appearance of limb buds. *Carnegie Contrib. Embryol.* **20**, 1–29.

Hodges, P. C. (1953). Ossification in the fetal pig. A radiographic study. *Anat. Rec.* **116**, 315–325.

Jung, P. (1937). Die Entwicklung des Schweine-Eierstockes bis zur Geburt. *Z. Mikro-Anat. Forsch.* **41**, 27–74.

Keibel, F. (1897). "Normaltafeln zur Entwicklungsgeschichte der Wirbeltiere," Vol. I, Normaltafel zur Entwicklungsgeschichte des Schweines *(Sus scrofa domesticus).* Fischer, Jena.

Kelly, G. L. (1928). Additional observations on internal migration of the ovum in the sow and in the ginea pig. *Anat. Rec.* **40**, 365–372.

Kemp, N. E. (1962). Development: Swine: *In* "Growth, Including Reproduction and Morphological Development" (P. L. Altman and D. S. Dittmer, eds.), pp. 299–303. Fed. of Amer. Soc. for Exp. Biol., Washington, D. C.

Kempermann, C. T. (1934). Beiträge zur Entwicklung des Genitaltraktus der Säuger. II. Die Entwicklung der Vagina des Hausschweines bis drei Tage nach dem Wurf. *Gegenb. Morphol. Jb.* **74**, 221–261.

Larsell, O. (1954). The development of the cerebellum of the pig. *Anat. Rec.* **118**, 73–107.

Lenkeit, W. (1927). Über das Wachstum des Bruskorbes und der Brustorgane (Herz, Lunge, Thymus) während der Entwicklung beim Schweine. *Z. Anat. Entwickl.-Gesch.* **82**, 605–642.

Lowrey, L. G. (1911). Prenatal growth of the pig. *Amer. J. Anat.* **12**, 107–138.

Marrable, A. W. (1971). "The Embryonic Pig, a Chronological Account." Pitman Publ., New York.

Marrable, A. W., and Ashdown, R. R. (1967). Quantitative observations on pig embryos of known ages. *J. Agr. Sci.* **69**, 443–447.

Mead, C. S. (1909). The chondrocranium of an embryo pig, *Sus scrofa. Amer. J. Anat.* **9**, 167–209.

Patten, B. M. (1948). *"Embryology of the Pig,"* 3rd ed. Blakiston, New York.

Perry, J. S., and Rowell, J. G. (1969). Variations in foetal weight and vascular supply along the uterine horn of the pig. *J. Reprod. Fertil.* **19**, 527–534.

Rugh, R. (1964). "Vertebrate Embryology: The Dynamics of Development," Chapter 7, The pig: a diffuse placentate, pp. 305–377. Harcourt, New York.

Sabin, F. R. (1911). A critical study of the evidence presented in several recent articles on the development of the lymphatic system. *Anat. Rec.* **5**, 417–446.

Sabin, F. R. (1917). Origin and development of the primitive vessels of the chick and pig. *Carnegie Contrib. Embryol.* **6**, 61–124.

Sajonski, H., Smollich, A., and Suckow, M. (1965). Beitrag zur quantitativen Organentwicklung (Herz, Lunge, Leber, Niere, Milz) des Schweines während der Fetalzeit. *Mh. Vet. Med.* **20**, 696–703.

Shanklin, W. M. (1944). Histogenesis of the pig neurohypophysis. *Amer. J. Anat.* **74**, 327–353.

Thyng, F. W. (1911). The anatomy of a 7.8 mm pig embryo. *Anat. Rec.* **5**, 17–45.

Ulbrey, D. E., Sprague, J. I., Becker, D. E., and Miller, E. R. (1965). Growth of the swine fetus. *J. Anim. Sci.* **24**, 711–717.

Vogler, A. (1926). Intrauterine Verknöcherung der Ossa faciei des Schweines. *Gegenb. Morphol. Jb.* **55**, 568–606.

Waldorf, D. P., Foote, W. C., Self, H. L., Chapman, A. B., and Casida, L. E. (1957). Factors affecting fetal pig weight late in gestation. *J. Anim. Sci.* **16**, 976–985.

Warwick, B. L. (1928). Prenatal growth of the swine. *J. Morphol. Physiol.* **46**, 59–84.

Wenham, G., McDonald, I., and Elsley, F. W. H. (1969). A radiographic study of the skeleton of the fetal pig. *J. Agr. Sci.* **72**, 123–130.

VII. Sheep

Abeloos, M. (1946). Foetal growth plans in calf and lamb. *C. R. Acad. Sci. Paris.* **222**, 342–343.

Aitken, R. N. C. (1959). Observations on the development of the seminal vesicles, prostate and bulbourethral glands in the ram. *J. Anat.* **93**, 43–51.

Barcroft, J. (1946). Growth and development. "Researches on Prenatal Life", Chapter 3. Blackwell, Oxford.

Batten, E. H. (1958). The origin of the acoustic ganglion in the sheep. *J. Embryol. Exp. Morphol.* **6**, 597–613.

Batten, E. H. (1960). The placodal relations of the glossopharyngeal nerve in the sheep: a contribution to the early development of the carotid body. *J. Comp. Neurol.* **114**, 1–37.

Benzie, D. (1950). Growth of the skeleton of the foetal sheep. *Brit. Vet. J.* **106**, 231–234.

Blin, P. C., and Bossavy, A. (1963). Dynamique topographique du foie, des estomac et de l'intestin du foetus et periodisation foetale chez le mouton de lacaune. *Econ. Med. Anim.* **4**, 69–93, 141–160.

Bogolyubskiy, S. N. (1959). (Intrauterine formation and development of body structure of Merion and Precoce sheep). *Acad. Sci. U.S.S.R.* **23**, 277–339.

Bonnet, T. (1889). Beiträge zur Embryologie der Wiederkäuer, gewonnen am Schafe. *Arch. Anat. Physiol. Leipzig* 1–106.

Bossavy, A. (1963). Dynamique topographique et pondérale du foies, des estomacs et de l'intestin chez le foetus de Mouton. Thesis, Alfort.

Bryden, M. M. (1969). Prenatal developmental anatomy of the sheep, with particular reference to the period of the embryo (11 to 34 days). Thesis, Cornell Univ.

Bryden, M. M., Evans, H. E., and Binns, W. (1972). Embryology of the sheep: 1. Extraembryonic membranes and development of body form. 2. The alimentary tract and associated glands. *J. Morphol.* **138**, 169–185.

Bulmer, D. (1956). The early stages of vaginal development in the sheep. *J. Anat.* **90**, 123–134.

Chang, T. K. (1949). Calcification in the fetus of normal and Ancon sheep. *Anat. Rec.* **105**, 723–735.

Clark, R. T. (1934). Studies on the physiology of reproduction in the sheep. II. The cleavage stages of the ovum. *Anat. Rec.* **60**, 135–159.

Cloete, J. H. L. (1939). Prenatal growth in the Merino sheep. Onderst. *J. Vet. Sci. An. Ind.* **13**, 417–546.

Danilova, L. V. (1962). (Somite differentiation in the Karakul sheep embryo.) *Izv. Akad. Nauk S.S.S.R. Ser. Biol.* **1**, 70–83 (English summary p. 83) *English transl. Fed. Proc.* **22**, T677–T689 (1963).

Davletova, L. V. (1959). The growth and development of the gastrointestinal tract in the Soviet Merino breed. *Tr. Inst. Morfol. Zhiv. Akad. Nauk S.S.S.R.* **23**, 188–230.

Eaton, O. N. (1952). Weight and length measurements of fetuses of Karakul sheep and goats. *Growth* **16**, 175–187.

Gerneke, W. H. (1963). The embryological development of the pharyngeal region of the sheep. *Onderst. J. Vet. Res.* **30**, 191–250.

Green, W. W. (1946). Comparative growth of the sheep and bovine animal during prenatal life. *Amer. J. Vet. Res.* **7**, 395–402.

Green, W. W., and Winters, L. M. (1945). Prenatal development of the sheep. *Univ. Minn. Agr. Exp. Sta. Tech. Bull.* No. 169, 1–36.

Hafez, E. S. E. (1963). Symposium on Growth: physiogenetics of prenatal and post-natal growth. *J. Anim. Sci.* **22**, 779–791.

Hafez, E. S. E. (1968). Gestation, prenatal development and parturition. *In* "Reproduction in Farm Animals," 2nd ed., Chapter 10. Lea and Febiger, Philadelphia, Pennsylvania.

Kemp, N. E. (1962). Development: Swine. In "Growth, Including Reproduction and

Harris, H. (1937). The foetal growth of sheep. *J. Anat.* **71**, 516–527.

Harvey, E. B. (1959). Implantation, development of the fetus, and fetal membranes. *In* "Reproduction in Domestic Animals," (H. H. Cole and P. T. Cupps, eds.), Vol. 1, Chapter 13. Academic Press, New York.

Joubert, D. M. (1956). A study of prenatal growth and development in the sheep. *J. Agr. Sci.* **47**, 382–428.

Lascelles, A. K. (1959). The time of appearance of ossification centres in the Peppin-type Merino. *Aust. J. Zool.* **7**, 79–86.

Lubberhuizen, H. W. (1931). Entwicklung der Hypophys beim Schaf. *Z. Anat. Entwickl.-Gesh.* **96**, 1–53.

Malon, A. P., and Curson, H. H. (1936). Studies in sex physiology. No. 15. Further observations on the body weight and crown-rump length of Merino fetuses. *Onderst. J. Vet. Sci. An. Ind.* **7**, 239–249.

Mukhamedgaliev, F. M., and Baimukhambetov, K. (1964). (Embryogenesis in fine-wooled sheep.) *Tr. Alma-Atinck Zoovet. Inst.* **13**, 199–219.

Pitkjanen, I. G. (1958). (Fertilization and early stages of embryonic development in the sheep.) *Izv. Akad. Nauk S.S.S.R. Ser. Biol.* No. 3, 291–298.

Romanes, G. J. (1947). The prenatal medullation of the sheep's nervous system. *J. Anat.* **81**, 64–81.

Rowson, L. E. A., and Moor, R. M. (1966). Development of the sheep conceptus during the first fourteen days. *J. Anat.* **100**, 777–785.

Schmidt, G. A. (1963). Phases of the blastocyst and trophoblastic capsule in the Karakul sheep. *Dokl. Akad. Nauk S.S.S.R. Biol. Sci. Sect. Transl.* **147**, 1298–1300.

Schwarztrauber, J. (1903). Kloake und Phallus des Schafes und Schweines. *Gegenb. Morphol. Jb.* **32**, 23–57.

Stephenson, S. K., and Lambourne, L. J. (1960). Prenatal growth in Romney and Southdown cross and Australian Merino sheep. I. Introduction and external growth patterns in the two breeds. *Aust. J. Agr. Res.* **11**, 1044–1062.

Tretyakov, N. N. (1959). Ossification of the skeleton of sheep of the Soviet Merino breed in the course of intrauterine development. Acad. Sci. U.S.S.R. Severtzev Inst. Anim. Morphol. 23: 146–187.

Winters, L. M., and Feuffel, G. (1936). Studies on the physiology of reproduction in sheep. IV. Foetal development. Tech. Bull. Univ. Minnesota No. 118.

218APPENDIX I

VIII. Ferret

Chang, M. C. (1950). Cleavage of unfertilized ova in immature ferrets. *Anat. Rec.* **108**, 31–44.
Donovan, B. T. (1964). Gonadal hormones and the control of ovarian function in the ferret. *Anat. Rec.* **148**, 277.
Hamilton, W. J. (1934). The early stages in the development of the ferret. Fertilization to the formation of the prochordal plate. *Tr. Roy. Soc. Edinburgh* **58**, 251–278.
Hamilton, W. J. (1936). The early stages in the development of the ferret. The formation of the mesoblast and notochord. *Tr. Roy. Soc. Edinburgh* **59**, 165–193.
Hammond, J., and Marshall, F. H. A. (1930). Oestrus and pseudopregnancy in the ferret. *Proc. Roy. Soc. London Sect. B.* **105**, 607–629.
Hammond, J., and Walton, A. (1934). Notes on ovulation and fertilization in ferrets. *J. Exp. Biol.* **11**, 307.
Hart, D. S. (1951). Photoperiodicity in the female ferret. *J. Exp. Biol.* **28**, 1–12.
Hill, M., and Parkes, A. S. (1930). On the relation between the anterior pituitary body and the gonads. II. The induction of ovulation in the anestrus ferret. *Proc. Roy. Soc. London Sect. B* **107**, 39–48.
Marshall, F. H. A., and Hammond, J. (1945). Experimental control by hormone action of the oestrous cycle in the ferret. *J. Endocrinol.* **4**, 159–168.
Steffek, A. J., Fabiyi, A., and King, C. T. G. (1968). Chlorcyclizine produced cleft palate in the ferret. *Arch. Oral Biol.* **13**, 1281–1283.
Wang, C. (1917). The earliest stages of the development of the blood vessels and of the heart in ferret embryos. *J. Anat.* **62**, 107–185.

IX. Cat

Coulter, C. B. (1909). The early development of the aortic arches of the cat, with especial reference to the presence of a fifth arch. *Anat. Rec.* **3**, 578–592.
Dawson, A. B. (1950). The domestic cat. *In* "The Care and Breeding of Laboratory Animals" (E. J. Farris, ed.), pp. 202–233. Wiley, New York.
Drews, M. (1933). Über Ossifikationsvorgänge am Katzen- und Hundeschädel. *Gegenb. Morphol. Jb.* **73**, 185–237.
Durbeck, W. (1907). Die äusseren Genitalien der Hauskatze. *Gegenb. Morphol. Jb.* **36**, 544–565.
Gilbert, P. W. (1947). The origin and development of the extrinsic ocular muscles in the domestic cat. *J. Morphol.* **81**, 151–193.
Halley, G. (1955). The placodal relations of the neural crest in the domestic cat. *J. Anat.* **89**, 133–152.
Hammond, W. S. (1941). The development of the aortic arch bodies in the cat. *Amer. J. Anat.* **69**, 265–293.
Hill, J. P., and Tribe, M. (1924). The early development of the cat *(Felis domestica)*. *Quart. J. Microsc. Sci.* **68**, 513–602.
Hoogeweg, H., and Folkers, E. R., Jr. (1970). Superfetation in a cat. *J. Amer. Vet. Med. Ass.* **156**, 73–75.
Huntington, G. S. (1911). "The Anatomy and Development of the Systemic Lymphatic Vessels in the Domestic Cat." Lippincott, Philadelphia, Pennsylvania.

Huntington, G. S., and McClure, C. F. W. (1920). The development of the veins in the domestic cat *(Felis domestica)* with especial reference, 1) to the share taken by the supracardinal veins in the development of the postcava and azygos veins and 2) to the interpretation of the variant conditions of the postcava and its tributaries, as found in the adult. *Anat. Rec.* **20**, 1–30.

Latimer, H. B. (1931). The prenatal growth of the cat. II. The growth of the dimensions of the head and trunk. *Anat. Rec.* **50**, 311–332.

Latimer, H. B. (1935). The prenatal growth of the cat. VI. Changes in the relative proportions. *Univ. Kansas Sci. Bull.* XXII (4), 61–77.

Marin-Padilla, M. (1971). Early prenatal ontogenesis of the cerebral cortex (neocortex) of the cat *(Felis domestica)*. A Golgi study. I. The primordial neocortical organization. *Z. Anat. Entwickl.-Gesch.* **134**, 117–145.

Murray, C. B. (1951). The mechanism of attachment of the blastocyst in the cat. *J. Anat.* **85**, 431.

Pohlmann, E. H. (1910). Die embryonale Metamorphose der Physiognomie und der Mundhöhle des Katzenkopfes. *Gegenb. Morphol. Jb.* **41**, 615–680.

Schaeffer, H. (1932). Die Ossifikationvorgänge im Gliedmassenskelett der Hauskatze. *Gegenb. Morphol. Jb.* **70**, 548–600.

Terry, R. J. (1917). The primordial cranium of the cat. *J. Morphol.* **29**, 281–433.

Troger, C.-P. (1969). Zur Störung von Fertilität und Gravidität bei der Katze. *Berl. Muenchener Tieraerzt. Wochens.* **82**, 477–480.

Turner, C. W., and Demoss, W. R. (1934). The normal and experimental development of the mammary gland. I. The male and female domestic cat. Res. Bull. Mo. Agr. Exp. Sta. No. 207.

Windle, W. F., and Griffin, A. M. (1931). Observations of embryonic and fetal movements of the cat. *J. Comp. Neurol.* **52**, 149–188.

X. Dog

Anderson, A. C., and Goldman, M. (1970). Growth and development. *In* "The Beagle as an Experimental Dog," 43–105. Iowa State Univ. Press, Ames.

Bischoff, T. L. W. (1845). "Entwicklungsgeschichte des Hundes." Braunschweig.

Bonnet, T. (1897). Beiträge zur Embryologie des Hundes. *Anat. Hefte* **9**, 419–512.

Bonnet, T. (1901). Beiträge zur Embryologie des Hundes. *Anat. Hefte* **16**, 230–232.

Bonnet, T. (1902). Beiträge zur Embryologie des Hundes. *Anat. Hefte* **20**, 323–499.

Drews, M. (1933). Über Ossifikationsvorgänge am Katzen- und Hundeschädel. *Morphol. Jahrb.* **73**, 185–237.

Evans, H. E. (1956). A dog comes into being. *Gaines Dog Res. Progr.* 1–3.

Evans, H. E. (1958). Prenatal ossification in the dog. *Anat. Rec.* **130**, 406.

Evans, H. E. (1962). Fetal growth and skeletal development in the dog. *Amer. Zool.* **2**, 521.

Evans, H. E. (1970). Development of the sphenoid bones in the dog. *Anat. Rec.* **166**, 303.

Gier, H. T. (1950). Early embryology of the dog. *Anat. Rec.* **108**, 561–562.

Hendrickx, A. G. (1964). The pharyngeal pouches of the dog. *Anat. Rec.* **149**, 475–483.

Holst, P. A., and Phemister, R. D. (1971). The prenatal development of the dog: Preimplantation events. *Biol. Reprod.* **5**, 194–206.

Houston, M. L. (1968). The early brain development of the dog. *J. Comp. Neurol.* **134**, 371–383.

Kanagasuntheram, R., and Anandaraja, S. (1960). Development of the terminal urethra and prepuce in the dog. *J. Anat.* **94**, 121–129.

Karbe, E. (1965). The development of the cranial lymph nodes in the dog. *Anat. Anz.* **116**, 155–164.

Kingsbury, B. F., and Roemer, F. J. (1940). The development of the hypophysis in the dog. *Amer. J. Anat.* **66**, 449–481.

Latimer, H. B., and Corder, R. L. (1948). The growth of the digestive system in the fetal dog. *Growth* **12**, 285–309.

Latimer, H. B. (1949). The prenatal growth of the heart and the lungs in the dog. *Anat. Rec.* **104**, 287–298.

Martin, E. W. (1960). The development of the vascular system in 5-21 somite dog embryos. *Anat. Rec.* **137**, 378.

Olmstead, M. (1911). Das Primordialcranium eines Hundeembryos *Anat. Hefte* **43**, 339–367.

Romanucci, D. (1950). Placentation in the dog. *Anat. Rec.* **108**, 562.

Sack, W. O. (1962). The development of the pharyngeal region of the dog. Ph.D. Thesis. Univ. of Edinburgh.

Sack, W. O. (1964). The early development of the embryonic pharynx of the dog. *Anat. Anz.* **115**, 59–80.

Schaeffer, H. (1934). Die Ossifikationsvorgänge im Gliedmassenskelett des Hundes. *Gegenb. Morphol. Jb.* **74**, 472–514.

Schliemann, H. (1966). Zur Morphologie und Entwicklung des Craniums von *Canis lupus familiaris* L. *Morphol. Jahrb.* **109**, 501–603.

Tietz, W. J., and Seliger, W. G. (1967). Temporal relationship in early canine embryogenesis. *Anat. Rec.* **157**, 333–334.

Turner, C. W., and Gomez, E. T. (1934). The normal and experimental development of the mammary gland. II. The male and female dog. Res. Bull. Mo. Agr. Exp. Sta. #207.

Whitney, L. F. (1940). The gestation period in the bitch. *Vet. Med.* **35**, 59–60.

XI. Rhesus Monkey and Baboon

Asling, C. W., and van Wagenen, G. (1967). A note on development of the secondary palate in the rhesus monkey *(Macaca mulatta)*. *Arch. Oral Biol.* **12**, 909–910.

Bollert, J. A., and Hendrickx, A. G. (1969). Morphogenesis of palate in baboon *(Papio* sp.). *Teratology* **2**, 258.

Dede, J. A., Liley, A. W., and Plentl, A. A. (1965). Vascular studies of the conceptus in the macaque. *Surg. Forum, Amer. College Surg.* **16**, 400–402.

Fujikura, T., and Niemann, W. H. (1967). Birth weight, gestational age, and type of delivery in rhesus monkeys. *Amer. J. Obstet. Gynecol.* **97**, 76–80.

Gasser, R. F., and Hendrickx, A. G. (1967). The development of the facial nerve in baboon embryos *(Papio* sp.). *J. Comp. Neurol.* **129**, 203–218.

Gilbert, C., and Heuser, C. H. (1954). Studies in the development of the baboon *(Papio ursinus)*. *Anat. Rec.* **94**, 553–568.

Gilbert, C., and Heuser, C. H. (1954). Studies on the development of the baboon *(Papio ursinus)*. A description of two presomite and two late somite stage embryos. *Carnegie Contrib. Embryol.* **35**, 11–54.

Glaser, D. (1970). Über die Ossifikation der Extremitäten bei neugeborenen Primaten (Mammalia). *Z. Morphol. Tiere* **68**, 127–139.

Hartman, C. G., Heuser, C. H., and Streeter, G. L. (1934). The 10-day macaque embryo. *Anat. Rec. Suppl.* **58**, 16.

Heintz, N. P.-M. (1970). Morphogenese du crane des primates. *C. R. Acad. Sci. Paris* **D271**, 1384–1386.

Hendrickx, A. G. (1965). Observations on the development of the thyroid and parathyroid glands in the baboon. *Pan Amer. Congr. Endocrinol., 6th, Excerpta Medica* No. 99, 122.

Hendrickx, A. G. (1966). A description of baboon embryos with 13–20 pairs of somites. *Anat. Rec.* **154**, 356.

Hendrickx, A. G. (1967). Studies in the development of the baboon embryo. *In* "The Baboon in Medical Research" (H. Vagtborg, ed.), Vol. II. Univ. Texas Press, Austin, Texas.

Hendrickx, A. G. (1970). Developmental stages of baboon embryo *(Papio* sp.). *Anat. Rec.* **166**, 318.

Hendrickx, A. G., and Houston, M. L. (1967). Observation on amniogenesis in baboon embryos during the third week of development. *Anat. Rec.* **157**, 363.

Hendrickx, A. G., and Houston, M. L. (1969). Observations of baboon embryos during the early period of somite formation. *Proc. Int. Congr. Primatol., 2nd* **2**, 61–65.

Hendrickx, A. G., Houston, M. L., Kraemer, D. C., Gasser, R. F., and Bollert, J. A. (1971). "Embryology of the Baboon." Univ. of Chicago Press, Chicago, Illinois.

Hendrickx, A. G., and Kraemer, D. C. (1967). Observations on ova and preimplantation embryos of the baboon *Papio* sp. *Anat. Rec.* **157**, 398–399.

Hendrickx, A. G., and Kraemer, D. C., (1968). Preimplantation stages of baboon embryos *(Papio* sp.). *Anat. Rec.* **162**, 111–119.

Heuser, C. H. (1932). An intrachorionic mesothelial membrane in young stages of the monkey. *Anat. Rec. Suppl.* **52**, 15–16.

Heuser, C. H. (1936). The origin of the yolk sac in the rhesus monkey. *Anat. Rec. Suppl.* **64**, 20.

Heuser, C. H., and Streeter, G. L. (1941). Development of the macaque embryo. *Carnegie Contrib. Embryol.* **29**, 15–55.

Kraemer, D. C. (1968). Further observations on preimplantation embryos of the baboon *(Papio* sp.). *Anat. Rec.* **160**, 514.

Lewis, W. H., and Hartman, C. G. (1941). Tubal ova of the rhesus monkey. *Carnegie Contrib. Embryol.* **29**, 7–14.

Luckett, W. P. (1971). Origin of extraembryonic mesoderm in early human and rhesus monkey embryos. *Abstr. Anat. Rec.* **169**, 369.

Marston, J. H., and Kelly, W. A. (1968). Time relationships of spermatozoon penetration into the egg of the rhesus monkey. *Nature (London)* **217**, 1073–1074.

Parer, J. T., and Behrman, R. E. (1967). The oxygen consumption of the pregnant uterus and fetus of *Macaca mulatta*. *Resp. Physiol.* **3**, 288–301.

Reinhard, W. (1958). Cranium of a 33 mm. long embryo of *Papio hamadryas* L. (Contribution to the knowledge of the crania of primates). *Z. Anat. Entwickl.-Gesch.* **120**, 427–455.

Schultz, A. H. (1937). Fetal growth and development of the rhesus monkey. *Carnegie Contrib. Embryol.* **26**, 71–97.

Short, R. V. (1969). Implantation and the maternal recognition of pregnancy. *In* "Foetal Autonomy" (G. E. W. Wolstenholme and M. O'Connor, eds.), pp. 2–31. Churchill, London.

Steffek, A. J., Verrusio, A. C., and King, C. T. G. (1968). The histology of palatal closure in the rhesus monkey *(Macaca mulatta). Teratology* 1, 425–430.

van Wagenen, G., and Asling, C. W. (1964). Ossification in the fetal monkey *(Macaca
mulatta).* Estimation of age and progress of gestation in roentgenography. *Amer.
J. Anat.* 114, 107–132.

van Wagenen, G., and Catchpole, H. R. (1965). Growth of the fetus and placenta of
the monkey. *Amer. J. Phys. Anthrop.* 23, 1–11.

SOME HIGH POINTS IN EARLY EMBRYOLOGY OF THE RAT

The rat is widely used in embryologic and teratologic research but many aspects of its early intrauterine development are not fully covered in scientific literature, or are only sketchily covered. Figures AII-1 through AII-4 were developed in the author's laboratory for use in familiarizing graduate students and research trainees with some of the key events and relationships of early embryogenesis in this experimental animal.

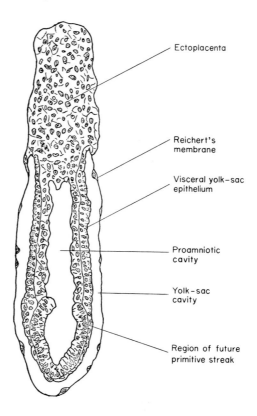

Ectoplacenta

Reichert's
membrane

Visceral yolk–sac
epithelium

Proamniotic
cavity

Yolk–sac
cavity

Region of future
primitive streak

FIG. AII-1. A composite drawing of the typical rat embryo at day 8½ of gestation. This is prior to the beginning of organogenesis and at this stage embryos subjected to adverse environmental influences tend to react mainly by embryolethality, although teratogenesis may be produced with certain agents. The embryo proper is a thimble-like configuration consisting of the two layers of primitive ectoderm and endoderm occupying the lower fifth of the elongated egg cylinder shown here. (Drawn by Charles Theisen, after Huber, 1915.)

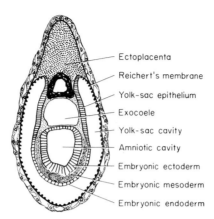

Ectoplacenta

Reichert's membrane

Yolk-sac epithelium

Exocoele

Yolk-sac cavity

Amniotic cavity

Embryonic ectoderm

Embryonic mesoderm

Embryonic endoderm

FIG. AII-2. Diagram of the typical rat embryo early in day 9 of gestation. Organogenesis is about to begin as evidenced by the presence of three germ layers, ectoderm, mesoderm, and endoderm. The longitudinal axis of the future embryo will soon be indicated by the primitive streak at the lowermost part of the egg cylinder, where ectoderm and mesoderm appear to be intimately joined. At this stage the embryo is probably at the peak of its teratogenic susceptibility.

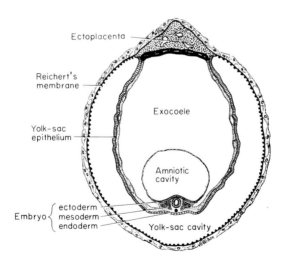

Ectoplacenta

Reichert's membrane

Exocoele

Yolk-sac epithelium

Amniotic cavity

Embryo { ectoderm / mesoderm / endoderm

Yolk-sac cavity

FIG. AII-3. Diagram of the rat embryo early in day 10 of gestation. Organogenesis is well under way in the nervous and cardiovascular systems and somites are beginning to appear in the mesoderm. The embryo proper represents only a small part of this embryonic vesicle, being confined to the ectoderm, mesoderm, and endoderm underlying the amniotic cavity. Teratogenic susceptibility is still high although the peak of responsiveness for many types of agents may already have passed.

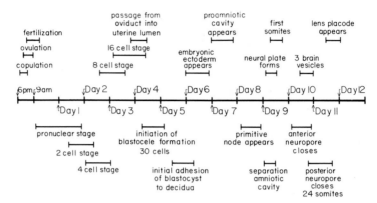

Fig. AII-4. Scale representing some of the major events of embryogenesis during the first 12 days of rat intrauterine development. Timing is represented as a range rather than a mean to indicate the degree of interlitter variation known or presumed to apply to most developmental events in this species. (Prepared by Charles Theisen.)

ATLAS OF FREEHAND (RAZOR BLADE) SECTIONS OF THE NORMAL 20-DAY RAT FETUS

Details of methods for removing, examining, and preserving 20-day rat fetuses have been presented elsewhere (Wilson, 1965). The cutting and examination of 1-mm freehand sections was also described but the quality of the photographic reproductions and the lack of identifying labels made the earlier illustrations less than ideal. Improved photography with key structures clearly labeled are presented here (Figs. AIII-1–AIII-15.) in the hope that this method will continue to be useful to those who must examine large numbers of fetuses in search of developmental abnormality in internal organs.

The method has been effectively used in near-term fetuses from mice, hamsters, and rabbits, as well as rats. There is every reason to expect that it could also be adapted to the study of other species such as guinea pigs, ferrets, dogs, cats, and pigs if fetuses were removed somewhat earlier than term, as suggested in Chapter 10 for dogs and pigs. The main consideration is that fetuses be allowed to remain *in utero* until ossification of the skeleton is sufficiently advanced to permit evaluation of major bony structures in a portion of the fetuses in each litter.

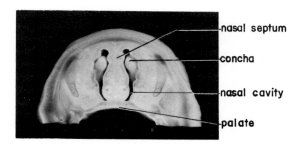

FIG. AIII-1. Palate.

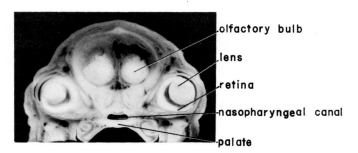

FIG. AIII-2. Eyes.

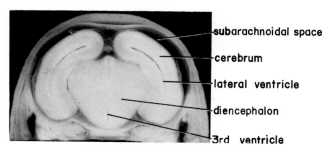

FIG. AIII-3. Brain ventricles.

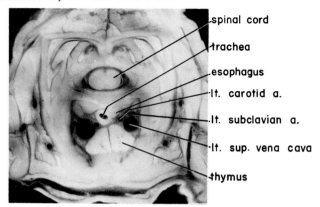

- spinal cord
- trachea
- esophagus
- lt. carotid a.
- lt. subclavian a.
- lt. sup. vena cava
- thymus

FIG. AIII-4. Neck.

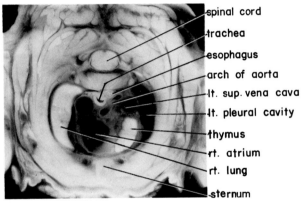

- spinal cord
- trachea
- esophagus
- arch of aorta
- lt. sup. vena cava
- lt. pleural cavity
- thymus
- rt. atrium
- rt. lung
- sternum

FIG. AIII-5. Arch of aorta.

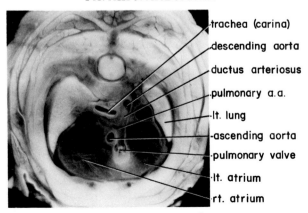

- trachea (carina)
- descending aorta
- ductus arteriosus
- pulmonary a.a.
- lt. lung
- ascending aorta
- pulmonary valve
- lt. atrium
- rt. atrium

FIG. AIII-6. Ductus arteriosus.

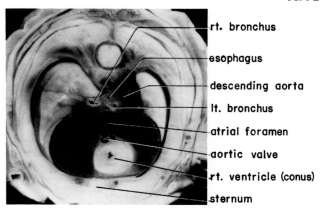

rt. bronchus

esophagus

descending aorta

lt. bronchus

atrial foramen

aortic valve

rt. ventricle (conus)

sternum

FIG. AIII-7. Aortic valve.

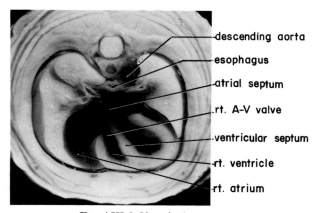

descending aorta

esophagus

atrial septum

rt. A-V valve

ventricular septum

rt. ventricle

rt. atrium

FIG. AIII-8. Ventricular septum.

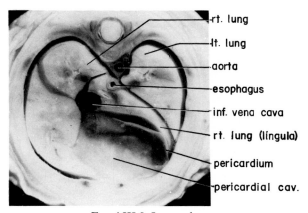

rt. lung

lt. lung

aorta

esophagus

inf. vena cava

rt. lung (lingula)

pericardium

pericardial cav.

FIG. AIII-9. Lower thorax.

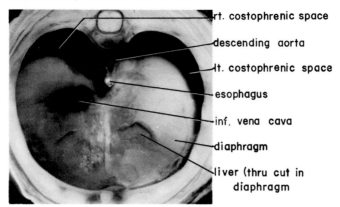

rt. costophrenic space

descending aorta

lt. costophrenic space

esophagus

inf. vena cava

diaphragm

liver (thru cut in
diaphragm

FIG. AIII-10. Dome of diaphragm.

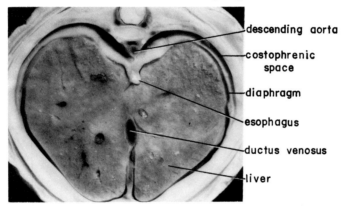

descending aorta

costophrenic
space

diaphragm

esophagus

ductus venosus

liver

FIG. AIII-11. Attachment of diaphragm.

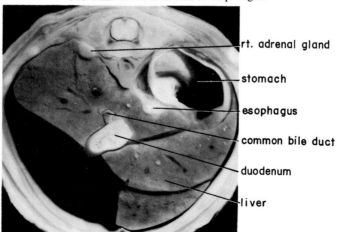

rt. adrenal gland

stomach

esophagus

common bile duct

duodenum

liver

FIG. AIII-12. Stomach.

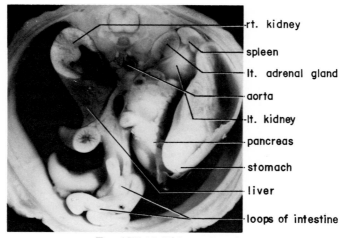

rt. kidney

spleen

lt. adrenal gland

aorta

lt. kidney

pancreas

stomach

liver

loops of intestine

FIG. AIII-13. Kidney-adrenal.

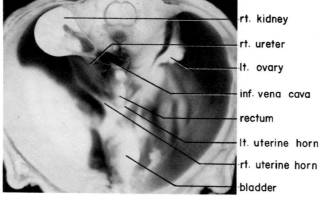

rt. kidney

rt. ureter

lt. ovary

inf. vena cava

rectum

lt. uterine horn

rt. uterine horn

bladder

FIG. AIII-14. Female pelvis.

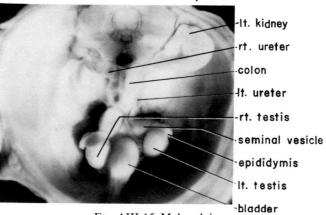

lt. kidney

rt. ureter

colon

lt. ureter

rt. testis

seminal vesicle

epididymis

lt. testis

bladder

FIG. AIII-15. Male pelvis.

BIBLIOGRAPHY

Abercrombie, M. (1970). Cellular interactions. *In* "Congenital Malformations" (F. C. Fraser and V. A. McKusick, eds.), pp. 111–114. Excerpta Medica, Amsterdam.

Adams, C. E. (1960). Embryonic mortality induced experimentally in the rabbit. *Nature (London)* **188**, 332–333.

Adamsons, K. (1965). Transport of organic substances and oxygen across the placenta. *In Symp. Placenta.* (D. Bergsma, ed.), Vol. 1, pp. 27–34. Nat. Foundation March of Dimes.

Aeppli, V. L. (1969). Teratologische Studien mit Imipramin an Ratte und Kaninchen. *Arzneim. Forsch.* **19**, 1617–1640.

Ahvenainen, E. K. (1959). A study of causes of neonatal deaths. *J. Pediatr.* **55**, 691–705.

Aksu, O., Mackler, B., Shepard, T. H., and Lemire, R. J. (1968). Studies on the development of congenital anomalies in embryos of riboflavin-deficient, galactoflavin fed rats. II. Role of terminal electron transport systems. *Teratology* **1**, 93–102.

Aladjem, S. (1970). The early placenta, structure and function. *In* "Congenital Malformations" (F. C. Fraser and V. A. McKusick, eds.), pp. 117–146. Excerpta Medica, Amsterdam.

Altman, J. (1971). Retardation of cerebellar and motor development by low level focal x-irradiation during infancy. *Teratology* **4**, 227.

Alzamora-Castro, V., Battilana, G., Abugattas, R., and Sialer, S. (1960). Patent ductus arteriosus and high altitude. *Amer. J. Cardiol.* **5**, 761–763.

Ancel, P. (1950). "La Chimiotératogenèse chez les Vertébrés." Doin, Paris.

Ancel, P. (1958). Recherches sur l'action tératogène du refroidissement temporaire de l'oeuf de Poule au cours de l'incubation. *J. Embryol. Exp. Morphol.* **6**, 335–345.

Andersen, D. H. (1949). Effects of diet during pregnancy upon the incidence of congenital hereditary diaphragmatic hernia in the rat. *Amer. J. Pathol.* **25**, 163–185.

Andersen, N. B. (1966). The effect of CNS depressants on mitosis. *Acta Anaesthesiol. Scand., Suppl.* **22**, 1–36.

Antonov, A. N. (1947). Children born during the siege of Leningrad in 1942. *J. Pediatr.* **30**, 250–259.

Apgar, V. (1964). Drugs in pregnancy. *J. Amer. Med. Ass.* **190**, 840–841.

Apgar, V. (1966). The drug problem in pregnancy. *Clin. Obstet. Gynecol.* **9**, 623–630.

233

Asling, C. W. (1969). Nutrition and teratogenesis. *In* "Methods for Teratological Studies in Experimental Animals and Man" (H. Nishimura and J. R. Miller, eds.), pp. 76–90. Igaku Shoin Ltd., Tokyo.

Assali, N. S. (1968). "Biology of Gestation. The Fetus and Neonate," Vol. 2. Academic Press, New York.

Assali, N. S., Dilts, P. V., Plentl, A., Kirschbaum, T. H., and Gross, S. J. (1968). Physiology of the placenta. *In* "Biology of Gestation" (N. S. Assali, ed.), Vol. 1, pp. 186–288. Academic Press, New York.

Auerbach, C. (1967). Chemical production of mutations. *Science* **158**, 1141–1147.

Bačič, M., Wesselius de Casparis, A., and Diczfalusy, E. (1970). Failure of large doses of ethinyl estradiol to interfere with early embryonic development in human species. *Amer. J. Obstet. Gynecol.* **107**, 531–534.

Baker, T. G. (1971). Radiosensitivity of mammalian oocytes with particular reference to the human female. *Amer. J. Obstet. Gynecol.* **110**, 746–761.

Balis, M. C. (1968). "Antagonists and Nucleic Acids." North-Holland Publ., Amsterdam.

Ballantyne, J. W. (1902). "Manual of Antenatal Pathology and Hygiene. I. The Fetus, II. The Embryo." Green, Edinburgh.

Barker, C. A. (1970). Anti-gestational and teratogenic effects of aimax (Methallibure) in gilts. *Can. Vet. J.* **11**, 39–40.

Barker, C. A. (1971). Teratogenic effect of Methallibure in swine. *Can. Vet. J.* **12**, 125–128.

Barnes, A. C. (1968). "Intra-Uterine Development." Lea and Febiger, Philadelphia, Pennsylvania.

Baron, J., Youngblood, L., Siewers, C. M. F., and Madearis, D. N. (1969). The influence of cytomegalovirus, herpes simplex, rubella and toxoplasma antibodies in microcephalic, mentally retarded and normocephalic children. *Pediatrics* **44**, 932–939.

Barrow, M. V., and Taylor, W. J. (1971). The production of congenital heart defects with the use of antisera of rat kidney, placenta, heart and lung homogenates. *Amer. Heart J.* **82**, 199–206.

Barson, A. J. (1972). Malformed infant. *Brit. Med. J.* **2**, 45.

Bass, N. H. (1971). The effect of neonatal undernutrition and subsequent rehabilitation on developing rat cerebrum. *Teratology* **4**, 228.

Bateman, A. J., and Epstein, S. S. (1971). Dominant lethal mutations in mammals. *In* "Chemical Mutagens" (A. Hollaender, ed.), Vol. 2, pp. 541–568. Plenum Press, New York.

Battinich, W. R. (1971). Effects of thalidomide on early limb development in rhesus monkey *(Macaca mulatta). Anat. Rec.* **169**, 274.

Baxter, H., and Fraser, F. C. (1950). Production of congenital defects in offspring of female mice treated with cortisone. *McGill Med. J.* **19**, 245–249.

Beaudoin, A. R. (1962). Interference of Niagara blue 2B with the teratogenic action of trypan blue. *Proc. Soc. Exp. Biol. Med.* **109**, 709–711.

Beaudoin, A. R., and Roberts, J. M. (1966). Teratogenic action of the thyroid stimulating hormone and its interaction with trypan blue. *J. Embryol. Exp. Morphol.* **15**, 281–289.

Beck, F. (1971). Personal communication.

Beck, F., and Lloyd, J. B. (1963). An investigation of the relationship between foetal death and foetal malformation. *J. Anat.* **97**, 555–564.

Beck, F., and Lloyd, J. B. (1965). Embryological principles of teratogenesis. *In* "Embryopathic Activity of Drugs" (J. M. Robson, F. Sullivan and R. L. Smith, eds.), pp. 1–20. Churchill, London.

Beck, F., Lloyd, J. B., and Griffiths, A. (1967a). Lysosomal enzyme inhibition by trypan blue: A theory of teratogenesis. *Science* **157**, 1180–1182.

Beck, F., Lloyd, J. B., and Griffiths, A. (1967b). A histochemical and biochemical study of some aspects of placental function in the rat using maternal injection of horseradish peroxidase. *J. Anat.* **101**, 461–478.

Beck, S. L. (1967). Effects of position in the uterus on foetal mortality and on response to trypan blue. *J. Embryol. Exp. Morphol.* **17**, 617–624.

Beck, S. L., and Smith, N. J. (1972). Cryptic skeletal variation correlated with selected response to trypan blue. *Teratology* **5**, 250.

Berendes, H. W., and Weiss, W. (1970). The NIH collaborative study. A progress report. *In* "Congenital Malformations" (F. C. Fraser and V. A. McKusick, eds.), pp. 293–298. Excerpta Medica, Amsterdam.

Biggs, R., and Rose, E. (1947). The familial incidence of adrenal hypertrophy and female pseudohermaphroditism. *J. Obstet. Gynacol. Brit. Emp.* **54**, 369–374.

Binns, W., Ceuto, C., Eliason, B. C., Heggestad, H. E., Hepting, G. H., Sand, P. F., Stephes, R. F., and Tschirley, F. H. (1970). Investigation of spray project near Globe, Arizona. Investigation conducted February, 1970.

Biological Handbook (various contributors). "Growth, Including Reproduction and Morphological Development." (P. L. Altman and D. S. Dittmer, eds.). Fed. of Amer. Soc. for Exp. Biol., Washington, D. C.

Birch, H. G., Piñeiro, C., Alcalde, E., Toca, T., and Cravioto, J. (1971). Relation of kwashiorkor in early childhood and intelligence at school age. *Pediatr. Res.* **5**, 579–585.

Bird, A. V. (1969). Anticonvulsant drugs and congenital abnormalities. *Lancet* **1**, 311.

Blandau, R. J. (1955). Ovulation in the living albino rat. *Fertil. Steril.* **6**, 391–404.

Bloom, A. D. (1972). Induced chromosomal aberrations: Biological and clinical significance. *J. Pediatr.* **81**, 1–8.

Bloom, F. (1965). Spontaneous renal lesions. *In* "The Pathology of Laboratory Animals" (W. E. Ribelin and J. R. McCoy, eds.) Thomas, Springfield, Illinois.

Boletti, M., and Croatto, L. (1958). Deafness in a 5-year-old girl resulting from streptomycin therapy during pregnancy. *Acta Pediatr.* **11**, 1.

Bolognese, R. J., Corson, S. L., Sever, J. L., Fuccillo, D. A., Lakoff, K. M., and Klein, J. (1972). Rubella vaccination during pregnancy. *Amer. J. Obstet. Gynecol.* **112**, 903–907.

Bongiovanni, A. M., and McFadden, A. J. (1960). Steroids during pregnancy and possible fetal consequences. *Fertil. Steril.* **11**, 181–186.

Bongiovanni, A. M., Di George, A. M., and Grumbach, M. M. (1959). Masculinization of the female infant associated with estrogenic therapy alone during gestation. *J. Clin. Endocrinol. Metab.* **19**, 1004–1010.

Bonnevie, K. (1934). Embryological analysis of gene mutations in Little and Bagg's abnormal mouse tribe. *J. Exp. Zool.* **67**, 443–520.

Boon, A. R., Farmer, M. B., and Roberts, D. F. (1972). A family study of Fallot's tetralogy. *J. Med. Genet.* **9**, 179–192.

Borisy, G. G., and Taylor, E. W. (1967a). The mechanism of action of colchicine. I. Binding of colchicine-^{3}H to cellular protein. *J. Cell. Biol.* **34**, 525–534.

Borisy, G. G., and Taylor, E. W. (1967b). The mechanism of action of colchicine. II. Binding of colchicine-³H to sea urchin eggs and the mitotic apparatus. *J. Cell. Biol.* **34**, 535–548.

Bornstein, S., Trasler, D. G., and Fraser, F. C. (1970). Effect of the uterine environment on the frequency of spontaneous cleft lip in CL/Fr mice. *Teratology* **3**, 295–298.

Bowler, K. (1972). The effect of repeated applications of heat on spermatogenesis in the rat: a histological study. *J. Reprod. Fertil.* **28**, 325–333.

Bowman, P. (1967). The effect of 2,4-dinitrophenol on the development of early chick embryos. *J. Embryol. Exp. Morphol.* **17**, 425–431.

Boyd, J. D., and Hamilton, W. J. (1970). "The Human Placenta." Heffer, Cambridge.

Bradford, G. E. (1972). Genetic control of litter size in sheep. *J. Reprod. Fertil., Suppl.* **15**, 23–41.

Brambell, F. W. R. (1957). The development of fetal immunity. *In Conf. Gestat., 4th,* Josiah Macy, Jr. Foundation.

Brandner, M., and Nusslé, D. (1969). Foetopathie due a l'aminoptérine avec sténose congénitale de l'espace médullaire des os tubulares longs. *Ann. Radiol.* **12**, 703–710.

Brent, R. L. (1964a). Effects of proteins, antibodies and autoimmune phenomena upon conception and embryogenesis. *In* "Teratology, Principles and Techniques" (J. G. Wilson and J. Warkany, eds.), pp. 215–250. Univ. Chicago Press, Chicago, Illinois.

Brent, R. L. (1964b). Drug testing in animals for teratogenic effects: thalidomide in pregnant rats. *J. Pediatr.* **64**, 762–770.

Brent, R. L. (1969). Direct and indirect effects of irradiation upon mammalian zygote, embryo and fetus. *In* "Methods for Teratological Studies in Experimental Animals and Man" (H. Nishimura and J. R. Miller, eds.), pp. 63–73. Igaku Shoin, Tokyo.

Brent, R. L. (1971a). Antibodies and malformations. *In* "Malformations Congénitales des Mammifères" (H. Tuchmann-Duplessis, ed.), pp. 187–220. Masson, Paris.

Brent, R. L. (1971b). Testimony before the Senate Subcommittee on Executive Reorganization and Government Research. Federal Registry, April, 1971.

Brent, R. L. (1972a). Protecting the public from teratogenic and mutagenic hazards. *J. Clin. Pharmacol.* **12**, 61–70.

Brent, R. L. (1972b). Irradiation in pregnancy. *In* "Davis' Gynecology and Obstetrics," Vol. 2. Harper, New York.

Brent, R. L. (1973). Radiation and teratogenesis in pregnancy. *In* "Pathobiology of Development." pp. 76–96. Williams and Wilkins, Baltimore, Maryland.

Brent, R. L., and Averich, E. (1961). The production of congenital malformations using tissue antibodies. I. Kidney Antisera. *Amer. J. Dis. Child.* **102**, 689–691.

Brent, R. L., and Franklin, J. B. (1960). Uterine vascular clamping: a new procedure for the study of congenital malformations. *Science* **132**, 89–91.

Brent, R. L., Johnson, A. J., and Jensen, M. (1971). The production of congenital malformations using tissue antisera. VII. Yolk-sac antiserum. *Teratology* **4**, 255–275.

Brent, R. L., Leung, C., London, W., and Whittingham, D. (1972). The demise of another vestigal organ. *Teratology* **5**, 251.

Brinsmade, A. B., and Rübsaamen, H. (1957). Zur teratogenetischen Wirkung von unspezifischem Fieber auf den sich entwickelnden Kaninchenembryo. *Beitr. Pathol. Anat.* **117**, 154–164.

Brown, G. C., and Karunas, R. S. (1972). Relationship of congenital anomalies and maternal infection with selected enteroviruses. *Amer. J. Epidemiol.* **95**, 207–217.

Burke, B. S., Beal, V. A., Kirkwood, S. B., and Steuart, H. C. (1943). The influence of nutrition during pregnancy upon the condition of the infant at birth. *J. Nutr.* **26**, 569–583.

Burns, J. J. (1970). Pharmacological aspects of teratology. *In* "Congenital Malformations" (F. C. Fraser and V. A. McKusick, eds.), pp. 173–179. Excerpta Medica, Amsterdam.

Burnside, B. (1971). Microtubules and microfilaments in newt neurulation. *Develop. Biol.* **26**, 416–441.

Butler, N. R., Goldstein, H., and Ross, E. M. (1972). Cigarette smoking in pregnancy: its influence on birth weight and perinatal mortality. *Brit. Med. J.* **2**, 127–130.

Butt, E. M., and Simonsen, D. G. (1950). Mercury and lead storage in human tissues. *Amer. J. Clin. Pathol.* **20**, 716.

Cahen, R. L. (1964). Evaluation of the teratogenicity of drugs. *Clin. Pharmacol. Ther.* **5**, 480–514.

Cahen, R. L. (1966). Experimental and clinical chemoteratogenesis. *Advan. Pharmacol.* **4**, 263–334.

Cahen, R., and Fave, A. (1970). Y a't'il une relation entre l'effet tératogène et le passage transplacentaire d'un médicament? *C. R. Soc. Biol.* **164**, 610–616.

Caldera, R. (1970). Carbutamide et malformations chez l'enfant. *Ann. Pediatr.* **17**, 432–436.

Calkins, E., Kahn, D., and Diner, W. C. (1956). Idiopathic familial osteoporosis in dogs: osteogenesis imperfecti. *Ann. N.Y. Acad. Sci.* **64**, 410–423.

Campbell, G. D. (1961). Possible teratogenic effect of tolbutamide in pregnancy. *Lancet* **1**, 891–892.

Campbell, G. D. (1963). Chlorpropamide and foetal damage. *Brit. Med. J.* **1**, 59–60.

Carswell, F., Kerr, M. M., and Hutchison, J. H. (1970). Congenital goitre and hypothyroidism produced by maternal ingestion of iodides. *Lancet* **1**, 1241–1243.

Carter, M. P. (1965). Discussion of a paper by B. C. S. Slater. *In* "Embryopathic Activity of Drugs" (J. M. Robson, F. M. Sullivan, and R. L. Smith, eds.), pp. 253–260. Little, Brown, Boston, Massachusetts.

Carter, M. P., and Wilson, F. (1965). Antibiotics in early pregnancy and congenital malformations. *Develop. Med. Child Neurol.* **7**, 353–359.

Caspersson, T., Lindsten, J., Zech, L., Buckton, K. E., and Price, W. H. (1972). Four patients with trisomy 8 identified by fluorescence and Giemsa bonding techniques. *J. Med. Genet.* **9**, 1–7.

Cattanach, B. M. (1971). Specific locus mutation in mice. *In* "Chemical Mutagens" (A. Hollaender, ed.), Vol. 2, pp. 535–539. Plenum Press, New York.

Cella, F. (1948). Congenital cystic microphthalmia in a litter of eight pigs. *Nuova Vet.* **24**, 145–148.

Chamberlain, J. G., and Nelson, M. (1963). Multiple congenital abnormalities in the rat resulting from acute maternal niacin deficiency during pregnancy. *Proc. Soc. Exp. Biol. Med.* **112**, 836–840.

Chase, H. P., Dalrere, C. S., Welch, N. N., and O'Brien, D. (1971). Intra-uterine undernutrition and brain development. *Pediatrics* **47**, 491–500.

Chaube, S., and Murphy, M. L. (1968). The teratogenic effects of the recent drugs active in cancer chemotherapy. *Advan. Teratol.* **3**, 181–237.

Cheng, D. W., Chang, L. F., and Bairnson, T. A. (1957). Gross observations on developing abnormal embryos induced by maternal vitamin E deficiency. *Anat. Rec.* **129**, 167–186.

Chepenik, K. P., Johnson, E. M., and Kaplan, S. (1969). Energy metabolism in normal and abnormal rat embryos. *Teratology* **2**, 259.

Chow, T. L., Melello, J. A., and Owen, N. V. (1964). Abortion experimentally induced in cattle by infectious bovine rhinotracheitis virus. *J. Amer. Vet. Med. Ass.* **144**, 1005–1007.

Clegg, D. J. (1971). Teratology. *Annu. Rev. Pharmacol.* **11**, 409–424.

Clemmer, T. P., and Telford, I. R. (1966). Abnormal development of the rat heart during prenatal hypoxic stress. *Proc. Soc. Exp. Biol. Med.* **121**, 800–803.

Coates, J. B., III (1970). Obstetrics in the very young adolescent. *Amer. J. Obstet. Gynecol.* **108**, 68–72.

Cohlan, S. Q. (1953). Excessive intake of vitamin A as a cause of congenital anomalies in the rat. *Science* **117**, 535–536.

Cohlan, S. Q. (1954). Congenital anomalies in the rat produced by excessive intake of vitamin A during pregnancy. *Pediatrics* **13**, 556–567.

Cohlan, S. Q. (1964). Fetal and neonatal hazards from drugs administered during pregnancy. *N.Y. Med. J.* **64**, 493–499.

Collaborative Study of 16 Laboratories (1966). The evaluation of drugs for foetal toxicity and teratogenicity in the rat. *Excerpta Med. Int. Congr., Ser. 115. Proc. Eur. Soc. Study. Drug. Tox.* **7**, 216–228.

Conney, A. H., and Burns, J. J. (1972). Metabolic interactions among environmental chemicals and drugs. *Science* **178**, 576–586.

Cook, M. J., Fairweather, F. A., and Hardwick, M. (1969). Further thoughts on teratogenic testing. *Teratology, Proc. Int. Symp. Teratol. Como, Italy.* (A. Bertelli, ed.), pp. 34–42. Excerpta Medica, Amsterdam.

Coopersmith, H., and Kerbel, N. C. (1962). Drugs and congenital anomalies. *Can. Med. Ass. J.* **87**, 193.

Corner, G. W. (1923). The problem of embryonic pathology in mammals with observations upon intra-uterine mortality in the pig. *Amer. J. Anat.* **31**, 523–545.

Courtney, K. D., Gaylor, D. W., Hogan, M. D., Falk, H. L., Bates, R. R., and Mitchell, I. A. (1970a). Teratogenic evaluation of pesticides: a large-scale screening study. *Teratology* **3**, 199.

Courtney, K. D., Gaylor, D. W., Hogan, M. D., Falk, H. L., Bates, R. R., and Mitchell, I. A. (1970b). Teratogenic evaluation of 2,4,5-T. *Science* **168**, 864–866.

Cowen, D., and Wolf, A. (1950). Experimental congenital toxoplasmosis. III. Toxoplasmosis in the offspring of mice infected by the vaginal route. Incidence and manifestations of the disease. *J. Exp. Med.* **92**, 417–429.

Coyle, C. F. V. (1959). A survey of 1,100 stillbirths. *Irish J. Med. Sci.* 6th ser., #400, 175.

Cravioto, J., and Delicardie, E. R. (1970). Mental performance in school age children. Findings after recovery from early severe malnutrition. *Amer. J. Dis. Child.* **120**, 405–410.

Creger, W. P., and Steele, M. R. (1957). Human fetomaternal passage of erythrocytes. *N. England J. Med.* **256**, 158–161.

Crichton, J. U., Dunn, H. G., McBurney, A. K., Robertson, A-M, and Tredger, E. (1972). Minor congenital defects in children of low birth weight. *J. Pediatr.* **80**, 830–832.

Crombie, D. L., Pinsent, R. J. F. H., and Fleming, D. (1972). Imipramine in pregnancy. *Brit. Med. J.* **1**, 745.

Crombie, D. L., Pinsent, R. J. F. H., Slater, B. C., Fleming, D., and Cross, K. W. (1970). Teratogenic drugs—R.C.G.P. Survey. *Brit. Med. J.* **4**, 178–179.

Cutting, R. T., Phuoc, T. H., Ballo, J. M., Benenson, M. W., and Evans, C. H. (1970). Congenital malformations, hydatidiform moles, and stillbirths in the Republic of Vietnam 1960–1969. Govt. Printing Office, Washington, D.C.

Dagg, C. P. (1967). Combined action of fluorouracil and two mutant genes on limb development in the mouse. *J. Exp. Zool.* **164**, 479–490.

Dagg, C. P., and Karnofsky, D. A. (1955). Teratogenic effects of azaserine on the chick embryo. *J. Exp. Zool.* **130**, 555.

Dagg, C. P., Doerr, A., and Offutt, C. (1966). Incorporation of 5-fluorouracil-2-C^{14} by mouse embryos. *Biol. Neonate* **10**, 32–46.

Dailey, M. E., and Benson, R. C. (1952). Hyperthyroidism in pregnancy. *Surg. Gynecol. Obstet.* **94**, 103–109.

Dancis, J., Money, W. L., Springer, D., and Levitz, M. (1968). Transport of amino acids by placenta. *Amer. J. Obstet. Gynecol.* **101**, 820–829.

Davey, J. R., and Stevenson, J. W. (1963). Pantothenic acid requirement of swine for reproduction. *J. Anim. Sci.* **22**, 9–13.

David, G., Mercier-Parot, L., and Tuchmann-Duplessis, H. (1963). Action tératogène d'hetero-anticorps tissulaires. I. Production de malformations chez la rat par action d'un sérum anti-rein. *C. R. Soc Biol.* **157**, 939–942.

Davidson, J. G., Fraser, F. C., and Schlager, G. (1969). A maternal effect on the frequency of spontaneous cleft lip in the A/J mouse. *Teratology* **2**, 371–376.

Davis, S. D., Nelson, T., and Shepard, T. H. (1970). Teratogenicity of vitamin B_6 deficiency: omphalocele, skeletal and neural defects and splenic hypoplasia. *Science* **169**, 1329–1330.

Dawes, G. S. (1968). "Foetal and Neonatal Physiology." Yearbook Publ., Chicago, Illinois.

de Alvarez, R. (1962). Discussion of paper: Goetsch, C. *Amer. J. Obstet. Gynecol.* **83**, 1474–1477.

Dean, J. R. (1927). Goiter and pregnancy. *Can. Med. Ass. J.* **17**, 1355–1356.

De Costa, E. J., and Abelman, M. A. (1952). Cortisone and pregnancy. An experimental and clinical study of the effects of cortisone on gestation. *Amer. J. Obstet. Gynecol.* **64**, 746–767.

Degenhardt, K. H. (1960). Cranio-facial dysplasia induced by oxygen-deficiency in rabbits. *Biol. Neonatorum* **2**, 94–104.

Degenhardt, K. H., and Knoche, E. (1959). Analysis of intrauterine malformations of the vertebral column induced by oxygen deficiency. *Can. Med. Ass. J.* **80**, 441–445.

De Haan, R. L. (1958). Cell migration and morphogenetic movements. *In* "The Chemical Basis of Development" (W. D. McElroy and B. Glass, eds.). Johns Hopkins Press, Baltimore, Maryland.

Dekaban, A. S. (1969). Differential vulnerability to irradiation of various cerebral structures during prenatal development. *In* "Radiation Biology of the Fetal and Juvenile Mammal" (M. R. Sikov and D. D. Mahlum, eds.), pp. 769–778. U.S. Atomic Energy Commission.

de la Cruz, M. V., Campillo-Sainz, C., and Munoz-Armas, A. (1966). Congenital heart defects in chick embryos subjected to temperature variations. *Circ. Res.* **18**, 257–261.

Delahunt, C. S., and Lassen, L. J. (1964). Thalidomide syndrome in monkeys. *Science* **146**, 1300–1305.

Delahunt, C. S., and Rieser, N. (1967). Rubella-induced embryopathies in monkeys. *Amer. J. Obstet. Gynecol.* **99**, 580–588.

Delatour, P., Dams, R., and Favre-Tissot, M. (1965). Thalidomide: embryopathies chez le chien *Thérapie* **20**, 573–589.

Dennis, S. M., and Leipold, H. W. (1972). Agnathia in sheep: external observations. *Amer. J. Vet. Res.* **33**, 339–347.

Deren, J. J., Padykula, H. A., and Wilson, H. (1966). Development of structure and function in the mammalian yolk sac. III. The development of amino acid transport by rabbit yolk sac. *Develop. Biol.* **13**, 370–384.

Desai, R. G., and Creger, W. P. (1963). Transplacental passage of formed elements of blood in guinea pigs. *Clin. Res. Proc.* **11**, 191.

Dewey, W. C., Miller, H. H., and Leeper, D. B. (1971). Chromosomal aberrations and mortality of x-irradiated mammalian cells: emphasis on repair. *Proc. Nat. Acad. Sci.* **68**, 667–671.

Diamond, I., Anderson, M. M.., and McCreadie, S. R. (1960). Transplacental transmission of Busulfan (Myleran) in a mother with leukemia: production of fetal malformation and cytomegaly. *Pediatrics* **25**, 85–90.

DiPaolo, J. A., and Kotin, P. (1966). Teratogenesis-oncogenesis: a study of possible relationships. *Arch. Pathol.* **81**, 3–23.

DiPaolo, R. V., and Newberne, P. M. (1971). The effects of copper deficiency, in utero, on newborn rats. *Teratology* **4**, 230.

Dishotsky, N. I., Loughman, W. K., Mogar, R. E., and Lipscomb, W. R. (1971). LSD and genetic damage. Is LSD chromosome damaging, carcinogenic, mutagenic, or teratogenic? *Science* **172**, 431–440.

Dobbing, J. (1970). Undernutrition and the developing brain. *Amer. J. Dis. Child* **120**, 411–415.

Doig, R. K., and Coltman, O. McK. (1956). Cleft palate following cortisone therapy in early pregnancy. *Lancet* **2**, 730.

Dolger, H., Baskman, J. J., and Nechemias, C. (1969). Tolbutamide in pregnancy and diabetes. *J. Mt. Sinai Hosp.* **36**, 471–474.

Dolnick, E. H., Lindahl, I. L., and Terrill, C. E. (1970). Treatment of pregnant ewes with cyclophosphamide. *J. Anim. Sci.* **31**, 944–946.

Domock, W. W. (1940). The diagnosis of virus abortion in mares. *J. Amer. Vet. Med. Ass.* **96**, 665.

Dudgeon, J. A. (1967). Maternal rubella and its effect on the foetus. *Arch. Dis. Child.* **42**, 110–125.

Dumars, K. W. (1971). Parental drug usage: effect upon chromosomes of progeny. *Pediatrics* **47**, 1037–1041.

Dunn, P. M. (1964). Congenital malformations and maternal diabetes. *Lancet* **2**, 644–645.

Dwornik, J. J., and Moore, K. L. (1965). Skeletal malformations in the Holtzman rat embryo following the administration of thalidomide. *J. Embryol. Exp. Morphol.* **13**, 181–193.

Dyban, A. P., Baranov, V. S., and Akimova, I. M. (1970). Basic methodic approaches to testing chemicals for teratogenic activity. *Arkh. Anat. Gistol. Embriol.* **59**, 89–100.

Earl, F. L., Tegeris, A. S., Whitmore, G. E., Morison, R., and Fitzhugh, O. G. (1964). The use of swine in drug toxicity studies. *Ann. N.Y. Acad. Sci.* **111**, 671–688.

Earl, F. L., Miller, E., and Van Loon, E. J. (in press) Teratogenic research in beagle dogs and miniature swine. *Proc. 5th Meeting Int. Committee Lab. Anim.*

Ebbs, J. H., Tisdall, F. F., and Scott, W. A. (1941). The influence of prenatal diet on the mother and child. *J. Nutr.* **22**, 515–526.

Ede, D. A., and Agerbak, G. S. (1968). Cell adhesion and movement in relation to the developing limb pattern in normal and talpid mutant chick embryos. *J. Embryol. Exp. Morphol.* **20**, 81–100.

Edmonds, L. D., Selby, L. A., and Case, A. A. (1972). Poisoning and congenital malformations associated with consumption of poison hemlock by sows. *J. Amer. Vet. Med. Ass.* **160**, 1319–1324.

Edwards, J. A. (1968). The external development of the rabbit and rat embryos. *Advan. Teratol.* **3**, 239–263.

Edwards, J. H. (1964). The epidemiology of congenital malformations. *In* "Congenital Malformations" (M. Fishbein, ed.). Int. Med. Congr., New York.

Edwards, M. J. (1968). Congenital malformations in the rat following induced hyperthermia during gestation. *Teratology* **1**, 173–178.

Edwards, M. J. (1969). Congenital defects in guinea pigs: fetal resorptions, abortions, and malformations following induced hyperthermia during early gestation. *Teratology* **2**, 313–328.

Ehling, U. H., Cumming, R. B., and Malling, H. V. (1968). Induction of dominant lethal mutations by alkylating agents in male mice. *Mutat. Res.* **5**, 417–428.

Eichenwald, H. F. (1965). The placental "barrier" and infections of the fetus. *Birth Defects Original Article Ser.* **1**, 74–76.

Eliason, B. C., and Posner, H. S. (1971). Placental passage of ^{14}C-Dieldren altered by gestational age and plasma protein. *Amer. J. Obstet. Gynecol.* **111**, 925–929.

Elshove, J., and van Eck, J. H. M. (1971). Aangeboren misvormingen, met name gespleten lip met of zonder gespleten verhemelte, bij kinderen van moeders met epilepsie. *Ned. Tijdchr Geneesk.* **115**, 1371–1375.

Emerson, D. J. (1962). Congenital malformations due to attempted abortions with aminopterin. *Amer. J. Obstet. Gynecol.* **84**, 356–357.

Emerson, J. L., and Delez, A. L. (1965). Cerebellar hypoplasia, hypomyelinogenesis, and congenital tumors in pigs, associated with prenatal hog cholera vaccination of sows. *J. Amer. Vet. Med. Ass.* **147**, 47–54.

Ercanbrack, S. K., and Price, D. A. (1971). Frequencies of various birth defects in Rambouillet sheep. *J. Hered.* **62**, 223–227.

Erickson, B. H., and Murphree, R. L. (1964). Limb development in prenatally irradiated cattle, sheep and swine. *J. Anim. Sci.* **23**, 1066–1071.

Evans, H. E., Ingalls, T. H., and Binns, W. (1966). Teratogenesis of craniofacial malformations in animals. III. Natural and experimental deformities in sheep. *Arch. Environ. Health* **13**, 706–714.

Everett, J. W. (1935). Morphological and physiological studies of the placenta in the albino rat. *J. Exp. Zool.* **70**, 243–284.

Farkas, G. (1969). Teratogenic effect of hyperemesis gravidarum and of the drugs used in its therapy. *In Proc. Int. Conf. Congenital Malformations, 3rd* **191**, 40. Excerpta Medica, Amsterdam.

Farquhar, H. G., and Turner, W. M. L. (1949). Congenital toxoplasmosis. Report of two cases. *Arch. Dis. Child.* **24**, 137–142.

Fave, A. (1964). Les embryopathies provoquées chez les mammifères. *Extrait Thérap.* no 1.

Fave, A. (1971). Techniques de controle toxicologique dans le domaine de la reproduction. *In* "Malformations Congénitales des Mammifères" (H. Tuchmann-Duplessis, ed.), Pp. 293–312. Masson, Paris.

Feckheimer, N. S. (1972). Causal basis of chromosome abnormalities. *J. Reprod. Fertil. Suppl.* **15**, 79–98.

Fedrick, J., Alberman, E. D., and Goldstein, H. (1971). Possible teratogenic effect of cigarette smoking. *Nature (London)* **231**, 529–530.

Ferm. V. H. (1964). Teratogenic effects of hyperbaric oxygen. *Proc. Soc. Exp. Biol. Med.* **116**, 975–976.

Ferm, V. H. (1965). The rapid detection of teratogenic activity. *Lab. Invest.* **14**, 1500–1505.

Ferm, V. H. (1966). Congenital malformations induced by dimethyl sulphoxide in the golden hamster. *J. Embryol. Exp. Morphol.* **16**, 49–54.

Ferm, V. H., and Kilham, L. (1963). Rat virus (RV) infection in fetal and pregnant hamsters. *Proc. Soc. Exp. Biol. Med.* **112**, 623–626.

Filippi, B. (1967). Antibiotics and congenital malformations: evaluation of the teratogenicity of antibiotics. *Advan. Teratol.* **2**, 239–256.

Fingl, E., and Woodbury, D. M. (1965). General principles. *In* "Pharmacological Basis of Therapeutics" (L. S. Goodman and A. Gilman, eds.), Chapter 1. Macmillan, New York.

Fish, S. A. (1966). Organophosphorus cholinesterase inhibitors and fetal development. *Amer. J. Obstet. Gynecol.* **96**, 1148–1154.

Fishbein, L., Flamm, W. G., and Falk, H. L. (1970). "Chemical Mutagens Environmental Effects on Biological Systems." Academic Press, New York.

Flickinger, R. A., Miyagi, M., Moser, C. R., and Rollins, E. (1967). The relation of DNA synthesis to RNA synthesis in developing frog embryos. *Develop. Biol.* **15**, 414–431.

Flynt, J. W., Ebbin, A. E., Oakley, G. P., Falek, A., and Heath, C. W. (1971). Metropolitan Atlanta Congenital Defects Program. *In* "Monitoring, Birth Defects and Environment" (E. B. Hook, D. T. Janerich and I. H. Porter, eds.). Academic Press, New York.

Forsberg, J-G. (1967). Studies on the cell degeneration rate during the differentiation of the epithelium in the uterine cervix and Mullerian vagina of the mouse. *J. Embryol. Exp. Morphol* **17**, 433–440.

Fox, B. W., and Fox, M. (1967). Biochemical aspects of the actions of drugs on spermatogenesis. *Pharmacol. Rev.* **19**, 21–57.

Fox, M. W. (1963). Inheritance of inguinal hernia and midline defects in the dog. *J. Amer. Vet. Med. Ass.* **143**, 602–604.

Franz, J. (1971). Cytological aspects of embryotoxicity and teratogenicity. *In* "Malformations Congéneitales des Mammifères" (H. Tuchmann-Duplessis, ed.), pp. 151–158. Masson, Paris.

Fraser, A., and Burnell, D. (1970). "Computer Genetics." McGraw–Hill, New York.

Fraser, F. C. (1959). Causes of congenital malformations in man. *J. Chronic Dis.* **10**, 97–110.

Fraser, F. C. (1963). Methodology of experimental mammalian teratology. *In* "Methodology in Mammalian Genetics" (W. J. Burdette, ed.) Holden-Day, San Francisco, California.

Fraser, F. C. (1969). Gene-environment interactions in the production of cleft palate. *In* "Methods for Teratological Studies in Experimental Animals and Man" (H. Nishimura and J. R. Miller, eds.), pp. 34–49. Igaku Shoin, Tokyo.

Fraser, F. C. (1971). The epidemiology of common major malformations as related to environmental monitoring. *In* "Monitoring, Birth Defects and Environment" (E. B. Hook, D. T. Janerich and I. H. Porter, eds.). Academic Press, New York.

Fraser, F. C., and Fainstat, T. D. (1951). Production of congenital defects in the offspring of pregnant mice treated with cortisone. *Pediatrics* **8**, 527–533.

Fraser, F. C., Walker, B. E., and Trasler, D. G. (1957). The experimental production of congenital cleft palate: genetic and environmental factors. *Pediatrics* **19**, 782–787.

Freeden, K. T. and Jarmoluk, L. (1963). Skeletal anomalies in swine. *Can. J. Anim. Sci.* **43**, 143.

Freese, E. (1971). Molecular mechanisms of mutations. *In* "Chemical Mutagens. Principles and Methods for their Detection" (A. Hollaender, ed.), Vol. 1, pp. 1–56. Plenum Press, New York.

Friedman, G. D. (1972). Screening criteria for drug monitoring. The Kaiser-Permanente drug reaction monitoring system. *J. Chronic Dis.* **25**, 11–20.

Friedman, M. H. (1957). Effect of O-diazoacetyl on the pregnancy of the dog. *J. Amer. Vet. Med. Ass.* **130**, 159–162.

Friedman, W. F., and Roberts, W. C. (1966). Vitamin D and the supravalvular aortic stenosis syndrome. The transplacental effects of vitamin D of the aorta of the rabbit. *Circulation* **34**, 77–86.

Friedmann, I., and Wright, M. I. (1966). Histopathological changes in the foetal and infantile inner ear caused by maternal rubella. *Brit. Med. J.* **2**, 20–23.

Frisch, R. E. (1970). Present status of the supposition that malnutrition causes permanent mental retardation. *Amer. J. Clin. Nutr.* **23**, 189–195.

Fritz, H., and Hess, R. (1970). Ossification of the rat and mouse skeleton in the perinatal period. *Teratology* **3**, 331–338.

Froehlich, L. A., and Fujikura, T. (1970). Placental hemangioma in relation to neonatal thrombocytopenic purpura, vascular nevi, and other perinatal effects. *Teratology* **3**, 200.

Frohberg, H., and Oettel, H. (1966). Method of testing for teratogenicity in mice. *Ind. Med. Surg.* **35**, 113–120.

Furchtgott, E., and Walker, S. F. (1969). Conditioning studies with prenatally irradiated rats. *In* "Radiation Biology of the Fetal and Juvenile Mammal" (M. R. Sikov and D. D. Mahlum, eds.), pp. 301–312. U.S. Atomic Energy Commission.

Gardner, D. L. (1959). Familial canine chondrodystrophia faetalis (achondroplasia). *J. Pathol.* **77**, 243–247.

Geller, L. M. (1959). Failure of nicotine to affect development of offspring when administered to pregnant rats. *Science* **129**, 212–214.

Genther, I. T. (1934). X-irradiation of the ovaries of guinea pigs and its effects on subsequent pregnancies. *Amer. J. Anat.* **55**, 1–45.

German, J. A. (1968). Mongolism, delayed fertilization and human sexual behavior. *Nature (London)* **217**, 516–518.

German, J., Kowal, A., and Ehlers, K. H. (1970). Trimethadione and human teratogenesis. *Tetatology* **3**, 349–362.

Gerrits, R. J., and Johnson, L. A. (1964). The effect of an orally administered nonsteroid on estrus, ovulation and fertility in gilts. *Proc. Int. Congr. Anim. Reprod. 5th* **2**, 455.

Gessner, I. H. (1970). Oxygen consumption and growth in chick embryos with mechanically induced heart defects. *Teratology* **3**, 201.

Gessner, I. H., and Bostrom, H. (1965). In vitro studies on ^{35}S-sulfate incorporation into the acid mucopolysaccharides of chick embryo cardiac jelly. *J. Exp. Zool.* **160**, 283–290.

Gibson, J. E., and Becker, B. A. (1968). Effect of phenobarbital and SKF 525-A on the teratogenicity of cyclophosphamide in mice. *Teratology* **1**, 393–398.

Gibson, J. P., Staples, R. E., and Newberne, J. W. (1966). Use of the rabbit in teratogenicity studies. *Toxicol. Appl. Pharmacol.* **9**, 398–408.

Ginsburg, J. (1968). Breakdown in maternal protection: drugs. *Proc. Roy. Soc. Med.* **61**, 1244–1247.

Ginsburg, J. (1971). Placental drug transfer. *Annu. Rev. Pharmacol.* **11**, 387–408.

Giroud, A. (1955). Les malformations congénitales et leur causes. *Biol. Med.* **44**, 1–86.

Giroud, A. (1971). L'équilibre nutritif et ses diverses dépendances au cours de la gestation. *In* "Malformations Congénitales des Mammifères" (H. Tuchmann-Duplessis, Ed.), pp. 223–241. Masson, Paris.

Giroud, A., and Martinet, M. (1950). Action de la sufaguanidine sur le développement del l'embryon. *Arch. Fr. Pédiatr.* **7**, 180–184.

Giroud, A., and Martinet, M. (1955). Malformations diverses du foetus de rat suivant les stades d'administration de vitamine A en exces. *C. R. Soc. Biol.* **149**, 1088–1090.

Giroud, A., Giroud, P., Martinet, M., and Vargues, R. (1951). Répercussions graves des maladies inapparentes. *Bull. Soc. Pathol. Exot.* **44**, 563–570.

Giroud, A., Lefebvres, J., and Dupuis, R. (1956). Carence en biotine et reproduction chez la Ratte. *C. R. Soc. Biol.* **150**, 2066–2067.

Giroud, P., Giroud, A., and Martinet, M. (1954). Répercussions de l'inoculation de toxoplasme a des rattes gestantes. *C. R. Soc. Biol.* **148**, 1030–1031.

Giroux, J., Boucard, M., Beaulatoin, S. *et al.* (1967). Difficulties in interpreting the results of studies on teratogenic risks. Experimental conditions and spontaneous malformations in the mouse. *Thérapie* **22**, 469–484.

Globus, M., and Gibson, M. A. (1968). A histological and histochemical study of the development of the sternum in thalidomide-treated rats. *Teratology* **1**, 235–256.

Goetsch, C. (1962). An evaluation of aminopterin as an abortifacient. *Amer. J. Obstet. Gynecol.* **83**, 1474–1477.

Goldschmidt, R. B. (1957). Problematics of the phenomenon of phenocopy. *J. Madras Univ.* **B27**, 17–24.

Goldstein, L., and Murphy, D. P. (1929). Etiology of ill-health in children born after maternal pelvic irradiation. II. Defective children born after postconception pelvic irradiation. *Amer. J. Roentgenol. Radium Ther. Nucl. Med.* **22**, 322–331.

Gottschewski, G. H. M. (1965). Konnen Tierversuche zur Losung der Frage nach der teratogenen Wirkung von Medikamenten auf den meschlichen Embryo beitragen? *Arzneim. Forsch.* **15**, 97–104.

Gottschewski, G. H. M. (1971). Voraussetzungen und Empfehlungen fur das teratologische Experiment. *Arzneim. Forsch.* **21**, 1269–1272.

Gould, S. M., and Pyle, W. L. (1896). "Anomalies and Curosities of Medicine." Saunders, Philadelphia, Pennsylvania (reprinted in 1956).

Grabowski, C. T. (1964). The etiology of hypoxia-induced malformations in the chick embryo. *J. Exp. Zool.* **157**, 307–326.

Grabowski, C. T. (1966). Physiological changes in the bloodstream of chick embryos exposed to teratogenic doses of hypoxia. *Develop. Biol.* **13**, 199–213.

Grabowski, C. T. (1970). Embryonic oxygen deficiency—a physiological approach to analysis of teratological mechanisms. *Advan. Teratol.* **4**, 125–167.

Grabowski, C. T., and Parr, J. (1958). The teratogenic effects of graded doses of hypoxia on the chick embryo. *Amer. J. Anat.* **103**, 313–348.

Grabowski, C. T., and Tsai, E. N. C. (1968). The effects of teratogenic doses of hypoxia on the blood pressure of 3-day chick embryos. *Teratology* **1**, 215.

Grauwiler, J. (1969). Variations in physiological reproduction data and frequency of spontaneous malformations in teratological studies with rats and rabbits. *In Proc. Int. Symp. Teratol. Como, Italy* (A. Bertelli, ed.), pp. 129–135. Excerpta Medica, Amsterdam.

Green, C. R. (1964). The frequency of maldevelopment in man. *Amer. J. Obstet. Gynecol.* **90**, 994–1013.

Greenberg, L. H., and Tanaka, K. R. (1964). Congenital anomalies probably induced by cyclophosphamide. *J. Amer. Med. Ass.* **188**, 423–426.

Greene, R. R., Burrill, M. W., and Ivy, A. C. (1939). Experimental intersexuality: the effect of antenatal androgens on sexual development of female rats. *Amer. J. Anat.* **65**, 415–469.

Greene, R. R., Burrill, M. W., and Ivy, A. C. (1940). Experimental intersexuality: the effects of estrogens on the antenatal sexual development of the rat. *Amer. J. Anat.* **67**, 305–345.

Greenwald, P., Barlow, J. J., Nasca, P. C., and Burnett, W. S. (1971). Vaginal cancer after maternal treatment with synthetic estorgens. *N. England J. Med.* **285**, 390–392.

Greenwood, R. D., and Sommer, A. (1971). Monosomy G: case report and review of literature. *J. Med. Genet.* **8**, 496–500.

Gregg, N. McA. (1941). Congenital cataract following German measles in the mother. *Trans. Ophthalmol. Soc. Aust.* **3**, 35.

Grisolia, S., Santos, I., and Mendelson, J. (1968). Inactivation of enzymes by aspirin and salicylate. *Nature (London)* **219**, 1252.

Gross, P. R. (1967). RNA metabolism in embryonic development and differentiation. II. Biosynthetic patterns and their regulation. *N. England J. Med.* **276**, 1297–1305.

Gruenwald, P. (1947). Mechanisms of abnormal development. *Arch. Pathol.* **44**, 398–664.

Gruenwald, P. (1958). Malformations caused by necrosis in the embryo. *Amer. J. Pathol.* **34**, 77–103.

Gruenwald, P. (1961). Abnormalities of placental vascularity in relation to intrauterine deprivation and retardation of fetal growth. *N.Y. State J. Med.* **61**, 1508–1517.

Gruenwald, P. (1966a). Growth of the human fetus. I. Normal growth and its variation. *Amer. J. Obstet. Gynecol.* **94**, 1112–1119.

Gruenwald, P. (1966b). Growth of the human fetus. II. Abnormal growth in twins and infants of mothers with diabetes, hypertension or isoimmunization. *Amer. J. Obstet. Gynecol.* **94**, 1120–1132.

Grumbach, M. M., and Ducharme, J. R. (1960). The effects of androgens on fetal sexual development; androgen-induced female pseudohermaphroidism. *Fertil. Steril.* **11**, 157–180.

Grüneberg, H. (1952). "The Genetics of the Mouse," 2nd ed. Nijhoff, The Hague.

Grüneberg, H. (1963). "The Pathology of Development. A study of Inherited Skeletal Disorders in Animals." Wiley, New York.

Gumpel, S. M., Hayes, K., and Dudgeon, J. A. (1971). Congenital perceptive deafness: role of intrauterine rubella. *Brit. Med. J.* **2**, 300–304.

Gunberg, D. L. (1958). Variations in the teratogenic effects of trypan blue administered to pregnant rats of different strain and substrain origin. *Anat. Rec.* **130**, 310.

Gustafsson, B. and Gledhill, B. L. (1966). Vagina, developmental abnormalities. *In "International Encyclopedia of Vet. Med."* Dalling *et al.* eds., pp. 3012–3015.

Haddad, R. K., Rabe, A., Laqueur, G. L., Spatz, M., and Valsamis, M. P. (1969). Intellectual deficit associated with transplacentally induced microcephaly in the rat. *Science* **163**, 88–90.

Hakosalo, J., and Saxén, L. (1971). Influenza epidemic and congenital defects. *Lancet* **2**, 1346–1347.

Hale, F. (1933). Pigs born without eyeballs. *J. Hered.* **24**, 105.

Hamburgh, M., Herz, R., and Landa, G. (1970). The effect of trypan blue on expressivity of the brachyury gene "T" in mice. *Teratology* **3**, 11–118.

Hamlin, R. L., Smelzer, D. L., and Smith, R. C. (1964). Interventricular septal defect (Roger's disease) in the dog. *J. Amer. Vet. Med. Ass.* **145**, 331–340.

Hansen, H. (1970). Epidemiologic considerations on maternal hyperphenylalaninemia. *Amer. J. Dent Defic.* **75**, 22–26.

Hanshaw, J. B. (1970). Developmental abnormalities associated with congenital cytomegalovirus infection. *Advan. Teratol.* **4**, 64–93.

Harada, Y. (1968). Congenital Minamata Disease. *In* Minamata Disease, pp. 73–91. Kumanoto Univ. Study Group of Minamata Disease.

Harbison, R. D., and Becker, B. A. (1969). Relation of dosage and time of administration of diphenylhydantoin to its teratogenic effect in mice. *Teratology* **2**, 305–312.

Haring, O. M., and Polli, J. F. (1957). Experimental production of cardiac malformations. *Arch. Pathol.* **64**, 290–296.

Harris, J. W., and Ross, I. P. (1956). Cortisone therapy in early pregnancy: relation to cleft palate. *Lancet* **1**, 1045–1047.

Harris, S. B., Wilson, J. G., and Printz, R. H. (1972). Embryotoxicity of methyl mercuric chloride in golden hamsters. *Teratology* **6**, 139–142.

Härtel, A., and Härtel, G. (1960). Experimental study of teratogenic effects of emotional stress in rats. *Science* **132**, 1483–1484.

Hawkins, R. J., and Meckel, R. S. (1950). A study of neonatal deaths. A six-year review. *Amer. J. Obstet. Gynecol.* **59**, 609–617.

Hay, S. (1971). Sex differences in the incidence of certain congenital malformations: a review of the literature and some new data. *Teratology* **4**, 277–286.

Hazzard, D. G., and Budd, R. A. (1969). Effect of in utero x-irradiation on the peripheral blood of the newborn rat. *In* "Radiation Biology of the Fetal and Juvenile Mammal" (M. R. Sikov and D. D. Mahlum, eds.), pp. 357–364. U.S. At. Energy Commission, Washington, D.C.

Helmsworth, B. N. (1968). Embryopathies in the rat due to alkane sulfonates. *J. Reprod. Fertil.* **17**, 325–334.

Hendrickx, A. G. (1966). Teratological findings in a baboon colony. *In* "Food and Drug Administration Conference on Nonhuman Primate Toxicology." Airlie House, Virginia.

Hendrickx, A. G. (1971a). "Embryology of the Baboon." Univ. of Chicago Press, Chicago, Illinois.

Hendrickx, A. G. (1971b). Teratogenic effects of thalidomide in bonnet monkey *(Macaca radiata)* and cynomolgus monkey *(Macaca irus)*. *Teratology* **4**, 231.

Hendrickx, A. G., Axelrod, L. R., and Clayborn, L. D. (1966). 'Thalidomide' syndrome in baboons. *Nature (London)* **210**, 958–959.

Herbst, A. L., Ulfelder, H., and Poskanzer, D. C. (1971). Adenocarcinoma of the vagina. *New England J. Med.* **284**, 878–881.

Hertig, A. T., and Rock, J. (1941). Two human ova of the pre-villous stage, having an ovulation age of about eleven and twelve days respectively. *Carnegie Contrib. Embryol.* **29**, 127–156.

Hertig, A. T., and Rock, J. (1945). Two human ova of the pre-villous stage, having a developmental age of about seven and nine days respectively. *Carnegie Contrib. Embryol.* **31**, 65–84.

Hertig, A. T., Rock, J., Adams, E. C., and Mulligan, W. J. (1954). On preimplantation stages of human ovum: description of 4 normal and 4 abnormal specimens ranging from second to fifth day of development. *Carnegie Contrib. Embryol.* **35**, 199–220.

Hertig, A. T., Rock, J., and Adams, E. C. (1956). Description of 34 human ova within first 17 days of development. *Amer. J. Anat.* **98**, 435–493.

Hertzig, M. E., Birch, H. G., Richardson, S. A., and Trzard, J. (1972). Intellectual levels of school children severely malnourished during the first two years of life. *Pediatrics* **49**, 814–824.

Heuser, C. H. (1932). A presomite human embryo with a definite chorda canal. *Carnegie Contrib. Embryol.* **23**, 251–267.

Heuser, C. H., Rock, J., and Hertig, A. T. (1945). Two human embryos showing early stages of the definitive yolk sac. *Carnegie Contrib. Embryol.* **31**, 85–99.

Heuser, C. H., and Streeter, G. L. (1941). Development of the Macaque embryo. *Carnegie Contrib. Embryol.* **29**, 15–55.

Hickey, M. F. (1953). Genes and mermaids: changing theories of the causation of congenital abnormalities. *Med. J. Aust.* **1**, 649–667.

Hicks, S. P. (1953). Developmental malformations produced by radiation. A timetable of their development. *Amer. J. Roentgenol.* **69**, 272–293.

Hicks, S. P. (1954). The effects of ionizing radiation, certain hormones, and radiomimetic drugs on the developing mouse embryo. *J. Cell. Comp. Physiol. Suppl. 1* **43**, 151–178.

Hicks, S. P., and D'Amato, C. J. (1966). Radiosensitivity at various stages of the mitotic cycle and cellular differentiation. *Advan. Teratol.* **1**, 215–227.

Hicks, S. P., D'Amato, C. J., Klein, S. J., Austin, L. L., and French, B. C. (1969). Effects of regional irradiation or ablation of the infant rat cerebellum on motor development. *In* "Radiation Biology of the Fetal and Juvenile Mammal" (M. R. Sikov and D. D. Mahlum, eds.), pp. 739–754. U. S. At. Energy Commission, Washington, D.C.

Hoar, R. M. (1962). Similarity of congenital malformations produced by hydrocortisone to those produced by adrenalectomy in guinea pigs. *Anat. Rec.* **144**, 155–164.

Hodges, R. C., Hamilton, H. E., and Keettel, W. C. (1952). Pregnancy in myxedema. *Arch. Int. Med.* **90**, 863–868.

Höglund, N. J. (1952). Effects of ethylmethane on reproduction in mice. *Acta Pharmacol. Toxicol.* **8**, 82–84.

Hollaender, A. (1971). "Chemical Mutagens. Principles and Methods for Their Detection," Vol. 1 and 2. Plenum Press, New York.

Hollaender, A., and Stapleton, G. E. (1959). Ionizing radiation and the cell. *Sci. Amer.* 2–8.

Holt, K. S., and Coffey, V. P. (1968). "Some Recent Advances in Inborn Errors of Metabolism." Livingstone, Edinburgh.

Holtfreter, J. (1945). Differential inhibition of growth and differentiation by mechanical and chemical means. *Anat. Rec.* **93**, 59–74.

Hook, E. B., Janerich, D. T., and Porter, I. H. (1971). "Monitoring Birth Defects and Environment." Academic Press, New York.

Hoover, E. A., and Grusemer, R. A. (1971). Experimental feline herpes virus infection in the pregnant cat. *Amer. J. Pathol.* **65**, 173–188.

Hoskins, D. (1948). Some effects of nitrogen mustard on the development of external body form in the rat. *Anat. Rec.* **102**, 493–512.

Howe, W. L., and Parsons, P. A. (1967). Genotype and environment in the determination of minor skeletal variants and body weight in mice. *J. Embryol. Exp. Morphol.* **17**, 283–292.

Hurley, L. S. (1967). Studies on nutritional factors in mammalian development. *J. Nutr.* **91**, 27–38.

Hurley, L. S. (1968a). Approaches to the study of nutrition in mammalian development. *Fed. Proc.* **27**, 193–198.

Hurley, L. S. (1968b). The consequences of fetal impoverishment. Nutrition Today, pp. 3–10.

Hurley, L. S. (1969). Nutrients and genes: interactions in development. Nutr. Rev., 27:3–6.

Hurley, L. S., and Cosens, G. (1970). Teratogenic magnesium deficiency in pregnant rats. *Teratology* **3**, 202.

Hurley, L. S., Everson, G. J., and Geiger, J. F. (1958). Manganese deficiency in rats: congenital nature of ataxia. *J. Nutr.* **66**, 309–320.

Hurley, L. S., Gowan, J., and Swenerton, H. (1971). Teratogenic effects of short-term and transitory zinc deficiency in rats. *Teratology* **4**, 199–204.

Idänpään-Heikkilä, J. E., Fritchie, G. E., Ho, B. T., and McIsaac, W. M. (1971). Placental transfer of C14-ethanol. *Amer. J. Obstet. Gynecol.* **110**, 426–428.

Idänpään-Heikkilä, J. E., Jonppila, P. I., Puolakka, J. O., and Vorne, M. S. (1971). Placental transfer and fetal metabolism of diazepan in early human pregnancy. *Amer. J. Obstet. Gynecol.* **109**, 1011–1016.

Iffy, L., Shepard, T. H., Jakobovits, R. J., Lemire, R. J., and Kerner, P. (1967). The rate of growth in young human embryos of Streeter's horizons XIII to XXIII. *Acta Anat.* **66**, 178–186.

Ihara, T. (1970). Comparative study of developmental progress in the mouse, rat and rabbit in their stages of organogenesis. *Congr. Anom.* **10**, 67–81.

Ingalls, N. W. (1920). A human embryo at the beginning of segmentation, with special reference to the vascular system. *Carnegie Contrib. Embryol.* **11**, 61–90.

Ingalls, T. H., and Curley, F. J. (1957). Principles governing the genesis of congenital malformations induced in mice by anoxia. *New England J. Med.* **257**, 1121–1127.

Ingalls, T., and Klingberg, M. A. (1965). Implications of epidemic embryopathy for public health. *Amer. J. Public Health* **55**, 200–208.

Ingram, D. L. (1958). Fertility and oocyte numbers after x-irradiation of the ovary. *J. Endocrinol.* **17**, 81–90.

Jacobs, P. A. (1970). Chromosome abnormalities and population studies. *In* "Congenital Malformations" (F. C. Fraser and V. A. McKusick, eds.), pp. 284–292. Excerpta Medica, Amsterdam.

Jacobsen, L. (1970). Radiation induced foetal damage. A quantitative analysis of seasonal influence and possible threshold effect following low dose x-irradiation. *Advan. Teratol.* **4**, 95–123.

James, L. F. (1972). Effect of locoweed on fetal development: preliminary study in sheep. *Amer. J. Vet. Res.* **33**, 835–840.

James, L. F., and Keeler, R. F. (1968). Teratogenic effects of aminopterin in sheep. *Teratology* **1**, 407–412.

Janz, D., and Fuchs, U. (1964). Sind antiepileptische Medikamente wahrend der Schwangerschaft sehadlich? *Deutsch. Med. Wochenschr.* **89**, 241–243.

Jensh, R. P., and Brent, R. L. (1967). An analysis of the growth retarding effects of trypan blue in the albino rat. *Anat. Rec.* **159**, 453–458.

Jensh, R. P., Brent, R. L., and Barr, M. (1970). The litter effect as a variable in teratologic studies of the albino rat. *Amer. J. Anat.* **128**, 185–192.

Jick, H., Miethnen, O. S., Shapiro, S., Lewis, G. P., Suskind, V., and Sloane, D. (1970). Comprehensive drug surveillance. *J. Amer. Med. Ass.* **213**, 1455–1460.

Johnson, E. M. (1965). Electrophoretic analysis of abnormal development. *Proc. Soc. Exp. Biol. Med.* **118**, 9–11.

Johnson, E. M., and Lambert, C. (1968). Effects of N-nitroso-N-methylurea on enzymatic ontogeny associated with teratogenesis. *Teratology* **1**, 179–192.

Johnson, E. M., Nelson, M. M., and Monie, I W. (1963). Effects of transitory pteroylglutamic acid (PGA) deficiency on embryonic and placental development in rat. *Anat. Rec.* **146**, 215–224.

Johnson, R. T., Johnson, K. P., and Edmonds, C. J. (1967). Virus-induced hydrocephalus: development of aqueductal stenosis in hamsters after mumps infection. *Science* **157**, 1066–1067.

Jones, D. C. (1969). Persistent and late effects of whole-body irradiation in juvenile male rats. *In* "Radiation Biology of the Fetal and Juvenile Mammal" (M. R. Sikov and D. D. Mahlum, eds.) pp. 439–447. U.S. At. Energy Commission, Washington, D.C.

Jones, H. W., and Scott, W. W. (1958). "Hermaphroditism, Genital Anomalies and Related Endocrine Disorders." Williams and Wilkins, Baltimore, Maryland.

Jordan, R. L., and Wilson, J. G. (1970). Radioautographic study of RNA synthesis in normal and actinomycin D treated rat embryos. *Anat. Rec.* **164**, 549–563.

Juchau, M. R. (1972). Mechanisms of drug biotransformation reactions in the placenta. *Fed. Proc.* **31**, 48–51.

Jukes, T. H. (1966). Mutations. *In* "Molecules and Evolution," pp. 100–145. Columbia Univ. Press, New York.

Kafotos, F. C., and Reich, J. (1968). Stability of differentiation-specific and nonspecific messenger RNA in insect cells. *Proc. Nat. Acad. Sci.* **60**, 1458–1465.

Källén, B. (1956). Contribution to the knowledge of the regulation of the proliferation processes in the vertebrate brain during ontogenesis. *Acta Anat.* **27**, 351–360.

Källén, B., and Winberg, J. (1968). A Swedish register of congenital malformations. *Pediatrics* **41**, 765–776.

Kalter, H. (1954). The inheritance of susceptibility to the teratogenic action of cortisone in mice. *Genetics* **39**, 185.

Kalter, H. (1957). Factors influencing the frequency of cortisone-induced cleft palate in mice. *J. Exp. Zool.* **134**, 449–468.

Kalter, H. (1960). Teratogenic action of a hypocaloric diet and small doses of cortisone. *Proc. Soc. Exp. Biol. Med.* **104**, 518–520.

Kalter, H. (1965). Interplay of intrinsic and extrinsic factors. *In* "Teratology: Principles and Techniques" (J. G. Wilson and J. Warkany, eds.), pp. 57–93. Univ. of Chicago Press, Chicago, Illinois.

Kalter, H. (1968). "Teratology of the Central Nervous System." Univ. of Chicago Press, Chicago, Illinois.

Kalter, H. (1969). The influence of some non-genetic features on the teratogenic response to triamcinolone in mice. *In Proc. Int. Conf. Congenital Malf., 3rd* (F. C. Fraser and F. J. G. Ebling, eds.), **191**, 53. Excerpta Medica, Amsterdam.

Kalter, H. (1971). Correlation between teratogenic and mutagenic effects of chemicals in mammals. *In* "Chemical Mutagens" (A. Hollaender, ed.), Vol. 1, pp. 57–82. Plenum Press, New York.

Kalter, H., and Warkany, J. (1959). Experimental production of congenital malformations in mammals by metabolic procedures. *Physiol. Rev.* **39**, 69–115.

Kaplan, S., and Grabowski, C. T. (1967). Analysis of trypan blue-induced rumplessness in chick embryos. *J. Exp. Zool.* **165**, 325–336.

Karlsson, K., and Kjellmer, I. (1972). The outcome of diabetic pregnancies in relation to the mother's blood sugar level. *Amer. J. Obstet. Gynecol.* **112**, 213–220.

Karnofsky, D. A. (1965a). Drugs as teratogens in animals and man. *Annu. Rev. Pharmacol.* **5**, 447–472.

Karnofsky, D. A. (1965b). Mechanisms of action of certain growth-inhibiting drugs. *In* "Teratology, Principles and Techniques" (J. G. Wilson and J. Warkany, eds.), pp. 185–213. Univ. of Chicago Press, Chicago, Illinois.

Kato, T., Jarvik, L. F., Roizin, L., and Moralishvili, E. (1970). Chromosome studies in pregnant rhesus macaque given LSD-25. *Dis. Nerv. Syst.* **31**, 245–250.

Kaufmann, A. F. (1972). The effects of spontaneous disease during quarantine, conditioning and reproduction of nonhuman primates for scientific use following importation. *In Int. Symp. Health Aspects of Int. Movement Anim.* WHO Sci. Publ. No. 235.

Kaven, A. (1938). Das Auftreten von Gehirnmissbildungen nach Röntgenbestrahlung von Mäuseembryonen *Z. Menschl. Vererb.-U. Konst. Lehre* **22**, 247–257.

Keeler, R. F., and Binns, W. (1968). Teratogenic compounds of Veratrum californicum. *Teratology* **1**, 5–10.

Kemp, N. E. (1962). Development: swine. *In* "Growth: Reproduction and Morphological Development" (P. L. Altman and D. S. Dittmer, eds.), pp. 300–303. Fed. Amer. Soc. Exp. Biol.

Kendrick, F. J., and Field, L. E. (1967). Congenital anomalies induced in normal and adrenalectomized rats by amniocentesis. *Anat. Rec.* **159**, 353–356.

Kennedy, W. P. (1967). Epidemiologic aspects of the problem of congenital malformations. *Birth Defects Orig. Art. Ser.* **3**, 1–18.

Kerschbaum, T. H., Dilts, P. V., and Brinkman, C. R. (1970). Some acute effects of smoking in sheep and their fetuses. *Obstet. Gynecol.* **35**, 527–536.

Keys, A., Brozek, J., Henschel, A., Mickelsen, O., and Taylor, H. L. (1950). Growth and development. *In* "The Biology of Human Starvation," Vol. 2, pp. 974–987. Univ. of Minneapolis Press, Minneapolis, Minnesota.

Khera, K. S., and Clegg, D. J. (1969). Perinatal toxicity of pesticides. *Can. Med. Ass. J.* **100**, 167–172.

Kilham, L., and Ferm, V. H. (1964). Rat virus (RV) infections of pregnant, fetal and newborn rats. *Proc. Soc. Exp. Biol. Med.* **117**, 874–879.

Kilham, L., and Margolis, G. (1966). Viral etiology of spontaneous ataxia of cats. *Amer. J. Pathol.* **48**, 991–1011.

Kimmel, C. A., and Wilson, J. G. (in press) Skeletal deviations in rats: malformations or variations. *Teratology.*

Kimmel, C. A., Wilson, J. G., and Schumacher, H. J. (1971). Studies on metabolism and identification of the causative agent in aspirin teratogenesis in the rat. *Teratology* **4**, 15–24.

King, C. T. G., Weaver, S. A., and Narrod, S. A. (1965). Antihistamines and teratogenicity in the rat. *J. Pharmacol. Exp. Ther.* **147**, 391–398.

King, G. J. (1969). Deformities in piglets following administration of methallibure during specific stages of gestation. *J. Reprod. Fertil.* **20**, 551–553.

Klemetti, A., and Saxén, L. (1967). Prospective versus retrospective approach in the search for environmental causes of malformations. *Amer. J. Publ. Health,* **57**, 2071–2075.

Klemetti, A., and Saxén, L. (1970). The Finnish register of congenital malformations. Organization and six years of experience. Health Serv. Res. of the Nat. Board of Health in Finland, Helsinki.

Klevit, H. K. (1960). Congenital virilizing adrenal hyperplasia. *Amer. J. Dis. Child.* **100**, 415–423.

Knelson, J. H. (1971). Environmental influence on intrauterine lung development. *Arch. Int. Med.* **127**, 421–425.

Kochhar, D. M. (1967). Teratogenic activity of retinoic acid. *Acta Pathol. Microbiol. Scand.* **70**, 398–404.

Kochhar, D. M., Larsson, K. S., and Bostrom, H. (1968). Embryonic uptake of S^{35}-sulfate: change in level following treatment with some teratogenic agents. *Biol. Neonate* **12**, 41–53.

Körner, W. F., and Nowak, H. (1971). The influence of vitamin B_6 deficiency during pregnancy on the fetal postnatal development of the rat. "Malformations Congénitales des Mammifères" (H. Tuchmann-Duplessis, ed.). Masson, Paris.

Krafka, J. (1941). The Torpin ovum, a presomite human embryo. *Carnegie Contrib. Embryol.* **29**, 167–193.

Krakoff, I. H., Brown, N. C., and Reichard, P. (1968). Inhibition of ribonucleoside diphosphate reductase by hydroxyurea. *Cancer Res.* **28**, 1559–1565.

Kučera, J. (1968). Exposure to fat solvents: a possible cause of sacral agenesis in man. *J. Pediatr.* **72**, 857–859.

Kučera, J. (1971a). Patterns of conenital anomalies in the offspring of women exposed to different drugs and/or chemicals during pregnancy. *Teratology* **4**, 492.

Kučera, J. (1971b). Down's syndrome and infective hepatitis in Bohemia. *Teratology* **4**, 492.

Kučera, J., Lenz, W., and Maier, W. (1965). Malformations of the lower limbs and the caudal part of the spinal column in children of diabetic mothers. *Ger. Med. Mon.* **10**, 393–396.

Kuenssberg, E. V., and Knox, J. D. E. (1972). Imipramine in pregnancy. *Brit. Med. J.* **2**, 292.

Laird, A. K. (1966). Dynamics of embryonic growth. *Growth* **30**, 263–275.

Landauer, W. (1954). On the chemical production of developmental abnormalities and of phenocopies in chicken embryos. *J. Cell. Physiol.* **43**, 261–305.

Landauer, W. (1957). Phenocopies and genotype, with special reference to sporadically-occurring developmental variants. *Amer. Natur.* **91**, 79–90.

Landauer, W. (1958). On phenocopies, their developmental physiology and genetic meaning. *Amer. Natur.* **92**, 201–213.

Landauer, W. (1960). Nicotine-induced malformations of chicken embryos and their bearing on the phenocopy problem. *J. Exp. Zool.* **143**, 107–122.

Landauer, W., and Clark, E. M. (1963). Interaction of insulin and chlorpromazine in teratogenesis. *Nature (London)* **198**, 215–216.

Landauer, W., and Clark, E. M. (1964). Uncouplers of oxidative phosphorylation and teratogenic activity of insulin. *Nature (London)* **204**, 285–286.

Landauer, W., and Sopher, D. (1970). Succinate, glycerophosphate and ascorbate as sources of cellular energy and as antiteratogens. *J. Embryol. Exp. Morphol.* **24**, 187–202.

Landauer, W., and Wakasugi, N. (1968). Teratological studies with sulphonamides and their implications. *J. Embryol. Exp. Morphol.* **20**, 261–284.

Landtman, B. (1948). On the relationship between maternal conditions during pregnancy and congenital malformations. *Arch. Dis. Child.* **23**, 237–246.

Langman, J., and Shimada, M. (1970). Developmental abnormalities of the cerebellum caused by postnatal treatment with 5-fluorodeoxyuridine. *Teratology* **3**, 204.

Langman, J., and Shimada, M. (1971). Neuronal deficits and abnormalities caused by prenatal treatment of neuroepithelium. *Anat. Rec.* **169**, 363.

Langman, J., Shimada, M., and Webster, W. (1972). The influence of FUdR and BUdR on development of the mouse neocortex. *Teratology* **5**, 260.

Lapinleimu, K., Koskimies, O., Cantell, K., and Saxén, L. (1972). Viral antibodies in mothers of defective children. *Teratology* **5**, 345–352.

Lapshin, S. A. (1968). Effect of manganese sulfate supplement feeding on the intrauterine development of sheep. *Uch. Zap. Mord. Gos. Univ.* 29–33.

Larsson, K. S., and Eriksson, M. (1966). Salicylate-induced fetal death and malformations in two mouse strains. *Acta Pediatr. Scand.* **55**, 569–576.

Larsson, K. S., Bostrom, H., and Erickson, B. (1963). Salicylate-induced malformations in mouse embryos. *Acta Pediatr. Scand.* **52**, 36–40.

Larsson, Y., and Sterky, G. (1961). Possible teratogenic effect of tolbutamide in a pregnant prediabetic. *Lancet* **2**, 1424–1425.

Layton, M. M., and Hallesy, D. W. (1965). Deformity of forelimb in rats: associated with high doses of acetazolamide. *Science* **149**, 306–308.

Lechner, G., and Leinzinger, E. (1965). The relationship between maternal toxoplasmosis and embryopathy. *Arch. Gynaekol.* **202**, 99–100.

Leck, I. (1966). Changes in the incidence of neural-tube defects (human). *Lancet* **2**, 791–793.

Lederberg, J. (1970). Genetic engineering and the amelioration of genetic defect. *Bioscience* **20**, 1307–1310.

Lederer, J. (1952). Traitement par les substances thyreostatiques de l'hyperthyroidie au cours de la grossesse, étude de 17 cas. *Ann. Endocrinol.* **13**, 697–704.

Lee, S. (1971). High incidence of true hermaphroditism in early human embryos. *Biol. Neonate* **18**, 418–425.

Lefebvres-Boisselot, J. (1951). Role tératogene de la déficience en acide pantothenique chez le rat. *Ann. Med.* **52**, 225–298.

Legator, M. S., and Malling, H. V. (1971). The host mediated assay, a practical procedure for evaluating potential mutagenic agents in mammals. *In* "Chemical Mutagens" (A. Hollaender, ed.), Vol. 2, pp. 569–589. Plenum Press, New York.

Lejour-Jeanty, M. (1966). Becs-de-lievre provoques chez le rat par un dérive de la penicilline, l'hadacidine. *J. Embryol. Exp. Morphol.* **15**, 193–211.

Lenz, W. (1961). Kindliche missbildungen nach medikament wahrend der draviditat? *Deutsch. Med. Wochenschr.* **86**, 2555–2556.

Lenz, W. (1964). Chemicals and malformations in man. *In* "Congenital Malformations." pp. 263–276. *Int. Med. Congr.,* New York.

Lenz, W. (1966). Malformations caused by drugs in pregnancy. *Amer. J. Dis. Child.* **112**, 99–106.

Lenz, W., and Maier, W. (1964). Congenital malformations and maternal diabetes. *Lancet* **2**, 1124–1125.

Lenz, W., Pfeiffer, R. A., and Tunte, W. (1967). Supernumerary chromosomes (trisomies) and maternal age. *Ger. Med. Mon.* **12**, 27–30.

Letavet, A. A., and Kurlyandskaya, E. B. (1970). The effect of uranous uranic oxide on the body of the pregnant female and the fetus. *In* "The Toxicology of Radioactive Substances," Vol. 4, Pergamon Press, Elmsford, New York.

Levin, J. N. (1971). Amphetamine ingestion with biliary atresia. *J. Pediatr.* **79**, 130–131.

Levy, G. (1965). Pharmacokinetics of salicylate elimination in man. *J. Pharm. Sci.* **54**, 959–967.

Lilienfeld, A. M. (1970). Population differences in frequency of malformations at birth. *In* "Congenital Malformations" (F. C. Fraser and V. A. McKusick, eds.), pp. 251–263. Excerpta Medica, Amsterdam.

Lillie, F. R. (1917). The free-martin: a study of the action of sex hormones in the fetal life of cattle. *J. Exp. Zool.* **23**, 371–452.

Lloyd, J. B., and Beck, F. (1969). The mechanism of teratogenic action of trypan blue. *In* "Teratology, Proceedings of the International Symposium on Teratology at Como, Italy" (A. Bertelli, ed.), pp. 145–151. Excerpta Medica, Amsterdam.

Long, S. Y. (1972). Does LSD induce chromosomal damage and malformations? A review of literature. *Teratology* **6**, 75–92.

Longo, L. D. (1972). Disorders of placental transfer. *In* "Pathophysiology of Gestation." (N. S. Assali, ed.), Vol. 2, pp. 1–76. Academic Press, New York.

Lowe, C. R. (1964). Congenital defects among children born to women under supervision or treatment for pulmonary tuberculosis. *Brit. J. Prev. Soc. Med.* **18**, 14–16.

Lucey, J. F. (1965). Drugs and the intrauterine patient. *In Symp. Placenta* (D. Bergsma, ed.), Vol. 1, pp. 46–51. Nat. Foundation-March of Dimes.

Lucey, J. F., and Behrman, R. E. (1963). Thalidomide: effect upon pregnancy in the rhesus monkey. *Science* **139**, 1295–1296.

Mabry, C. C. (1970). Maternal phenylketonuria. Known matings of women with phenylketonuria. Personal communication.

MacCready, R. A., and Levy, H. L. (1972). The problem of maternal phenylketonuria. *Amer. J. Obstet. Gynecol.* **113**, 121–128.

Mackler, B. (1969). Studies of the molecular basis of congenital malformations. *Pediatrics* **43**, 915–926.

MacMahon, B. (1962). Prenatal x-ray exposure and childhood cancer. *J. Nat. Cancer Inst.* **28**, 1173–1191.

Madearis, D. N. (1964). Mouse cytomegalovirus. III. Attempts to produce intrauterine infection. *Amer. J. Hyg.* **80**, 113–120.

Malamud, N. (1964). Neuropathology. *In* "Mental Retardation" (H. A. Stevens and R. Heber, eds.). Univ. of Chicago Press, Chicago, Illinois.

Malorny, G. (1969). Acute and chronic toxicity of formic acid and its formates. *Z. Ernaehrungswiss.* **9**, 332–339.

Malowista, S. E., Sato, H., and Bensch, K. G. (1968). Vinblastine and griseofulvin reversibly disrupt the living mitotic spindle. *Science* **160**, 770–771.

Marin-Padilla, M. (1966). Mesodermal alterations induced by hypervitaminosis A. *J. Embryol. Exp. Morphol.* **15**, 261–269.

Martin, P. G. (1969). Growth response of rats to prenatal irradiation as indicated by changes in DNA, RNA and protein. *In* "Radiation Biology of the Fetal and Juvenile Mammal" (M. R. Sikov and D. D. Mahlum, eds.), pp. 375–380. U.S. At. Energy Commission, Washington, D.C.

Mason, K. E. (1933). Differences in testis injury and repair after vitamin A deficiency, vitamin E deficiency and inanition. *Amer. J. Anat.* **52**, 153–239.

Matsumoto, H. G., Goyo, K., and Takevchi, T. (1965). Fetal Minamata disease. A neuropathological study of two cases of intrauterine intoxication by a methylmercury compound. *J. Neuropathol. Exp. Neurol.* **24**, 563–574.

McBride, W. G. (1961). Thalidomide and congenital abnormalities. *Lancet* **2**, 1358.

McBride, W. G. (1972). The teratogenic effects of imipramine. *Teratology* **5**, 262.

McIntosh, R., Merritt, K. K., Richards, M. R., Samuels, M. H., and Bellows, M. T. (1954). The incidence of congenital malformations: a study of 5,964 pregnancies. *Pediatrics* **14**, 505–521.

McKeown, T. (1961). Sources of variation in the incidence of malformations. *1st Int. Conf. Cong. Malf.* pp. 45–52. Lippincott, Philadelphia, Pennsylvania.

McKeown, T., and Record, R. C. (1963). Malformations in a population observed for five years after birth. *In* "Ciba Foundation Symposium on Congenital Malformations" (G. E. W. Wolstenholme and C. M. O'Connor, eds.), pp. 2–16. Little, Brown, Boston, Massachusetts.

McKeown, T., and Record, R. C. (1971). Early environmental influences on the development of intelligence. *Brit. Med. Bull.* **27**, 48–52.

McLaren, A., and Michie, D. (1963). Congenital runts. *In* "Ciba Foundation Symposium on Congenital Malformations" (G. E. W. Wolstenholme and C. M. O'Connor, eds.), pp. 178–194. Little, Brown, Boston, Massachusetts.

McLaughlin, J., Reynaldo, E. F., Lamar, J. K., and Marliac, J.-P. (1969). Teratology studies in rabbits with captan, folpet and thalidomide. *Toxicol. Appl. Pharmacol.* **14**, 59.

McMullin, G. P. (1971). Teratogenic effects of anticonvulsants. *Brit. Med. J.* **2**, 430.

Meadow, S. R. (1968). Anticonvulsant drugs and congenital abnormalities. *Lancet* **2**, 1296.

Meadow, S. R. (1970). Congenital abnormalities and anticonvulsant drugs. *Proc. Roy. Soc. Med.* **63**, 12–13.

Mellin, G. W. (1963). Fetal life study; a prospective epidemiologic study of prenatal influences in fetal development: meclizine and other drugs. *Bull. Soc. Roy. Belge Gynecol. Obstet.* **83**, 79.

Mellin, G. W. (1964). Drugs in the first trimester of pregnancy and the fetal life of Homo sapiens. *Amer. J. Obstet. Gynecol.* **90**, 1169–1180.

Mellin, G. W., and Katzenstein, M. (1964). Increased incidence of malformations—chance or change? *J. Amer. Med. Ass.* **187**, 570–573.

Meltzer, H. J. (1956). Congenital anomalies due to attempted abortion with 4-aminopteroylglutamic acid. *J. Amer. Med. Ass.* **161**, 1253.

Menges, R. W., Selby, L. A., Marienfeld, C. J., Aue, W. A., and Greer, D. L. (1970). A tobacco related epidemic of congenital limb deformities in swine. *Environ. Res.* **3**, 285–302.

Meniro, K. M. H., and Barnett, S. A. (1969). Variation of the lumbar vertebrae of mice at two environmental temperatures. *J. Embryol. Exp. Morphol.* **21**, 97–103.

Menkes, B., Sander, S., and Ilies, A. (1970). Cell death in teratogenesis. *Advan. Teratol.* **4**, 169–215.

Menser, M. A., Lorimer, D., and Harley, J. D. (1967). A twenty-five year follow-up of congenital rubella. *Lancet* **2**, 1347–1350.

Meselson, M. S., Westing, A. H., and Constable, J. D. (1970). Background material relevant to presentations at the 1970 annual meeting of the AAAS. Revised January 14, 1971. Herbicide Assessment Comm. of the Amer. Ass. for the Advan. of Sci.

Middlekamp, J., Reed, C., and Patrizi, G. (1967). Placental transfer of herpes simplex in pregnant rabbits. *Proc. Soc. Exp. Biol. Med.* **125**, 757–760.

Milham, S., and Elledge, W. (1972). Maternal methimazole and congenital defects in children. *Teratology* **5**, 125.

Miller, H. C. (1947). The effects of pregnancy complicated by alloxan diabetes on fetuses of dogs, rabbits and rats. *Endocrinology* **40**, 251–258.

Miller, H. C., and Hassanein, K. (1971). Diagnosis of impaired fetal growth in newborn infants. *Pediatrics* **48**, 511–522.

Miller, J. R. (1958). Experimental and clinical approaches to the biology of congenital defects. Thesis, Dept. of Genet., McGill Univ.

Miller, J. R. (1969). The use of a registry for the study of congenital defect. *In* "Methods for Teratological Studies in Experimental Animals and Man" (H. Nishimura and J. R. Miller, eds.), pp. 206–214. Igaku Shoin, Tokyo.

Miller, J. R., and Shapiro, S. (1972). Detection and evaluation of adverse drug reactions. *J. Amer. Med. Ass.* **220**, 1011.

Miller, R. W. (1956). Delayed effects occurring within the first decade after exposure of young individuals to the Hiroshima atomic bomb. *Pediatrics* **18**, 1–18.

Miller, R. W. (1969). Epidemiologic studies of congenital defects. *In* "Methods for Teratological Studies in Experimental Animals and Man" (H. Nishimura and J. R. Miller, eds.), pp. 158–166. Igaku Shoin, Tokyo.

Milunsky, A., Graef, J. W., and Gaynor, M. F. (1968). Methotrexate-induced congenital malformations, with a review of the literature. *J. Pediatr.* **72**, 790–795.

Mirkin, B. L. (1971). Placental transfer and neonatal elimination of diphenylhydantoin. *Amer. J. Obstet. Gynecol.* **109**, 930–933.

Miyamoto, K., Stephanides, L. M., and Bernsohn, J. (1967). Incorporation of (1-^{14}C) linoleate and linolenate into polyunsaturated fatty acids of phospholipids of the embryonic chick brain. *J. Neurochem.* **14**, 227–237.

Monie, I. W. (1965). Comparative development of rat, chick and human embryos. *Proc. Teratol. Workshop, 2nd, Berkeley, California.*

Monie, I. W., Kho, K., and Morgan, J. (1965). Dissection procedure for rat fetuses permitting alizarin red staining of skeleton and histological study of viscera. *Proc. Teratol. Workshop, 2nd, Berkeley, California.*

Monnet, P., Kalb, J. C., and Pujol, M. (1967). Harmful effects of isoniazid on the fetus and infants. *Lyon Med.* **217**, 431–455.

Morton, N. E. (1970). Birth defects in racial crosses. *In* "Congenital Malformations" (F. C. Fraser and V. A. McKusick, eds.), pp. 264–274. Excerpta Medica, Amsterdam.

Mosier, H. D., and Jansons, R. A. (1972). Fate of nicotine in the rat fetus. *Teratology* **5**, 263.

Moss, P. D. (1962). Phenmetrazine and foetal abnormality. *Brit. Med. J.* **2**, 1610.

Moya, F., and Thorndike, V. (1962). Passage of drugs across the placenta. *Amer. J. Obstet. Gynecol.* **84**, 1778–1798.

Mulvihill, J. J., and Priester, W. A. (1971). The frequency of congenital heart defects (CHD) in dogs. *Teratology* **4**, 236–237.

Murakami, U., and Kameyama, Y. (1963). Vertebral malformation in the mouse foetus caused by maternal hypoxia during early stages of pregnancy. *J. Embryol. Exp. Morphol.* **11**, 107–118.

Murphree, R. L., and Graves, R. B. (1969). Effect of dose rate on prenatally irradiated lambs. *In* "Radiation Biology of the Fetal and Juvenile Mammal" (M. R. Sikov and D. D. Mahlum, eds.), pp. 243–250. U.S. At. Energy Commission, Washington, D.C.

Murphy, M. L. (1959). A comparison of the teratogenic effects of five polyfunctional alkylating agents on the rat fetus. *Pediatrics* **23**, 231–244.

Murphy, M. L. (1965). Factors influencing teratogenic response to drugs. *In* "Teratology: Principles and Techniques" (J. G. Wilson and J. Warkany, eds.), pp. 145–184. Univ. of Chicago Press, Chicago, Illinois.

Murphy, M. L., Dagg, C. P., and Karnofsky, D. (1957). Comparison of teratogenic chemicals in the rat and chick embryos. *Pediatrics* **19**, 701–714.

Myers, R. C., Hill, D. E., Holt, A. B., Scott, R. E., Mellits, E. D. and Cheek, D. B. (1971). Fetal growth retardation produced by experimental placental insufficiency in the rhesus monkey. *Biol. Neonate* **18**, 379–394.

Myrianthopoulos, N.C. (1969). Role of maternal factors in the occurrence of congenital malformations and other abnormalities of childhood. *In Proc. Int. Conf. Congenital Malf., 3rd* **191**, 66. Excerpta Medica, Amsterdam.

Naeye, R. L. (1966). Abnormalities in infants of mothers with toxemia of pregnancy. *Amer. J. Obstet. Gynecol.* **95**, 276–283.

Naggan, L., and MacMahon, B. (1967). Ethnic differences in the prevalence of anencephaly and spina bifida in Boston, Massachusetts. *New England J. Med.* **277**, 1119–1123.

Nair, V. (1969). Effects of exposure to low doses of x-radiation during pregnancy on the development of biochemical systems in the offspring. *In* "Radiation Biology of the Fetal and Juvenile Mammal" (M. R. Sikov and D. D. Mahlum, eds.), pp. 899–911. U.S. At. Energy Commission, Washington, D.C.

Nair, V., and DuBois, K. P. (1968). Prenatal and early postnatal exposure to environmental toxicants. *Chicago Med. Sch. Quart.,* **27**, 75–89.

Navarette, V. N., Torres, I. H., Rivera, I. R., Shor, V. P., and Gracia, P. M. (1967). Maternal carbohydrate disorder and congenital malformations. *Diabetes* **16**, 127–129.

Navarette, V. N., Rojas, C. E., Algee, C. R., and Paniagua, N. E. (1970). Subsequent diabetes in mothers delivered of a malformed infant. *Lancet* **2**, 993–994.

Neel, J. V. (1958). A study of major congenital defects in Japanese infants. *Amer. J. Human Genet.* **10**, 398–445.

Neel, J. V. (1961). Some genetic aspects of congenital defect. *In Congenital Malformations, 1st Int. Conf.* pp. 63–69. Lippincott, Philadelphia, Pennsylvania.

Neel, J. V. (1963). "Changing Perspectives on the Genetic Effects of Radiation." Thomas, Springfield, Illinois.

Neel, J. V. (1971). The detection of increased mutation rates in human population. *Perspect. Biol. Med.* **14**, 522–537.

Nelson, M. M. (1963). Teratogenic effects of pteroylglutamic acid deficiency in the rat. *In Ciba Foundation Symp. Congenital Malformations* (G. E. W. Wolstenholme and C. M. O'Connor, eds.), pp. 134–151. Little, Brown, Boston, Massachusetts.

Nelson, M. M., and Forfar, J. O. (1971). Associations between drugs administered during pregnancy and congenital abnormalities of the fetus. *Brit. Med. J.* **1**, 523–527.

Nelson, M. M., Asling, C. W., and Evans, H. M. (1952). Production of multiple congenital abnormalities in young by maternal pteroylglutamic acid deficiency during gestation. *J. Nutr.* **48**, 61–80.

Nelson, M. M., Wright, H. V., Asling, C. W., and Evans, H. M. (1955). Multiple congenital abnormalities resulting from transitory deficiency of pteroylglutamic acid during gestation in the rat. *J. Nutr.* **56**, 349–370.

Nelson, M. M., Baird, C. D. C., and Wright, H. V. (1956). Multiple congenital abnormalities in the rat resulting from riboflavin deficiency induced by the antimetabolite galactoflavin. *J. Nutr.* **58**, 125–134.

Nelson, M. M., Wright, H. V., Baird, C. D. C., and Evans, H. M. (1957). Teratogenic effects of pantothenic acid deficiency in the rat. *J. Nutr.* **62**, 395–405.

Netzloff, M. L., Johnson, E. M., and Kaplan, S. (1968). Respiratory changes observed in abnormally developing rat embryos. *Teratology* **1**, 375–386.

Neurath, P. W. (1968). High gradient magnetic field inhibits embryonic development of frogs. *Nature (London)* **219**, 1358–1359.

Nichols, W. W. (1966). The role of viruses in the etiology of chromosomal abnormalities. *Amer. J. Human Genet.* **18**, 81–92.

Nicholson, H. O. (1968). Cytotoxic drugs in pregnancy. *J. Obstet. Gynecol. Brit. Commonw.* **75**, 307–312.

Nielsen, N. O. (1969). Teratogenic effects of hyperthermia in chick embryos. *In Teratol., Proc. Int. Symp. Teratol. Como, Italy* (A. Bertelli, ed.), pp. 102–107. Excerpta Medica, Amsterdam.

Nishimura, H. (1963). Interstrain differences in susceptibility to the teratogenic effects of mitomycin C in mice. Abstracts of Papers presented at 3rd annu. meeting of The Teratology Society. Ste. Adele, Quebec.

Nishimura, H. (1964). "Chemistry and Prevention of Congenital Anomalies." Thomas, Springfield, Illinois.

Nishimura, H. (1970). Incidence of malformations in abortions. *In* "Congenital Malformations" (F. C. Fraser and V. A. McKusick, eds.), pp. 275–283. Excerpta Medica, Amsterdam.

Nishimura, H., and Nakai, K. (1958). Developmental anomalies in offspring of pregnant mice treated with nicotine. *Science* **127**, 877–878.

Nishimura, H., and Yamamura, H. (1969). Comparison between man and some other mammals of normal and abnormal developmental processes. *In* "Methods for Teratological Studies in Experimental Animals and Man" (H. Nishimura and J. R. Miller, eds.), pp. 223–240. Igaku Shoin, Tokyo.

Nishimura, H., Takano, K., Tanimura, T., and Yasuda, M. (1968a). Normal and abnormal development of human embryos: first report of the analysis of 1,213 intact embryos. *Teratology* **1**, 281–290.

Nishimura, H., Takano, K., Tanimura, T., Yasuda, M., Tanaka, O., and Tonomura, A. (1968b). Embryonic wastage in clinically healthy women in early pregnancy. *Teratology* **1**, 219.

Noble, R. C., and Moore, J. H. (1967). Liver phospholipids of the developing chick embryo. *Can. J. Biochem.* **45**, 627–640.

Nolen, G. A. (1969). Variations in teratogenic response to hypervitaminosis A in three strains of the albino rat. *Food Cosmet. Toxicol.* **7**, 209–214.

Nolen, G. A. (1971). The effects of dietary protein levels on the teratogenesis of retinoic acid in rats. *Teratology* **4**, 237.

Nomura, T. (1969). Management of animals for use in teratological experiments. *In* "Methods for Teratological Studies in Experimental Animals and Man" (H. Nishimura and J. R. Miller, eds.), pp. 3–15. Igaku Shoin, Tokyo.

Nora, J. J., Trasler, D. G., and Fraser, F. C. (1965). Malformations in mice induced by dexamphetamine sulphate. *Lancet* **2**, 1021–1022.

Nora, J. J., McNamara, D. G., and Fraser, F. C. (1967a). Dexamphetamine sulphate and human malformations. *Lancet* **1**, 570–571.

Nora, J. J., Nora, A. H., Sommerville, R. J., Hill, R. M., and McNamara, D. G. (1967b). Maternal exposure to potential teratogens. *J. Amer. Med. Ass.* **202**, 1065–1069.

Nora, J. J., Vargo, T., Nora, A. H., Love, K. E., and McNamara, D. G. (1970). Dexamphetamine: a possible environmental trigger in cardiovascular malformations. *Lancet* **1**, 1290–1291.

Notter, A., and Delande, M. S. (1962). Prophylaric des exces de poids chez les gratantes d'apparence normale. *Gynecol. Obstet.* **61**, 359–377.

Ogawa, T. (1967). Comparative study on the development in the stage of organogenesis in the rat and mouse. *Cong. Anom.* **7**, 27–30.

O'Grady, D. J., Berry, H. K., and Sutherland, B. S. (1970). Phenylketonuria: intellectual development and early treatment. *Develop. Med. Child. Neurol.* **12**, 343–347.

Ohmori, K. (1968). Changes in incidence of the manifestations of anatomical variations of the vertebrae in the mouse fetus caused by x-radiation or maternal hypervitaminosis. *Cong. Anom.* **7**, 219–238.

Okuda, H., Yamashita, N., and Suzuki, K. (1968). Induction of anomalous fetuses in mice by injection of vitamin K. *In Proc. Cong. Anom. Res. Ass. Japan, 8th Annu. Meeting, Tokyo* p. 46.

Opitz, J. M., Grosse, F. R., and Haneberg, B. (1972). Congenital effects of bromism. *Lancet* **1**, 91–92.

Orlova, O. I. (1966). The health and development of children from mothers with thyrotoxicosis. *Akush. Ginekol.* **4**, 61–65 (cited from *Excerpta Medica* Sect. 21, 6: 609, No. 2749).

Ostertag, B. (1969). Behavior, motility, and anatomical findings in mice surviving prenatal irradiation. *In* "Radiation Biology of the Fetal and Juvenile Mammal" (M. R. Sikov and D. D. Mahlum, eds.), pp. 289–300. U.S. At. Energy Commission. Washington, D.C.

Otis, E. M., and Brent, R. (1954). Equivalent ages in mouse and human embryos. *Anat. Rec.* **120**, 33–64.

Ounsted, M., and Ounsted, C. (1968). Rate of intrauterine growth. *Nature* **220**, 599–600.

Packard, D. S., and Skalko, R. G. (1972). BUdR-induced growth retardation and cellular damage in mouse embryos. *Anat. Rec.* **172**, 378–379.

Padykula, H. A., Deren, J. J., and Wilson, T. H. (1966). Development of structure and function in the mammalian yolk sac. I. Development morphology and vitamin B_{12} uptake of the rat yolk sac. *Develop. Biol.* **13**, 311–348.

Paget, G. E., and Thorpe, E. (1964). A teratogenic effect of a sulphonamide in experimental animals. *Brit. J. Pharmacol.* **23**, 305–312.

Palludan, B. (1966a). "A-Avitaminosis in Swine." Munksgaard, Copenhagen.

Palludan, B. (1966b). Swine in teratological studies. *In* "Swine in Biomedical Research" (L. K. Bustad and R. O. McClellan, eds.), Frayn Printing, Seattle, Washington.

Palludan, B. (1970). The influence of A-avitaminosis on fetal development in swine at late stages of gestation. *Teratology* **3**, 207–208.

Palmer, A. K. (1968). Spontaneous malformations of the New Zealand white rabbit: the background to safety evaluation studies. *Lab. Anim.* **2**, 195–206.

Palmer, A. K. (1969a). The relationship between screening tests for drug safety and other teratological investigations. *In Teratol., Proc. Int. Symp. Teratol. Como, Italy.* (A. Bertelli, ed.), pp. 55–72. Excerpta Medica, Amsterdam.

Palmer, A. K. (1969b). The concept of the uniform animal relative to teratogenicity. *Carworth Eur. Coll. Papers* **3**, 101–113.

Palmer, A. K. (1971). Personal communication.

Palmisano, P. A., and Polhill, R. B. (1972). Fetal pharmacology. *Pediatr. Clin. North Am.* **19**, 3–20.

Palmisano, P. A., Sneed, R. C., and Cassady, G. (1969). Untaxed whiskey and fetal lead exposure. *J. Pediatr.* **75**, 869.

Panigel, M. (1971). La perméabilité du placenta chez l'homme et certains primates non humains. *In* "Malformations Congénitales des Mammifères" (H. Tuchmann-Duplessis, ed.), pp. 27–48. Masson, Paris.

Pashayan, H., Pruzansky, D., and Pruzansky, S. (1971). Are anticonvulsants teratogenic? *Lancet* **2**, 702–703.

Patten, B. M. (1948). "Embryology of the Pig," 3rd ed. Blakiston, Philadelphia, Pennsylvania.

Payne, F. (1925). General description of a 7-somite human embryo. *Carnegie Contrib. Embryol.* **16**, 115–123.

Payne, G. S., and Deuchar, E. M. (1972). An *in vitro* study of function of embryonic membranes in the rat. *J. Embryol. Exp. Morphol.* **27**, 533–542.

Pedersen, L. M., Trygstrup, I., and Pedersen, J. (1964). Congenital malformations in newborn infants of diabetic women. *Lancet* **1**, 1124–1126.

Peters, J. H. (1971). Observations on utility of subhuman primates as models of man for drug studies. *Proc. West. Pharmacol. Soc.* **14**, 72.

Pettersson, F., Olding, L., and Gustavson, K. H. (1970). Multiple severe malformations in a child of a diabetic mother treated with insulin and dibein during pregnancy. *Acta Obstet. Gynecol. Scand.* **49**, 385–387.

Pharoah, P. O. D., Battfield, I. H., and Helzel, B. S. (1971). Neurological damage to the fetus resulting from severe iodine deficiency during pregnancy. *Lancet* **1**, 308–310.

Phemister, R. D., Garner, R. J., Shively, J. N., and Tietz, W. J. (1969). Radiosensitivity of the developing beagle. *In* "Radiation Biology of the Fetal and Juvenile Mammal" (M. R. Sikov and D. D. Mahlum, eds.), pp. 395–406. U.S. At. Energy Commission, Washington, D.C.

Phemister, R. D., Holst, P. A., and Hopwood, M. L. (1972). Determination of ovulation time in the beagle bitch. *In* CSU-PHS Collaborative Radiolog. Health Lab., Annu. Rep. 1971. DHEW Publ. No. (FDA) 72–8032.

Pike, R. L. (1951). Congenital cataract in albino rats fed different amounts of tryptophan and niacin. *J. Nutr.* **44**, 191–204.

Piper, J., and Rosen, J. (1954). Management of hyperthyroidism during pregnancy. *Acta Med. Scand.* **150**, 215–222.

Pitkin, R. M., Reynolds, W. A., and Filer, L. J. (1970). Placental transmission and fetal distribution of cyclamate in early human pregnancy. *Amer. J. Obstet. Gynecol.* **108**, 1043–1050.

Platt, B. S., and Stewart, R. J. C. (1968). Effects of protein caloric deficiency in dogs. I. Reproduction, growth, and behavior. *Develop. Med. Child Neurol.* **10**, 3–24.

Polani, P. E., and Campbell, M. (1960). Factors in the causation of persistent ductus arteriosus. *Ann. Human Genet.* **24**, 343–357.

Pond, W. G., Strachan, D. N., Sinha, U. N., Walker, E. F., Dunn, J. A., and Barnes, R H. (1969). Effect of protein deprivation of swine during all or part of gestation on birth weight, postnatal growth rate and nucleic acid content of brain and muscle of progeny. *J. Nutr.* **99**, 61–67.

Popert, A. J. (1962). Pregnancy and adrenocortical hormones. Some aspects of their action in rheumatic disease. *Brit. Med. J.* **1**, 967–972.

Posner, H. (1971). Fluid imbalances in embryo and fetus. *In Proc. Conf. Toxicol.: Implications Teratol.* pp. 196–233. Nat. Inst. of Child Health and Human Develop., Bethesda, Maryland.

Posner, H. S., Graves, A., King, C. T. G., and Wilk, A. (1967). Experimental alteration of the metabolism of chlorcyclizine and the incidence of cleft palate in rats. *J. Pharmacol. Exp. Ther.* **155**, 494–505.

Poswillo, D. E., Hamilton, W. J., and Sopher, D. (1972). The marmoset as an animal model for teratological research. *Nature (London)* **239**, 460–462.

Potter, E. L. (1953). "Pathology of the Fetus and the Newborn." Yearbook Publ., Chicago, Illinois.

Potter, E. L. (1962). Defective babies that die before birth. *Clin. Pediatr.* **1**, 73–74.

Potworowska, M., Sianozecka, E., and Szufladowicz, R. (1966). Ethionamide treatment and pregnancy (including drug induced abnormalities). *Pol. Med. J.* **5**, 1152–1158.

Powell, P. D., and Johnstone, J. M. (1962). Phenmetrazine and foetal abnormalities. *Brit. Med. J.* **2**, 1327.

Qazi, Q. H., and Thompson, M. W. (1972). Genital changes in congenital virilizing adrenal hyperplasia. *J. Pediatr.* **80**, 653–654.

Ramsey, E. M., and Harris, J. W. S. (1966). Comparison of uteroplacental vasculature and circulation in the rhesus monkey and man. *Carnegie Contrib. Embryol.* **38**, 59–70.

Rane, A., and Sjöqvist, F. (1972). Drug metabolism in the human fetus and newborn infant. *Pediatr. Clin. North Amer.* **19**, 37–49.

Rapport fram en expert grupp (1971). Fenoxisyror, granskuing av aktuell information. Giftnämnden, Stockholm.

Reilly, W. A. (1958). Hormone therapy during pregnancy: effects on the fetus and newborn. *Quart. Rev. Pediatr.* **13**, 198–202.

Report of the 2,4,5-T Advisory Committee (1971). Submitted May 7, 1971, to William D. Ruckelshaus, Administrator, Environmental Protection Agency, Washington, D.C.

Report of the Committee on Adverse Drug Reactions (1971). Rep. 6th annu. of the New Zealand Committee on Adverse Drug Reactions. *NZ Med. J.* **74**, 184–191.

Report of the International Conference on Adverse Reactions Reporting Systems (1971). Drug Res. Board, Nat. Res. Council, Nat. Acad. of Sci., Washington, D.C.

Report of a WHO Meeting (1972). International drug monitoring: the role of national centres. Tech. Rep. 498, WHO, Geneva.

Report of a WHO Scientific Group (1967). Principles for the testing of drugs for teratogenicity. Tech. Rep. 364, WHO, Geneva.

Richards, L. D. G. (1969). Congenital malformations and environmental influences in pregnancy. *Brit. J. Prev. Soc. Med.* **23**, 218.

Rickenbacher, J. (1968). The importance of regulation for the normal and abnormal development. Experimental investigations on the limb buds of chick embryos. *Biol. Neonate* **12**, 65–68.

Ritter, E. J., Scott, W. J., and Wilson, J. G. (1971). Teratogenesis and inhibition of DNA synthesis induced in rat embryos by cytosine arabinoside. *Teratology* **4**, 7–14.

Ritter, E. J., Scott, W. L., and Wilson, J. G. (1973). Mechanisms of teratogenesis with inhibitors of DNA synthesis. Relationship of temporal patterns of cell death and development to malformations in the rat limb. *Teratology*. **7**, 219–225.

Robens, J. F. (1969). Teratologic studies of carbaryl, diazinon, norea, disulfiram and thiram in small laboratory animals. *Toxicol. Appl. Pharmacol.* **15**, 152–163.

Robertson, D. S. F. (1970). Selenium—a possible teratogen? *Lancet* **1**, 518–519.

Robinson, A. (1921). Prenatal death. (Struthers lecture of 1920). *Edinburg Med. J.* **137**, 209.

Robinson, A., and Puck, T. T. (1967). Studies on chromosomal nondisjunction in man. II. *Amer. J. Human. Genet.* **19**, 112–119.

Robinson, A., Good, W. B., Puck, T. T., and Harris, J. S. (1969). Studies on chromosomal nondisjunction in man. III. *Amer. J. Human Genet.* **21**, 466–485.

Robinson, G. C., and Cambon, K. G. (1964). Hearing loss in infants of tuberculous mothers treated with streptomycin during pregnancy. *New England J. Med.* **271**, 949–951.

Robson, J. M. (1970). Testing drugs for teratogenicity and their effects on fertility. The present position. *Brit. Med. Bull.* **26**, 212–216.

Robson, J. M., and Sullivan, F. M. (1963). The production of foetal abnormalities in rabbits by imipramine. *Lancet* **1**, 638–639.

Rorke, L. B., Fabiyi, A., Elizan, T. S., and Sever, J. L. (1968). Experimental cerebrovascular lesions in congenital and neonatal rubella virus infection in ferrets. *Lancet* **2**, 153–154.

Rosenfeld, I., and Beath, O. A. (1947). Congenital malformations of eyes of sheep. *J. Agr. Res.* **75**, 93–103.

Rosenkrantz, J. G., Lynch, F. P., and Frost, W. W. (1970). Congenital anomalies in the pig; teratogenic effects of trypan blue. *J. Pediatr. Surg.* **5**, 232–237.

Rosenquist, G. C. (1970). Cardia bifida in chick embryos: anterior and posterior defects produced by transplanting tritiated thymidine-labeled grafts medial to the heart-forming regions. *Teratology* **3**, 135–142.

Roszkowski, I., Iwanska, J., and Myszkowski, L. (1969). Amino acids in the blood serum of non-pregnant women who formerly gave birth to children with malformations (large). *In Proc. Int. Conf. Congenital Malformations, 3rd* (F. C. Fraser and F. J. G. Ebling, eds.), **191**, 75–76. Excerpta Medica, Amsterdam.

Roux, C., Emerit, I., and Taillemite, J. (1971). Chromosomal breakage and teratogenesis. *Teratology* **4**, 303–315.

Roux, J. M. (1971). Decrease in the rate of the deoxyribonucleic acid synthesis in newborn rats with intrauterine growth retardation. *Biol. Neonate* **18**, 463–467.

Rubin, A., and Murphy, D. P. (1958). Studies on human reproduction. III. The frequency of congenital malformations in the offspring of non-diabetic and diabetic individuals. *J. Pediatr.* **53**, 579–585.

Rugh, R. (1968). "The Mouse, Its Reproduction and Development." Burgess Publ., Minneapolis, Minnesota.

Runner, M. N. (1959). Inheritance of susceptibility to congenital deformity. Metabolic clues provided by experiments with teratogenic agents. *Pediatrics* **23**, 245–251.

Runner, M. N. (1967). Comparative pharmacology in relation to teratogenesis. *Fed. Proc.* **26**, 1131–1136.

Runner, M. N., and Dagg, C. P. (1960). Metabolic mechanisms of teratogenic agents during morphogenesis. *In* "Normal and Abnormal Differentiation and Development" (N. Kaliss, ed.), pp. 41–54. Nat. Cancer Inst. Monograph 2, U.S. Govt. Printing Office, Washington, D.C.

Runner, M. N., and Miller, J. R. (1956). Congenital deformity in the mouse as a consequence of fasting. *Anat. Rec.* **124**, 437.

Rush, D., and Kass, E. H. (1972). Maternal smoking: a reassessment of the association with perinatal mortality. *Amer. J. Epidemiol.* **96**, 183–196.

Rusnak, S. L., and Driscoll, S. G. (1965). Congenital spinal anomalies in infants of diabetic mothers. *Pediatrics* **35**, 989–995.

Russell, K. P., Harvey, R., and Starr, P. (1957). The effect of radioactive iodine on maternal and fetal thyroid function during pregnancy. *Surg. Gynecol. Obstet.* **104**, 560–564.

Russell, L. B. (1950). X-ray induced developmental abnormalities in the mouse and their use in the analysis of embryological patterns. I. External and gross visceral changes. *J. Exp. Zool.* **114**, 545–602.

Russell, L. B. (1956). X-ray induced developmental abnormalities in the mouse and their use in the analysis of embryological patterns. II. Abnormalities of the vertebral column and thorax. *J. Exp. Zool.* **131**, 329–390.

Russell, L. B. (1965). Death and chromosome damage from irradiation of preimplantation stages. *In Ciba Foundation Symp. Preimplantation Stages of Pregnancy* pp. 217–241. Churchill, London.

Russell, L. B., and Russell, W. L. (1954). An analysis of the changing radiation response of the developing mouse embryo. *J. Cell. Comp. Physiol. Suppl.* 1, **43**, 103–150.

Russell, W. L. (1951). X-ray induced mutations in mice. *Cold Spring Harbor Symp. Quant. Biol.* **16**, 327.

Rutter, W. J., Kemp, J. D., Bradshaw, W. S., Clark, W. R., Ronzio, R. A., and Sanders, T. G. (1968). Regulation of specific protein synthesis in cytodifferentiation. *J. Cell. Physiol. Suppl.* 1, **72**, 1–18.

Rychter, Z. (1960). The vascular system of the chick embryo. VII. The theory of the teratogenetic role of the local disturbance of the heart loop and aortic arches. *Excerpta Medica Abstr. Human Develop. Biol.* **1**, 664, #2612, 1961.

Sartori, E. (1971). On the pathogenesis of favism. *J. Med. Genet.* **8**, 462.

Saunders, J. W. (1966). Death in embryonic systems. *Science* **154**, 604–612.

Saunders, J. W., and Fallon, J. F. (1966). Cell death in morphogenesis. *In* "Major Problems in Developmental Biology" (M. Locke, ed.). Academic Press, New York.

Savini, E. C., Moulin, M. A., and Herrou, M. F. (1968). Effets tératogènes de l'oxytetracycline. *Thérapie* **23**, 1247–1260.

Sawin, P. B. (1955). Recent genetics of the domestic rabbit. *Advan. Genet.* **7**, 183-226.

Sawin, P. B. and Crary, D. (1964). Genetics of skeletal deformities in the domestic rabbit. *Clin. Orthop.* **33**, 71–90.

Sawin, P. B., and Gow, M. (1967). Morphogenetic studies of the rabbit. XXXVI. Effect of gene and genome interaction on homeotic variation. *Anat. Rec.* **157**, 425–435.

Sawin, P. B., Crary, D., Fox, R. R., and Wuest, H. M. (1965). Thalidomide malformations and genetic background in the rabbit. *Experentia* **21**, 672–677.

Saxén, L. (1972). Tissue interactions and teratogenesis. *In* "Pathobiology of Development" pp. 31–51. Williams and Wilkins, Baltimore, Maryland.

Saxén, L., and Rapola, J. (1969). "Congenital Defects." Holt, New York.

Saxén, L., and Toivonen, S. (1962). "Primary Embryonic Induction." Academic Press, New York.

Scanlon, F. J. (1969). Use of antidepressant drugs during the first trimester. *Med. J. Aust.* **2**, 1077.

Schiff, D., Aranda, J. V., and Stern, L. (1970). Neonatal thrombocytopenia and congenital malformations associated with administration of tolbutamide to the mother. *J. Pediatr.* **77**, 457–458.

Schnell, V., and Newberne, J. W. (1970). Accelerated clearing and staining of teratologic specimens by heat and light. *Teratology* **3**, 345–348.

Schnurrbusch, U., and Möckel, P. (1969). Experimental malformations in swine fetuses caused by intravenous administration of n-ethyl-n-nitroso-urea. *Arch. Geschwulstforsch.* **33**, 31–38.

Schultz, G., and Delay, P. D. (1955). Losses of newborn lambs associated with blue tongue vaccination of pregnant ewes. *J. Amer. Vet. Med. Ass.* **127**, 224–226.

Schumacher, H. J., Wilson, J. G., and Jordan, R. L. (1969). Potentiation of the teratogenic effects of 5-fluorouracil by natural pyrimidines. II. Biochemical aspects. *Teratology* **2**, 99–105.

Scott, W. J., Ritter, E. J., and Wilson, J. G. (1971). DNA synthesis inhibition and cell death associated with hydroxyurea teratogenesis in rat embryos. *Develop. Biol.* **26**, 306–315.

Scott, W. J., Butcher, R. L., Kindt, C. W., and Wilson, J. G. (1972). Greater sensitivity of female than male rat embryos to acetazolamide teratogenicity. *Teratology* **6**, 239–240.

Scott, W. J., Ritter, E. J., and Wilson, J. G. (1973). DNA synthesis inhibition cytotoxicity and their relationship to teratogenesis following administration of a nicotinamide antagonist, aminothiadiazole, to pregnant rats. *J. Embryol. Exp. Morphol.*, (in press).

Sechzer, J. A., Faro, M. D., Barker, J. N., Barsky, D., Gutieriez, S., and Windle, W. F. (1971). Developmental behaviors: delayed appearance in monkeys asphixiated at birth. *Science* **171**, 1173–1175.

Selby, L. A., Hopps, H. C., and Edmonds, L. D. (1971). Comparative aspects of congenital malformations in man and swine. *J. Amer. Vet. Med. Ass.*, **159**, 1485–1490.

Selby, L. A., Menges, R. W., Houser, E. C., Flatt, R. C., and Case, A. A. (1971). Outbreak of swine malformations associated with the wild black cherry, *Prunus serotina*. *Arch. Environ. Health* **22**, 496–501.

Sever, J. (1969). Viruses and embryos. *In* "Methods for Teratological Studies in Experimental Animals and Man." (H. Nishimura and J. R. Miller, eds.), pp. 92–100. Igaku Shoin, Tokyo.

Sever, J. (1970). Viruses and embryos. *In* "Congenital Malformations" (F. C. Fraser and V. A. McKusick, eds.), pp. 180–186. Excerpta Medica, Amsterdam.

Sever, J. (1971). Virus infections and malformations. *Fed. Proc.* **30**, 114–117.

Sever, J. L., and London, W. T. (1969). Viruses and embryos. *Teratology* **2**, 39–46.

Shaner, R. F. (1951). Complete and corrected transposition of the aorta, pulmonary artery and the ventricles in pig embryos, and a case of corrected transposition in a child. *Amer. J. Anat.* **88**, 35–62.

Shaw, E. B., and Steinbach, H. L. (1968). Aminopterin-induced fetal malformation. *Amer. J. Dis. Child.* **115**, 477–482.

Shaw, M. W. (1970). Human chromosome damage by chemical agents. *Annu. Rev. Med.* **21**, 409–432.

Shenefelt, R. E. (1972). Morphogenesis of malformations in hamsters caused by retinoic acid: relation to dose and stage of treatment. *Teratology* **5**, 103–118.

Shepard, T. H., Tanimura, T., and Robkin, M. (1969). In vitro study of rat embryos. I. Effects of decreased oxygen on embryonic heart rate. *Teratology* **2**, 107–109.

Shepard, T. H., Tanimura, T., and Robkin, M. (1970). Energy metabolism in early mammalian embryos. *In* "Changing Syntheses in Development" (M. N. Runner, ed.) pp. 42–58. Academic Press, New York.

Sheppard, M. (1951). Some observations on cat practice. *Vet Rec.* **63**, 685.

Shettles, L. B. (1955). Further observations on living human oocytes and ova. *Amer. J. Obstet. Gynecol.* **69**, 365–371.

Shimada, M., and Langman, J. (1970). Repair of the external granular layer of the hamster cerebellum after prenatal and postnatal administration of methylazoxymethanol. *Teratology* **3**, 119–134.

Shotten, D., and Monie, I. W. (1963). Possible teratogenic effect of chlorambucil on a human fetus. *J. Amer. Med. Ass.* **186**, 74–75.

Sigler, A. T., Lilienfeld, A. M., Cohen, B. H., and Westlake, J. E. (1965). Radiation exposure in parents of children with Mongolism (Down's syndrome). *Bull. Johns Hopkins Hosp.* **117**, 374–399.

Silver, P. H. S. (1959). Embryonic growth relative to the vitelline membrane and its role in determining the level of post-operative abnormality, as measured in the chick. *J. Embryol. Exp. Morphol.* **7**, 564–571.

Sim, M. (1972). Imipramine and pregnancy. *Brit. Med. J.* **2**, 45.

Sims, F. H. (1951). Methionine and choline deficiency in the rat with special reference to the pregnant state. *Brit. J. Exp. Pathol.* **32**, 481–492.

Sinclair, J. G. (1950). Specific transplacental effect of urethane in mice. *Tex. Rep. Biol. Med.* **8**, 623–632.

Skalko, R. G., and Morse, J. M. D. (1967). The response of the early mouse embryo to actinomycin D treatment in vitro. *Anat. Rec.* **157**, 322.

Skalko, R. G., and Packard, D. S. (1971). Dose-response phenomena in teratology; the relationship between fetal death and fetal malformation. *Teratology* **4**, 242.

Skalko, R. G., Packard, D. S., Schwendimann, R. N., and Raggio, J. F. (1971). The teratogenic response of mouse embryos to 5-bromodeoxyuridine. *Teratology* **4**, 87–94.

Slater, B. C. S. (1965). The investigation of drug embryopathies in man. *In* "Embryopathic Activity of Drugs" (J. M. Robson, F. M. Sullivan, and R. L. Smith, eds.), pp. 241–260. Little, Brown, Boston, Massachusetts.

Slotnick, V., and Brent, R. L. (1966). The production of congenital malformations using tissue antisera. V. Fluorescent localization of teratogenic antisera in the maternal and fetal tissues of the rat. *J. Immunol.* **96**, 606–610.

Smalley, H. E., Curtis, J. M., and Earl, F. L. (1968). Teratogenic action of carbaryl in beagle dogs. *Toxicol. Appl. Pharmacol.* **13**, 392–403.

Smith, A. U. (1957). The effects on foetal development of freezing pregnant hamsters *(Mesocricetus auratus).* *J. Embryol. Exp. Morphol.* **5**, 311–323.

Smith, C. (1972). Computer programme to estimate recurrence risks for multifactorial familial disease. *Brit. Med. J.* **1**, 495–497.

Smith, C. A. (1947). Effects of maternal undernutrition upon the newborn infant in Holland (1944–1945). *J. Pediatr.* **30**, 229–243.

Smith, C. C. (1968). Predicting drug metabolic pathways in man. *In* "Use of Nonhuman Primates in Drug Evaluation" (H. Vagtborg, ed.). Univ. of Texas Press, Austin, Texas.

Smith, C. C. (1969). Value of nonhuman primates in predicting disposition of drugs in man. *Ann. N.Y. Acad. Sci.* **162**, 604–609.

Smith, D. W. (1970). "Recognizable Patterns of Human Malformations." Saunders, Philadelphia, Pennsylvania.

Smith, D. W. (1971). Minor malformations: their relevance and significance. *In* "Monitoring, Birth Defects and Environment" (E. B. Hook, D. T. Janerich, and I. H. Porter, eds.), pp. 169–175. Academic Press, New York.

Smithberg, M. (1961). Teratogenic effects of some hypoglycemic agents in mice. *Univ. Minn. Med. Bull.* **33**, 62–72.

Smithberg, M. (1967). Inbred strains of mice in teratology. *Advan. Teratol.* **2**, 258–288.

Smithells, R. W. (1966). Drugs and human malformations. *Advan. Teratol.* **1**, 251–278.

Smithells, R. W., and Chinn, E. R. (1964). Meclozine and foetal malformations: a prospective study. *Brit. Med. J.* **1**, 217–218.

Snyder, R. D. (1971). Congenital mercury poisoning. *New England J. Med.* **284**, 1014–1016.

Sobel, D. E. (1960). Fetal damage due to ECT, insulin coma, chlorpromazine or reserpine. *Arch. Gen. Psychiat.* **2**, 606–611.

Sokal, J. E., and Lessman, E. M. (1960). Effects of cancer chemotherapeutic agents on human fetus. *J. Amer. Med. Ass.* **172**, 1765–1771.

Somers, G. F. (1962). Thalidomide and congenital abnormalities. *Lancet* **1**, 912–913.

Speidel, B. D., and Meadow, S. R. (1972). Maternal epilepsy and abnormalities of the fetus and newborn. *Lancet* **2**, 839.

Spooner, B. S., and Wessells, N. K. (1972). An analysis of salivary gland morphogenesis: role of cytoplasmic microfilaments and microtubules. *Develop. Biol.* **27**, 38–54.

Spyker, J. M., and Smithberg, M. (1972). Effects of methylmercury on prenatal development in mice. *Teratology* **5**, 181–189.

Spyker, J. M., Sparber, S. B., and Goldberg, A. M. (1972). Subtle consequences of methylmercury exposure: behavioral deviations in offspring of treated mothers. *Science* **177**, 621–623.

Steffek, A. J., and Verrusio, A. C. (1972). Experimentally induced oral-facial malformations in the ferret *(Mustela putorius furo). Teratology* **5**, 268.

Steffek, A. J., Fabiyi, A., and King, C. T. G. (1968). Chlorcyclizine produced cleft palate in the ferret. *Arch. Oral. Biol.* **13**, 1281–1283.

Stempak, J. G. (1964). Etiology of trypan blue induced antenatal hydrocephalus in the albino rat. *Anat. Rec.* **148**, 561–571.

Sterne, J. (1963). Antidiabetic drugs and teratogenicity. *Lancet* **1**, 1165.

Stevenson, A. C. (1969). Findings and lessons for the future from a comparative study of congenital malformations at 24 centres in 16 countries. *In* "Methods for Teratological Studies in Experimental Animals and Man" (H. Nishimura and J. R. Miller, eds.), pp. 195–205. Igaku Shoin, Tokyo.

Stevenson, S. S., Worcester, J., and Rice, R. G. (1950). 677 congenitally malformed infants and associated gestational characteristics. I. General considerations. *Pediatrics* **6**, 37–50.

Stiekle, G. (1968). Defective development and reproductive wastage in the United States. *Amer. J. Obstet. Gynecol.* **100**, 442–447.

Stiles, K. A., and Watterson, R. L. (1937). The effects of jarring upon the embryogeny of chick embryos. *Anat. Rec.* **70**, 7–12.

Stockard, C. R. (1921). Developmental rate and structural expression: an experimental study of twins, "double monsters" and single deformities, and the interaction among embryonic organs during their origin and development. *Amer. J. Anat.* **28**, 115–227.

Stoller, A. (1968). Virus-chromosome interaction as a possible cause of Down's syndrome (mongolism) and other congenital anomalies. *In Advan. Teratol.* **3**, 97–126.

Streeter, G. L. (1921). Weight, sitting height, head size, foot length and menstrual age of the human embryo. *Carnegie Contrib. Embryol.* **11**, 143–170.

Streeter, G. L. (1942). Developmental horizons in human embryos: age group XI, 13 to 20 somites and age group XII, 21 to 29 somites. *Carnegie Contrib. Embryol.* **30**, 211–245.

Streeter, G. L. (1945). Developmental horizons in human embryos. Descriptions of age group XIII, embryos about 4 or 5 millimeters long and age group XIV, period of indentation of the lens vesicle. *Carnegie Contrib. Embryol.* **31**, 29–63.

Streeter, G. L. (1948). Developmental horizons in human embryos. Description of age groups XV, XVI, XVII, XVIII. *Carnegie Contrib. Embryol.* **32**, 133–203.

Streeter, G. L. (1951). Developmental horizons in human embryos. Description of age groups XIX, XX, XXI, XXII, XXIII. *Carnegie Contrib. Embryol.* **34**, 165–196.

Streissguth, A. P., Vanderveer, B. B., and Shepard, T. H. (1970). Mental development of children with congenital rubella. *Amer. J. Obstet. Gynecol.* **108,**, 391–399.

Sutherland, J. M., and Light, I. J. (1965). The effects of drugs upon the developing fetus. *Pediatr. Clin. North Amer.* **12**, 781–806.

Suttle, N. F., Field, A. C., and Barlow, R. M. (1970). Experimental copper deficiency in sheep. *J. Comp. Pathol.* **80**, 151–162.

Sutton, H. S., and Harris, M. I. (1972). "Mutagenic Effects of Environmental Contaminants." Academic Press, New York.

Takano, K. (1969). Comparative teratological effects of metabolic diseases of the mother. *In* "Methods for Teratological Studies in Experimental Animals and Man" (H. Nishimura and J. R. Miller, eds.), pp. 103–114. Igaku Shoin, Tokyo.

Tanaka, S., Ihara, T., and Mizurani, M. (1968). Apical defects in rat fetuses observed after intraperitoneal injection of high concentration of sodium chloride. *Cong. Anom.* **8**, 197–209.

Tanimura, T. (1972). Effects on Macaque embryos of drugs reported or suspected to be teratogenic in humans. *In* "The Use of Non-human Primates in Research on Human Reproduction" (E. Diczfalusy and C. C. Standley, eds.), pp. 293–308. WHO Res. and Training Center on Human Reproduction, Stockholm.

Tanimura, T., Tanaka, O., and Nishimura, H. (1971). Effects of thalidomide and quinine dihydrochloride on Japanese and rhesus monkey embryos. *Teratology* **4**, 247.

Tapernoux, A., and Delatour, P. (1967). Quelques aspects de la tératologie médicamenteuse chez les carnivores et les primates. *Thérapie* **22**, 1055–1061.

Taylor, W. F. (1970). The probability of fetal death. *In* "Congenital Malformations" (F. C. Fraser and V. A. McKusick, eds.), pp. 307–322. Excerpta Medica, Amsterdam.

Thalhammer, O. (1967). "Pränatale Erkrankungen des Menschen." Georg Thieme Verlag, Stuttgart.

Thiersch, J. B. (1952). Therapeutic abortions with a folic acid antagonist, 4-aminopteroylglutamic acid (4-amino P.G.A.) administered by the oral route. *Amer. J. Obstet. Gynecol.* **63**, 1298–1304.

Thiersch, J. B. (1956). The control of reproduction in rats with the aid of antimetabolites and early experiments with antimetabolites as abortifacient agents in man. *Acta Endocrinol. Suppl.* **28** 23: 37–45.

Thiersch, J. B. (1957). Effect of 2,4,6, triamino-"S"-triazine (TR), 2,4,5 "tris" (ethyleneimino)-"S"-triazine (TEM) and N, N', N"-triethylenephosphoramide (TEPA) on rat litter in utero. *Proc. Soc. Exp. Biol. Med.* **94**, 36–40.

Thiersch, J. B. (1962). Effects of acetamides and formamides on the rat litter in utero. *J. Reprod. Fertil.* **4**, 219–220.

Tolmach, L. J., Weiss, B. G., and Hopwood, L. E. (1971). Ionizing radiations and the cell cycle. *Fed. Proc.* **30**, 1742–1751.

Töndury, G. (1969). The virus as a danger to human embryos. In *Teratol., Proc. Teratol. Como, Italy* (A. Bertelli, ed.), pp. 211–222. Excerpta Medica, Amsterdam.

Trasler, D. G. (1960). The influence of uterine site on the occurrence of spontaneous cleft lip in mice. Paper presented at the *Teratol. Conf. N. Y. April* 9–10.

Trasler, D. G. (1960). The influence of uterine site on the occurrence of spontaneous

Trasler, D. G., Walker, B. E., and Fraser, F. C. (1956). Congenital malformations produced by amniotic-sac puncture. *Science* **124**, 439.

Trinkaus, J. P. (1965). Mechanisms of morphogenetic movements. In "Organogenesis" (R. L. DeHaan and H. Urspring, eds.), pp. 55–104. Holt, New York.

Tuchmann-Duplessis, H. (1965). "Teratogenic Action of Drugs." Pergamon, Oxford.

Tuchmann-Duplessis, H. (1969). The action of anti-tumor drugs on gestation and on embryogenesis. In *Teratol., Proc. Int. Symp. Como, Italy.* (A. Bertelli, ed.), pp. 75–86. Excerpta Medica, Amsterdam.

Tuchmann-Duplessis, H. (1972). Teratogenic drug screening. Present procedures and requirements. *Teratology* **5**, 271–285.

Tuchmann-Duplessis, H., and Lefebvres-Boisselot, J. (1957). Les effects tératogènes de l'acide x-methyl folique chez la chatte. *C. R. Soc. Biol.* **151**, 2005–2008.

Tuchmann-Duplessis, H., and Mercier-Parot, L. (1958). Influence de trois sulfamides hypoglycémiants sur la ratte gestante. *C. R. Soc. Biol.* **247**, 1134–1137.

Tuchmann-Duplessis, H., and Mercier-Parot, L. (1960). A propos de l'action tératogène de l'actinomycine. *C. R. Soc. Biol.* **153**, 1697–1700.

Tuchmann-Duplessis, H., and Mercier-Parot, L. (1963). Production de malformations chez la souris et le lapin par administration d'un sulfamide hypoglycémiant, la carbutamide. *C. R. Soc. Biol.* **158**, 1193–1197.

Tuchmann-Duplessis, H., and Mercier-Parot, L. (1964a). Répercussions des neuroleptiques et des antitumoraux sur le développement prénatal. *Bull. Schweiz. Akad. Med. Wiss.* **35**, 490–526.

Tuchmann-Duplessis, H., and Mercier-Parot, L. (1964b). A propos des tests tératogènes malformations spontanees du lapin. *C. R. Soc. Biol.* **157**, 666–670.

Tuffrey, M., Bishun, N. P., and Barnes, R. D. (1969). Porosity of the mouse placenta to maternal cells. *Nature (London)* **221**, 1029–1030.

Uchida, I., and Curtis, E. J. (1961). A possible association between maternal irradiation and mongolism. *Lancet* **2**, 848–850.

Uchida, I. A., Holunga, R., and Lawler, C. (1968). Maternal radiation and chromosomal aberrations. *Lancet* **2**, 1045–1049.

Uhlig, H. (1959). Fehlbildungen nach Follikel-hormonen beim Menschen. *Geburt-schilfe Frauenheilkd.* **19**, 346–352.

Ullery, D. E., Becker, D. E., Terrill, S. W., and Notzold, R. A. (1955). Dietary levels of pantothenic acid and reproductive performance in female swine. *J. Nutr.* **57**, 401–414.

Valensi, G., and Nahum, A. (1958). Action de l'iode radio-actif sur le foetus humain. *Tunis. Med.* **36**, 69.

Van Loosli, R., and Theiss, E. (1964). "Methodik und Problematik der medikamen-tos-experimentellen Teratogenese." Schwabe, Basel.

van Wagenen, G., and Gardner, W. U. (1960). X-irradiation of the ovary in the monkey *(Macaca mulatta). Fertil. Steril.* **11**, 291–302.

van Wagenen, G., and Hamilton, J. B. (1943). The experimental production of pseu-dohermaphroditism in the monkey. *Essays Biol.* 583–607.

Various contributors (1962). Development of tissues and organs: man. In "Growth: Reproduction and Morphological Development" (P. L. Altman and D. S. Ditt-mer, eds.), pp. 275–298. Fed. Amer. Soc. Exp. Biol.

Varpela, E. (1964). On the effect exerted by first-line tuberculosis medicines on the foetus. *Acta Tuberc. Scand.* **35**, 53–69.

Verrusio, A. C., and Watkins, C. A. (1969). Effects of 6-aminonicotinamide on the mitochondria of C57BL/6J and A/J mice. *Teratology* **2**, 271–272.

Villee, C. A. (1965). Placental transfer of drugs. *Ann. N.Y. Acad. Sci.* **123**, 237–242.

Villee, C. A. (1967). Biochemical aspects of the mammalian placenta. *In "The Bio-chemistry of Animal Development."* (R. Weber, ed.). Academic Press, New York.

Villee, C. A. (1971). Species differences in transport. *In Proc. Conf. Toxicol.: Impli-cations Teratol.* (R. Newburgh, ed.), pp. 297–319. Nat. Inst. of Child Health and Human Develop., Bethesda, Maryland.

Vondruska, J. F., Fancher, O. E., and Calandra, J. C. (1971). An investigation into the teratogenic potential of captan, folpet, and difolatan in nonhuman primates. *Toxicol. Appl. Pharmacol.* **18**, 619–624.

Voorhess, M. L. (1967). Masculinization of the female fetus associated with norethin-dronemestranol therapy during pregnancy. *J. Pediatr.* **71**, 128–131.

Waddell, W. J. (1972). Localization and metabolism of drugs in the fetus. *Fed. Proc.* **31**, 52–61.

Waddington, C. H., and Carter, T. C. (1952). Malformations in mouse embryos in-duced by trypan blue. *Nature (London)* **169**, 27–28.

Waisman, H. A. (1966). Some newer inborn errors of metabolism. *Pediatr. Clin. North Amer.* **13**, 469–501.

Walker, B. E. (1966). Production of cleft palate in rabbits by glucocorticoids. *Abstr. Terat. Soc.* **6**, 27.

Warburton, D., and Fraser, F. C. (1964). Spontaneous abortion risks in man: data from reproductive histories collected in a medical genetics unit. *Amer. J. Human Genet.* **16**, 1.

Ward, C. O. (1968). Role of placenta in teratogenesis. *New England J. Med.* **279**, 720–721.

Waring, M. J. (1968). Drugs which affect the structure and function of DNA. *Nature (London)* **219**, 1320–1325.

Warkany, J. (1943). Effect of maternal rachitogenic diet on skeletal development of young rat. *Amer. J. Dis. Child.* **66**, 511.

Warkany, J. (1952–53). Congenital malformation induced by maternal dietary defi-ciency. The Harvey Lectures, Ser. XLVIII, 89–109.

Warkany, J. (1959). Congenital malformations in the past. *J. Chronic Dis.* **10**, 84–95.

Warkany, J. (1971). "Congenital Malformations, Notes and Comments." Yearbook Publ., Chicago, Illinois.

Warkany, J., and Kalter, H. (1962). Maternal impressions and congenital malformations. *Plast. Reconstr. Surg.*, **30**, 628–637.

Warkany, J., and Nelson, R. C. (1940). Appearance of skeletal abnormalities in the offspring of rats reared on a deficient diet. *Science* **92**, 383–384.

Warkany, J., and Schraffenberger, E. (1944). Congenital malformations induced in rats by maternal nutritional deficiency. VI. Preventive factor. *J. Nutr.* **27**, 477–484.

Warkany, J., and Schraffenberger, E. (1947). Congenital malformations induced in rats by roentgen rays. *Amer. J. Roentgenol. Radium Ther.* **57**, 455–463.

Warkany, J., and Takacs, E. (1959). Experimental production of congenital malformations in rats by salicylate poisoning. *Amer. J. Pathol.* **35**, 315–331.

Warkany, J., and Takacs, E. (1965). Congenital malformations in rats from streptonigrin. *Arch. Pathol.* **79**, 65–79.

Warkany, J., Roth, C. B., and Wilson, J. G. (1948). Multiple congenital malformations: a consideration of etiologic factors. *Pediatrics* **1**, 462–471.

Warkany, J., Beaudry, P. H., and Hornstein, S. (1959). Attempted abortion with aminopterin (4-aminopteroylglutamic acid). *Amer. J. Dis. Child.* **97**, 274–281.

Warrell, D. W., and Taylor, R. (1968). Outcome for the foetus of mothers receiving prednisolone during pregnancy. *Lancet* **1**, 117–118.

Warren, S., and Gates, O. (1969). Effects of continuous irradiation of mice from conception to weaning. *In* "Radiation Biology of the Fetal and Juvenile Mammal" (M. R. Sikov and D. D. Mahlum, eds.), pp. 419–438. U.S. At. Energy Commission. Washington, D.C.

Warwick, E. J., Chapman, A. B., and Ross, B. (1943). Some anomalies in pigs. *J. Hered.* **34**, 349–352.

Wasz-Höckert, O., Nummi, S., Vuopala, S., and Järvinen, P. A. (1970). Transplacental passage of azidocillin, ampicillin and penicillin G during early and late pregnancy. *Scand. J. Infect. Dis.* **2**, 125–130.

Watanabe, G., Yoshida, S., and Hirose, K. (1968). Teratogenic effect of benzol in pregnant mice. *In Proc. Cong. Anom. Res. Ass. Japan, 8th Annu. Meeting, Tokyo* p. 45.

Webster, D. A., and Gross, J. (1970). Studies on possible mechanisms of programmed cell death in chick embryo. *Develop. Biol.* **22**, 157–184.

Wegner, G. (1966). Autoradiographische Untersuchungen der DNA-Synthese und der Mitosehaufigkeit einiger Zellarten wahrend der ungestorten Embryonal und Fetalen wicklung der Ratte und Strahlenembryopalkien. Habilitationsschrift Freiburg im Breisgan, Universitat (cited by Franz, '71).

Weidman, W. H., Young, H. H., and Zollman, P. E. (1963). The effects of thalidomide on the unborn puppy. *Mayo Clin. Proc.* **38**, 518.

Wells, C. N. (1953). Treatment of hyperemesis gravidarum with cortisone. *Amer. J. Obstet. Gynecol.* **66**, 598–

Werboff, J., and Havlena, J. (1962). Postnatal behavioral effects of tranquilizers administered to the gravid rat. *Exp. Neurol.* **6**, 263–269.

Werthemann, A., and Reiniger, M. (1950). Uber augenentwicklungsstorungen bei Rattenembryonen durch sauerstoffmangel in der Fruhschwangerschaft. *Acta Anat.* **11**, 329–347.

Whitelaw, M. J. (1947). Thiouracil in the treatment of hyperthyroidism complicating pregnancy and its effect on the human fetal thyroid. *J. Clin. Endocrinol* **7**, 767–773.

Wickes, I. G. (1954). Foetal defects following insulin coma therapy in early pregnancy. *Brit. Med. J.* **2**, 1029.

Widdowson, E. M. (1968). Growth and composition of the fetus and newborn. *In* "Biology of Gestation." (N. S. Assali, ed.), Vol. 2, pp. 1–44. Academic Press, New York.

Widdowson, E. M. (1972). Intrauterine growth retardation in the pig. I. Organ size and cellular development at birth and after growth to maturity. *Biol. Neonate* **19**, 329–340.

Wilkins, L. (1960). Masculinization of female fetus due to use of orally given progestins. *J. Amer. Med. Ass.* **172**, 1028–1032.

Williamson, A. P., Blattner, R. J., and Robertson, G. G. (1967). Study of teratogenic effects of particulate compounds in the amniotic cavity of chick embryos. *Proc. Soc. Exp. Biol. Med.* **124**, 524–532.

Willis, R. A. (1958). "The Borderland of Embryology and Pathology." Butterworth, London and Washington, D.C.

Wilson, J. G. (1953). Influence of severe hemorrhagic anemia during pregnancy on development of the offspring in the rat. *Proc. Soc. Exp. Biol. Med.* **84**, 66–69.

Wilson, J. G. (1954a). Differentiation and the reaction of rat embryos to radiation. *J. Cell. Comp. Physiol. Suppl. 1*, **43**, 11–38.

Wilson, J. G. (1954b). Influence on the offspring of altered physiologic states during pregnancy in the rat. *Ann. N.Y. Acad. Sci.* **57**, 517–525.

Wilson, J. G. (1955). Teratogenic activity of several azo dyes chemically related to trypan blue. *Anat. Rec.* **123**, 313–334.

Wilson, J. G. (1957). Is there specificity of action in experimental teratogenesis? *Pediatrics* **19**, 755–763.

Wilson, J. G. (1959). Experimental studies on congenital malformations. *J. Chronic Dis.* **10**, 111–130.

Wilson, J. G. (1964a). Experimental teratology. *Amer. J. Obstet. Gynecol.* **90**, 1181–1192.

Wilson, J. G. (1964b). Teratogenic interaction of chemical agents in the rat. *J. Pharmacol. Exp. Ther.* **144**, 429–436.

Wilson, J. G. (1965a). Embryological considerations in teratology. *In* "Teratology: Principles and Techniques" (J. G. Wilson and J. Warkany, eds.), pp. 251–261. Univ. of Chicago Press, Chicago, Illinois.

Wilson, J. G. (1965b). Methods for administering agents and detecting malformations in experimental animals. *In* "Teratology: Principles and Techniques" (J. G. Wilson and J. Warkany, eds.), pp. 262–277. Univ. of Chicago Press, Chicago, Illinois.

Wilson, J. G. (1966). Effects of acute and chronic treatment with actinomycin D on pregnancy and the fetus in the rat. *Harper Hosp. Bull.* **24**, 109–118.

Wilson, J. G. (1968). Problems of teratological testing. *In* "Toxic Effects of Anesthetics" (B. R. Fink, ed.), pp. 259–268. The Williams and Wilkins Co., Baltimore, Maryland.

Wilson, J. G. (1970). Embryotoxicity of the folic antagonist methotrexate. *Anat. Rec.* **166**, 398.

Wilson, J. G. (1971). Use of rhesus monkeys in teratological studies. *Fed. Proc.* **30**, 104–109.

Wilson, J. G. (1972a). Environmental effects on development—teratology. *In* "Pathophysiology of Gestation." (N. S. Assali, ed.), Vol. 2, pp. 269–320. Academic Press, New York.

Wilson, J. G. (1972b). Abnormalities of intrauterine development in non-human primates. *In* "The Use of Non-human Primates in Research on Human Reproduction" (E. Diczfalusy and C. C. Standley, eds.), pp. 261–292. WHO Res. and Training Center on Human Reproduction, Stockholm.

Wilson, J. G. (1972c). Interrelations between carcinogeniticy, mutagenicity and teratogenicity. *In Proc. Conf. Mutagenic Effect Environ. Contaminants* (H. S. Sutton and M. I. Harris, eds.). Academic Press, New York.

Wilson, J. G., and Fradkin, R. (1969). Early diagnosis of pregnancy and abortion in the rhesus monkey. *Anat. Rec.* **163**, 286.

Wilson, J. G., and Gavan, J. A. (1967). Congenital malformations in nonhuman primates: spontaneous and experimentally induced. *Anat. Rec.* **158**, 99–110.

Wilson, J. G., and Warkany, J. (1949). Aortic arch and cardiac anomalies in the offspring of vitamin A deficient rats. *Amer. J. Anat.* **85**, 113–155.

Wilson, J. G., Brent, R. L., and Jordan, H. C. (1953). Differentiation as a determinant of the reaction of rat embryos to x-irradiation. *Proc. Soc. Exp. Biol. Med.* **82**, 67–70.

Wilson, J. G., Jordan, H. C., and Brent, R. L. (1953a). Effects of irradiation on embryonic development. II. X-rays on the ninth day of gestation in the rat. *Amer. J. Anat.* **92**, 153–187.

Wilson, J. G., Roth, C. B., and Warkany, J. (1953b). An analysis of the syndrome of malformations induced by maternal vitamin A deficiency. Effects of restoration of vitamin A at various times during gestation. *Amer. J. Anat.* **92**, 189–217.

Wilson, J. G., Maren, T. H., Takano, K., and Ellison, A. (1968). Teratogenic action of carbonic anhydrase inhibitors in the rat. *Teratology* **1**, 51–60.

Wilson, J. G., Jordan, R. L., and Schumacher, H. (1969). Potentiation of the teratogenic effects of 5-fluorouracil by natural pyrimidines. I. Biological aspects. *Teratology* **2**, 91–97.

Wilson, J. G., Fradkin, R., and Hardman, A. (1970). Breeding and pregnancy in rhesus monkeys used for teratological testing. *Teratology* **3**, 59–71.

Winckel, C. W. F. (1948). Quinine and congenital injuries of ear and eye of the foetus. *J. Trop. Med.* **51**, 2.

Windle, W. F. (1969). Brain damage by asphyxia at birth. *Sci. Amer.* **221**, 76–84.

Winfield, J. B., and Bennett, D. (1971). Gene-teratogen interaction: potentiation of actinomycin D teratogenesis in the house mouse by the lethal gene brachyury. *Teratology* **4**, 157–170.

Winick, M. (1969). Malnutrition and brain development. *J. Pediatr.* **74**, 667–679.

Winick, M. (1971). Cellular growth during early malnutrition. *Pediatrics* **47**, 967–977.

Witschi, E. (1962). Development: rat. *In* "Growth: Reproduction and Morphological Development" (P. L. Altman and D. S. Dittmer, eds.), pp. 304–314. Fed. Amer. Soc. Exp. Biol.

Witschi, E. (1970). Teratogenic effects from overripeness of the egg. *In* "Congenital Malformations" (F. C. Fraser and V. A. McKusick, eds.), pp. 157–169. Excerpta Medica, Amsterdam.

Wood, J. W., Johnson, K. G., and Omori, Y. (1967). In utero exposure to the Hiroshima atomic bomb. An evaluation of head size and mental retardation twenty years later. *Pediatrics* **39**, 385–392.

Woolf, C. M., Koehn, J. H., and Coleman, S. S. (1968). Congenital hip disease in Utah: the influence of genetic and non-genetic factors. *Amer. J. Human Genet.* **20**, 430–439.

Woollam, D. H. M., and Millen, J. W. (1960). The modification of the activity of certain agents exerting a deleterious effect on the development of the mammalian embryo. *In* "Ciba Foundation Symposium on Congenital Malformations" (G. E. W. Wolstenholme and C. M. O'Connor, eds.), pp. 158–172. Little, Brown, Boston, Massachusetts.

Woollam, D. H. M., Millen, J. W., and Fozzard, J. A. F. (1959). The influence of cortisone on the teratogenic activity of x-radiation. *Brit. J. Radiol.* **32**, 47–48.

Wright, S. (1934). Genetics of abnormal growth in the guinea pig. *Cold Spring Harbor Symp. Quant. Biol.* **2**, 137–147.

Wright, S. (1960). The genetics of vital characters of the guinea pig. *J. Cell. Comp. Physiol.* **56**, 123–125.

Yaktin, U. S., and McLaren, D. S. (1970). The behavioral development of infants recovering from severe malnutrition. *J. Mental Defic. Res.* **14**, 25–32.

Yamazaki, J. N. (1966). A review of the literature on the radiation dosage required to cause manifest central nervous system disturbances from in utero and postnatal exposure. *Pediatrics,* **27**, 877–903.

Yerushalmy, J. (1970). The California child health and development studies. Study design and some illustrative finds in congenital heart disease. *In* "Congenital Malformations" (F. C. Fraser and V. A. McKusick, eds.), pp. 299–306. Excerpta Medica, Amsterdam.

Yerushalmy, J., and Milkovich, L. (1965). Evaluation of the teratogenic effect of meclizine in man. *Amer. J. Obstet. Gynecol.* **93**, 553–562.

Young, G. A. (1967). Congenital and hereditary defects. *In* ARC Anim. Breeding Res. Organization Rep. 35–41.

Young, G. A., Kitchell, R. L., Luedke, A. J., and Sautter, J. H. (1955). The effect of viral and other infections of the dam on fetal development in swine. Modified hog colera virus. *J. Amer. Vet. Med. Ass.* **126**, 165–171.

Yu, J. S., and O'Halloran, M. T. (1970). Children of mothers with phenylketonuria. *Lancet* **1**, 210–212.

Zamenof, S., van Marthens, E., and Granel, L. (1971). Prenatal cerebral development: effect of restricted diet, reversal by growth hormone. *Science* **174**, 954–955.

Zeman, F. J. (1967). Morphological and histochemical changes in kidneys of newborn young of low-protein fed rats. *Fed. Proc.* **26**, 520.

Zimmerman, E. F., and Bowen, D. (1972). Distribution and metabolism of triamcinolone acetate in inbred mice with different cleft palate sensitivities. *Teratology* **5**, 335–344.

Zimmerman, W. (1964). Methoden fur experimentelle Untersuchungen am Kaninchen wahrend der fruhen Embryonalentwicklung. *Zentralbl. Bakteriol. Parasitenkunde, Infektionskrankheiten Hygiene* **194A**, 255–266.

Zwilling, E., and De Bell, E. (1950). Micromelia and growth retardation as independent effects of sulfanilimide in chick embryos. *J. Exp. Zool.* **115**, 59.

AUTHOR INDEX

Numbers in italics refer to the pages on which the complete references are listed.

SUBJECT INDEX

Nondisjunction, *see* Chromosomal
  aberrations
Nucleic acid
  altered metabolism, 39, 88-90
  DNA, 27
    growth retardation, 108
    interference with, 88, 89, 101
    nucleotide sequence, 84-86, 88-90
    somatic mutations, 4
  faulty genetic expression, 88-90
  metabolism, 89
  mutations, 84-86, 88, 89
  protein synthesis, 88-90
  RNA
    actinomycin D, 101, 115
    biosynthesis, 116
    interference with, 88, 89, 101
    organogenesis, 18
    protein synthesis, 88-90
Nutrients, analogs and antagonists to, 91
Nutrition, *see* Dietary deficiency

O

Oil of wintergreen, mammals, 39
Organogenesis, 15-23, 123, 135
  dietary imbalance, 40-42
  gross defects, 17
  lethality, 17, 148-154
  metabolic shift, 92
  radiation, 37, 38
  susceptibility, 19-22, 121-123
    man, 123
    monkeys, 153
    rats, 19, 149-154
    swine, 153
  teratogenicity in testing, 148-154
Osmolar imbalance, 25, 75, 93-94
Oxygen, hypoxia, 44

P

Pantothenic acid, 34, 40
Para-aminosalicylic acid, man, 70
Parathion, rats, 79
Pathogenesis (abnormal embryogenesis),
    23-26, 83, 84, 97-103, *see also*
    Developmental defects

definition, 7-8, 25
final common pathway, 25-26, 102-103
lethality, *see* Intrauterine death
refractory periods, 16, 17, 18
susceptible periods, 11-23, 31, 32, 33,
    121-136
PCNB (pesticide), laboratory mammals, 39
Penicillin, laboratory mammals, 39, 70
Pentobarbital, laboratory mammals, 39
Pesticides, *see also* individual listings, 39
  in various animals, 39, 79, 151
  man, 79-80
  use during testing, 160, 192
Phenmetrazine, man, 65
Phenobarbital, man, 57, 63
Phenocopies, 14
Phenylalanine, man, 56, 82
Phenylketonuria
  man, 30, 49, 82
  maternal, *see* Maternal phenylketonuria
  recessive gene, 109
Phosphorylation, uncoupling of oxidative,
    91
Pilonidal cysts, half-sibships, 56
Placenta, 26-28, 35, 111, 112-118, 156-158,
    161
  changes in structure, 113-114
  defenses, 113-118
    degradation of chemicals, 116
    embryo dose, 116-118
    transfer, 114-116, 118
  insufficiency, 108
  viruses, 42
  yolk sac placenta, 47-48, 95, 118-120,
      157, 162
    antibodies, 47, 91
    atypical transport, 113
Placental dysfunction, 95
Placental failure, 47-48, 90-91, 118
Placental transfer, 26-28, 40, 113-116, 157,
    161
  embryo to mother, 27, 28
  man and monkey, 170
  modes of, 114-116
  mother to embryo, 27, 28, 114-116
  rates, 26-28, 40, 116-118, 170
Plasma concentration, 111-113, 116-118
Podophyllin, mitotic interference, 88
Point mutations, 24, 36
Poliomyelitis, man, 53

Reporting
  centers for, 140, 145
  early warning system, 145
  hospital, 140-141
  medical literature, cases, 141-142
  monitoring developmental defects, 140
  spontaneous, 140-141
  uniformity, 141
Reserpine, laboratory mammals, 39
Resorption, *see* Intrauterine death
Retinoic acid, rats, 41, 149
Rh immunization, half-sibships, 56
  placental leakage, 116
Rhinotracheitis virus, cattle, 43
Riboflavin
  antagonists to, 34, 40, 91
  deficiency, 34, 40, 139
  as protective agent, 23
  rats, 91, 139
Ribonucleoside diphosphate reductase, 92
RNA, *see* Nucleic acid, RNA
Rodents, *see also* specific animals
  ambiguous genitalis, 45
  cleft palate, 45
  intrauterine death, 46
  malformation and lethality, 188-189
  teratogenic susceptibility, 158
  use in testing, 157, 159, 162-164, 193,
    197, 198-200
  yolk sac placenta, 47-48, 91, 95, 118, 157
Rubella, 10, 18, 52
  associated defects, 109, 138-139
  fetal susceptibility, 33, 42, 43
  man, 42, 49, 52-53
  monkey, 43
Rubeola, man, 53

S

Sacral agenesis, fat solvents, 79
Salicylates, *see also* Aspirin
  enzyme inhibition, 92
  man, 67
Saline
  hypertonic solution, 93-94, 102
  osmolar imbalance, 93-94
Serotonin, animals, 114
Sex hormones, 45, 59-61
Sheep
  embryology, 135, 166, 216-217
  use in testing, 166

Sickle cell trait, 50
Situs inversus, 102
Skeletal malformations, 19
  acetazolamide, 74, 75
  alkylating agents, 66
  aspirin, 67
  diabetes, 55
  hypoxia, 44
  imipramine, 71
  industrial solvents, 79
  irradiation, 37, 39
  minor, 37, 184-188
  physical trauma, 47
  thalidomide, 58-59
Skeleton, 178-180
  anatomic variants, 184-188
  cervical rib, 68
  retardation, 188
  ribs, 184-188
  sternebrae, 184-188
  vertebrae, 55, 184-188
Solvents, animals and man, 39, 78, *see also*
    specific substances
Species differences, 12, 146-171
Spinal cord, 20
Spontaneous malformations, *see*
    Manifestations
Stathmokinetic agents, *see* Mitosis
Steroid hormones, 45, 59-61
Stillbirth
  antibiotics, 70
  developmental defects, 104
  diabetes, 55
  nutritional deficiency, 41, 81
  recording of, 176
Strain differences, 12-13
Streptomycin
  man, 70
  RNA, 88, 89
  rats, 101
Streptonigrin
  DNA interference, 89
  laboratory mammals, 39
  rats, 24, 70
  rodents, 70
Sulfonamides, animals and man, 57, 74, 91
Sulfonylureas, man, rodents, rabbits, 46,
    65-66
Surveillance, 81, 137-171
  clinical trials, 144
  drugs and chemicals, 81
  famine areas, 81, 143

DENTAL SCHOOL LIBRARY

DENTAL SCHOOL LIBRARY

DENTAL SCHOOL LIBRARY

KU-288-439

Issues
in
Social
Policy

Kathleen Jones
John Brown
and
Jonathan Bradshaw

Routledge & Kegan Paul

London, Henley and Boston

First published in 1978
by Routledge & Kegan Paul Ltd
39 Store Street,
London WC1E 7DD,
Broadway House,
Newtown Road,
Henley-on-Thames,
Oxon RG9 1EN and
9 Park Street,
Boston, Mass. 02108, USA
Set in 10/12pt Press Roman by
Hope Services, Wantage
and printed in Great Britain by
Lowe & Brydone Printers Ltd
Thetford, Norfolk
© Kathleen Jones, John Brown and Jonathan Bradshaw 1978
No part of this book may be reproduced in
any form without permission from the
publisher, except for the quotation of brief
passages in criticism

British Library Cataloguing in Publication Data

Jones, Kathleen, b.1922

   Issues in social policy.
   1. Great Britain – Social policy
   I. Title   II. Brown, John, b.1948
   III. Bradshaw, Jonathan
   361.6'2'0941   HN385   78-40508

   ISBN 0 7100 8972 4
   ISBN 0 7100 8973 2 Pbk.

Contents

503656

'Life is a swallow, theory a snail.'
        R. H. Tawney

Introduction

H. M. Hyndman once remarked to Karl Marx that, as he got older, he grew more tolerant. 'Do you', said Marx, '*do* you?'[1] There are signs that the study of social policy is ageing like Marx rather than like Hyndman, for tolerance is on the wane. The liberal certainties of the first decades of the 'welfare state', the general consensus about the search for social justice, the faith in the ability of society to work towards humanitarian goals, have run into very sharp attacks from both extremes of the political spectrum. As late as 1965, T. H. Marshall could write that the existence of the welfare state was generally acceptable, and the remaining problems were those of social engineering rather than of ideology.[2] That is no longer true.

From the right comes a persistent barrage of anti-collectivism, characterised by the work of Milton Friedman and Hayek, and the many articles and pamphlets of the Institute of Economic Affairs. Their message is that collectivism has been tried, and has failed. It has failed because it ignores or obscures the profit motive which is the basic dynamic of human behaviour; because it removes free market choice, which is the best (and indeed the only rational) mode of allocating scarce resources; because it is inefficient, and lends to the creation of government bureaucracy; and because it centralises political power, whereas a free market economy distributes economic power as a counter-balance to the centralising tendencies of the state. This was the message of Hayek's *The Road to Serfdom,* published as early as 1944, and now enjoying a considerable revival. In the ensuing years, the battle has been fought over housing, health, education, pensions and other social services, the claim being made that the only sensible means of operation is through the basic mechanisms of supply and demand.[3]

The attack was relatively urbane in the affluent 1960s, when it was argued that a growth economy would of itself eliminate poverty, and that in time all would share in the pleasures of choice. It was even conceded that some basic services should be provided for those who had not yet reached this happy position. A modification of Charles Booth's doctrine of 'limited socialism' would provide residual services for those who lagged behind in the race to the consumer paradise. The rediscovery of poverty in the mid 1960s, the revelation that apparently affluent societies like Britain and the USA still rested on a base of underprivilege and constricted lives should have been enough to kill it; but the attack continued, now focusing on the evils of bureaucracy, now on the virtues of individualism; and paradoxically, in the stringent 1970s (when one might have expected right-wing economists to sing small, because they have been wrong about so many things, including the continuance of the growth economy) it became markedly more shrill. The explicit policy of the International Monetary Fund, which insisted on the cutting of public expenditure and the increase of unemployment as the price of a loan to Britain, made it plain once and for all that unrestricted capitalism can actually require a section of the community to live in economic hardship for the sake of its own operation. The lesson could hardly have been clearer. Yet the attacks on 'scroungers' and 'layabouts' continued, and acquired almost a moral fervour. The personal social services, which had expanded at an unprecedented rate in the early 1970s on the lines laid down by the Seebohm Report,[4] came to a full stop. Thus at a time when unemployment soared towards the two million mark, and the first to suffer were the more vulnerable sections of the community — school leavers, the elderly, the handicapped, those of Asian or West Indian origin, those in irregular or insecure employ ment — the social services which had been Britain's pride in the civilised world came to be regarded as Britain's liability.

If there is criticism from the extreme right, there has been an equal barrage from the extreme left. Marxists and neo-Marxists (the titles change, though the ideas remain relatively static) have as little use for the welfare state as Hayek and Friedman. Marx's withering contempt for the liberal reformers of his own day — for those who supported such movements as those for factory reform, political representation or women's suffrage — has been poured into the attack. To it has been added a mood of disillusion with the efforts of reformers, which follows Engels' celebrated attack on the middle classes:[5]

What have they ever done to prove their professed goodwill towards you? Have they ever paid any serious attention to your grievances? Have they ever done more than paying the expenses of half a dozen commisions of enquiry, whose voluminous reports are damned to everlasting slumber among heaps of waste paper on the shelves of the Home Office? Have they ever done as much as to compile from those rotting blue-books a single readable book from which everybody might easily get some information on the condition of the great majority of 'free-born Britons'? . . . they have left it to a foreigner to inform the civilised world of the degrading situation you live in.

To this impatience with the slow pace of reform, the multiplication of reports and blue-books, many of them still 'damned to everlasting slumber' on the shelves of this department of state or that, is now added a strong distrust of the professionalisation of social work, which seems to make social workers richer while their clients get poorer. The rapid build-up of local authority social services departments, since 1971 the main employers of qualified social workers, has been accompanied by a good deal of soul-searching about what social workers actually do, and what legitimates intervention into other people's lives. For some, this free-floating anxiety has fastened on 'the system', whether this is seen as the operation of a particular local authority in a particular town, or the way Britain is run, or the capitalist system as a whole. Those who create and maintain the social services are then open to Paolo Freire's charge of 'assistencialism';[6] that they are actually propping up 'the system' and delaying the day of its inevitable breakdown. Ideals of social justice and human rights, care and concern for individuals and groups in need, are simply 'false consciousness'. Those who believe in this approach must be 'unmasked' as dupes, if not agents, of social control.

The attack from the extreme right comes from outside the field of social policy studies. The attack from the extreme left comes from inside; but the two attacks, superficially so different, have a good deal in common. Both regard the study of social policy as unnecessary, the one because it allegedly supports collectivism, the other because it allegedly supports capitalism. One might have some grounds for thinking that a philosophy which can be so thoroughly abused from opposite points of view must, after all, have something in it. Both are based on economic determinism: the view that *only* the control of the means of production matters, and that one system or the other will inevitably produce the right kind of society (though they differ markedly as to what the right kind of society is). Both have a certain grandiosity, claiming that their analyses are relevant to all societies in all periods of history. The intellectual pretensions of the extreme right are now fairly threadbare, though the argument to what is seen as hard-headed realism has a certain persuasiveness in times of recession, and the fact that it is advanced by people who actually control the means of production gives it an added force. (If you are arguing with an international banker, it may be intellectually satisfying to point out that the quality of his

4   Introduction

theoretical constructs would not pass muster on an undergraduate course, but it is not likely to make much practical difference to the outcome of the argument.) The intellectual pretensions of the extreme left are founded on a very simplistic view of history — Marx stood Hegel's doctrine of the *Welthistorische Volksgeister* on its head to prove, not the inevitability of the glorious destiny of great nations, but the inevitability of the breakdown of capitalism, arguing that 'tendencies work out with an iron necessity towards an inevitable goal'.[7] That may have been a reasonable view for the editor of a radical journal to take of the state of affairs in France and Germany in the 1840s, but it has simply not stood the test of time. Marx was not to foresee the rise of the managerial class, the development of powerful trade unions, the effect of universal education — or, as Dahrendorf points out, the rise of the joint stock company.[8] All these factors, and many others, modify his simple division of society into the exploiters and the exploited. While there is now a range of Marxist and neo-Marxist thought, it is significant that Marx's ideas have taken hold, not in the industrially developed west, but in the relatively feudal societies of Russia, China, and Freire's Brazil, at periods when the gap between the social classes remained much as he described it. It seems unlikely that, during the thirty years when he lived in London 'like a frog in a swamp', working in the British Museum Library from nine till seven on *Das Kapital,* he saw much of the social change which was going on around him. The social achievements of mid-Victorian Britain, if slow, were real. Engels, returning to London as an old man in 1892, was forced to concede, rather against his own inclinations, that 'during the period of England's industrial monopoly the English working class have, to a certain extent, shared in the benefits of the monopoly', and to speak with some pride of the revival of the trade union movement in the East End — 'one of the greatest and most fruitful facts of the *fin de siècle,* and glad and proud I am to have lived to see it'.[9]

Both the extreme right and extreme left points of view are basically materialistic. Their explanations of human conduct leave no room for emotional satisfaction, for human achievement in art, culture or morality, for altruism, for community spirit, or for affection. Every aspect of human life is reducible to explanation in terms of control-over-the-means-of-production. Both take a uni-dimensional view of mankind as well as a uni-dimensional view of history, diminishing human beings to a level where they are seen as actuated only by the profit motive, or only by the class struggle.

Both points of view are basically pitiless. For the extreme right is prepared to sacrifice the underprivileged section of society in the name of economic progress (with the promise that it will all come right when we achieve infinite economic growth), while the extreme left is prepared to sacrifice them in the name of the destruction of the capitalist system (with the promise that it will all come right after the revolution). Neither is much use to the black teenager in Brent who needs a job, or the housebound old lady in Barnsley who needs a hot meal. Experience should by now have made us wary of infinitely receding carrots. The fully affluent society, or the revolution, may or may not come in our time. Meanwhile, there is a good deal to be said for getting on with the job.

For these reasons, and some others which will later become apparent, the essays which follow take what is fundamentally a reformist stance. We believe that there are many problems in British social policy, some of them old, some of them new. We do not share the easy Utopianism of the early post-war period, when the phrase 'the kingdom of heaven here on earth' was frequently heard in the drab meeting halls where the reforming enthusiasts gathered. Nor do we share the rather glib faith of the 1960s that the problems are merely questions of 'social engineering'. Some of them are extremely complex questions of value, and it is only when we abandon simplistic theories of history and simplistic theories of man that we can begin to tackle them in their own right. For history is not only about control-of-the-means-of-production. It is about many kinds of human endeavour, many aspirations, failures and achievements, and the kaleidoscope is changing all the time. Social policy does not develop in a linear way. In health, housing, education, social insurance, and any other field one cares to name there are experiments, false starts, twisted concepts, new interpretations, shifts of emphasis and of interest which require detailed analysis. No lofty 'macro' view can do justice to the complexities of hammering out policy, getting it implemented, testing it, and hammering it out again. And human beings are not simply animals with an economic sense. They are capable of some selfish actions, some unselfish actions, and a considerable amount of sheer muddle. They are Schopenhauer's 'freezing porcupines' — huddling together for warmth, shuffling apart when the prickles hurt, and huddling together for warmth again. They have a capacity for community, and a capacity for what the sociologists call 'privatisation'. But in some ways, at some times, they do progress. In any field of social policy, there have been enormous improvements in the past hundred years, and some in the past ten. And in this process, the patient accumulation of knowledge, even in the form of 'rotting blue-books' has played a part.

There are already several readable and informative texts on social policy. Most of them are primarily descriptive, and for that reason, soon date. The late Penelope Hall used to describe her *Social Services of Modern England* as ' the old man of the sea'. Like Sinbad, she carried her burden, which in her case was one of continuous up-dating. We think that the study of social policy is now getting beyond the purely descriptive stage, and we have tried to select some themes which are capable of a degree of conceptual analysis in order to pursue the subject at a more theoretical level. These are not the only 'issues in social policy', and many others might be selected for similar treatment; but they form a group which three of us, with some help from colleagues, have found fruitful for study.

We are conscious that, year by year, the amount of material available for courses in Social Policy and Administration expands, and that students' time does not. We have therefore tried to provide a short introductory text, but we hope that reading will not stop at the superficial level. The chapters can be used as a first guide to the problems involved. Each is very fully annotated, and the notes can be used as a guide to further study — the pursuit of ideas, themes and issues which contribute to the student's own understanding of the field of social policy. The book is meant to be a working document, not a definitive statement. It is something to be argued with and wrestled with.

Readers will find that, although the chapter headings appear to deal with discrete topics, the subjects of discussion are frequently contingent on one another. Thus the chapter on 'Universality and Selectivity' could be treated as a special case of the issues discussed in 'Equality and Equity'; 'Professionalisation' is the subject of Chapter 4, but the issue of professional people, the autonomy they possess, and the way they define their professional tasks come up in all the subsequent chapters. We can turn the spotlight here and there, but we cannot, except for limited and temporary purposes, create discrete areas of discussion in a growing and developing field.

We particularly wish to acknowledge the assistance of Ian Cole, who did much of the work for the chapter on 'Citizen Participation', and Richard Barker, who helped with legal material for the chapter on 'The Redress of Grievances'. We are also grateful to our own post-graduate students, who have worked over much of the material with us, and whose contributions have been frequently trenchant and occasionally hilarious.

York, December 1977   KJ
                                                                       JB
                                                                       JRB

References

1 H. M. Hyndman, *Record of an Adventurous Life*, quoted by Isaiah Berlin, *Karl Marx*, Oxford University Press, 3rd edn, 1963, p. 265.
2 T. H. Marshall, *Social Policy*, Hutchinson, 1965, 2nd edn, 1967, p. 89.
3 See e.g., M. Friedman, *Capitalism and Freedom*, University of Chicago Press, 1962; F. A. Hayek, *Individualism and the Economic Order*, Routledge & Kegan Paul, 1949; *The Constitution of Liberty*, Routledge & Kegan Paul, 1960; IEA pamphlets.
4 *Report of the Committee on Local Authority and Allied Personal Social Services*, Cmnd 3703, HMSO, 1968.
5 F. Engels, *The Condition of the Working Class in England* (1844), Panther edn, 1969, p. 324.
6 P. Freire, *Education: the Practice of Freedom*, Writers' and Readers' Publishing Co-operative, 1976, pp. 14-15, 15n.
7 From the foreword to *Das Kapital*.
8 R. Dahrendorf, *Class and Conflict in Industrial Society*, Routledge & Kegan Paul, 1963, pp. 41-2.
9 Engels, op. cit., pp. 34-5 (first published in the English edn of 1892).

Chapter one

Equality and Equity

[handwritten margin note: problems in formula "equal" pol.]

The terms 'equality' and 'equity' are often used interchangeably, but
they have very different meanings. 'Equality' means equal shares. 'Equity'
means fair shares. If three men have a cake, a policy of equality will give
each man one-third of it; but if one man is hungry and the other two
well-fed, a policy of equity would give the hungry man a larger slice.
The subject therefore introduces problems of *paradox* — it is impossible
to produce a policy which is egalitarian and equitable at the same time,
unless people's needs are equal; and problems of *degree* — if people's
needs are unequal, how unequal are they, and what kind of apportion-
ment will secure equity?

Viewed historically, the argument has four main phases:

(i) A very long period in which gross inequality (a situation in which
the rich or powerful appropriated the whole cake and decided its
distribution) was held to be not only inevitable but desirable.

(ii) A counter-assertion, most strongly articulated in the period of the
American and French Revolutions, that equality was both desirable
and attainable.

(iii) Growing doubts about equality on the grounds that it would lead
to an intolerable degree of uniformity, or that it would lead to new
forms of inequality.

(iv) The introduction of the idea of equity, and with it the concept of
positive discrimination for under-privileged groups.

Gross inequality — social, political and economic — has a very long
and respectable history. Most writers up to 200 or 300 years ago
assumed that it was an inescapable fact of society as they experienced
it, and a natural way of ordering human relationships. Aristotle set out
the advantages of an ordered, hierarchical society in which landowners
were superior to peasants, masters to slaves, men to women, and the old
to the young. Such patterns of superordination and subordination were
held to be socially cohesive. Dahrendorf uses 'the Aristotelian argument'
as shorthand for all treatments of the subject of inequality up to the
middle of the eighteenth century.[1] While there are earlier statements of
some sort of basic equality for some people — for instance in the works
of Cicero — one has to look fairly hard to find them. For the most part,

only the defenders of inequality had the education to develop their ideas, the leisure to record them, and means to afford scarce and expensive writing materials. And of course, most of the underprivileged could neither read nor write.

The stubborn view that gross inequality is wrong comes to us in the main from slave rebellions and peasant uprisings, in the form of rallying cries or bits of doggerel which were incorporated into oral tradition.[2] A full exposition of the case for equality had to wait on the spread of literacy and the commercial distribution of literature. Even as late as the seventeenth century, it is notable that Sir Robert Filmer, the author of *Patriarcha*, that most exhaustive of justifications for inequality, could afford to produce a weighty book, while Gerrard Winstanley, the Digger leader, could only express his views in pamphlets.[3]

Today, very few writers argue for inequality in the classic form, and few for equality in its eighteenth century form. Such defenders of the capitalist system as Friedman and Hayek are careful to phrase their arguments in semi-egalitarian terms — Friedman argues that capitalism has actually operated to reduce inequality,[4] while Hayek defends free enterprise on the grounds that it frees men to seek equality.[5] On the left, there is a certain Orwellian disenchantment with political systems which seem inevitably to make some men more equal than others, and a realisation that 'Liberty, Equality, Fraternity' may involve conflicting values unless each is carefully defined.

Schiller argued that inequality was a spur to progress, since it enabled man to leave 'the tranquil nausea of his paradise'. There is an echo of this thinking in Dahrendorf's ingenious formulation. He argues that total equality would lead to 'total terror or absolute boredom'. Any society, in order to organise itself, selects some values and norms from a potentially limitless range. This process in itself creates inequality, since some people will approximate closer to those norms and values than to others. But the formulation of social order contains the seeds of its own destruction, since the underprivileged will seek to change the norms in their own interest:[6]

> The very existence of social inequality . . . is an impetus towards liberty, because it guarantees a society's on-going, dynamic, historical quality. The idea of a perfectly egalitarian society is not only unrealistic, it is terrible.

This is a difficult position to maintain, for two reasons. First, few advocates of equality wish to push the idea to the extremes of uniformity. If human beings are born equal in some respects, they are manifestly different in mental and physical endowment, talents, energy, creativity, tastes and preferences. They are born with different life-chances, and meet different circumstances. As Tawney says, we all go to the doctor, but we do not all need the same treatment. Second, the idea of an 'on-going, dynamic, historical' struggle presupposes a conflict between parties with an equal chance of success. Groups like the poor, the old, the handicapped and immigrants have a less than equal chance, and no self-regulating mechanism is going to bring them to a position where they can become the norm-changers.

Jefferson, writing in the white heat of the controversy following the American Revolution, produced a relatively sophisticated formula in which he specified *in what respects* men ought to be considered equal. They were 'created equal', and among the 'rights inherent and inalienable' pertaining to this status were life, liberty and the pursuit of happiness.[7] There is a right to survive, a right to personal liberty, and a right to go on looking for happiness — whatever that means to each of us individually — though there is no automatic right to find it. The ideas of rights and equality are inextricably bound together, since it is in the recognition of certain basic rights that fundamental equality is guaranteed, and the limitation of these rights in turn prevents equality from degenerating into uniformity.

Tawney on inequality

In the late eighteenth and the nineteenth century, discussion of the concepts of equality and inequality centred on political rights. In the twentieth century, it has shifted to economic and social rights. R. H. Tawney wrote in the early 1930s of 'the ravages of the disease of inequality':[8]

> a perpetual misdirection of limited resources for the production and upkeep of costly futilities . . . the human energies which are the source of wealth are, in the case of the majority of the population, systematically under-developed from birth to maturity.

Tawney was prepared to acknowledge that equality was theoretically unattainable. It was an ideal rather than an realisable goal; but he pointed out that 'we do not use the impossibility of absolute cleanliness as an excuse for rolling on a manure heap.' The important thing is not that it should be completely attained but that it should be sincerely sought.[9]

The fundamental reasons for the search were both moral and practical: moral, because only working together for the common good held a people together and created genuine social bonds between then (a theme to be taken up later by Richard Titmuss in *The Gift Relationship*);[10] practical, because inequality led to 'power divorced from responsibility . . . the poison of states' and massive inefficiency. The redistribution of wealth would not make everybody rich, any more than levelling the Himalayas would add more than a few inches to the earth's surface, but gross inequalities were 'a source of torpor and stagnation . . . active irritation, inefficiency and confusion'. His attack was against the suppression and misdirection of social energy, and the touchstones of a good society were the distribution of wealth and income, and the expansion of collective provision for social needs.

Tawney takes for granted the importance and validity of moral imperatives in human affairs. In recent years, philosophers have sought to find a formulation which is valid on purely rational grounds. The outstanding theoretical work in this field is that of John Rawls, who has developed a complex variant of social contract theory.[11]

Rawls's theory of justice

Social contract theory, as developed by Locke and Rousseau, involves imagining a group of human beings of immense rationality and considerable political insight, but absolutely no political experience, who agree together on the best way to conduct their joint affairs. For Locke, this was a species of 'golden age' theory in which the free consent of individuals to safeguard their common interests made for majority rule and the preservation of a reasonable amount of personal property, though he offers some justification for regarding the contract as an historical possibility.[12] Rousseau seems less certain. For him the agonising paradox is that man is 'born free' but is somehow enchained by artificial constructs relating to social institutions such as property ownership, slavery and political oppression for which he can see no good reason.[13] Both views should be clearly distinguished from the type of 'primal horde' theory used by Freud, who relates basic decisions about power and authority to a definite period of human history (when the Asian hordes first swept across Europe) and comes to very different conclusions — a highly inegalitarian form of social relationship based on a crude struggle for power in which envy plays a major part.[14] Rawls derives his model from Locke and Rousseau, but states very clearly that it is an artificial model. It has no historical basis, and it is never likely to happen in practice. That would be 'to stretch fantasy too far', and the device is purely expository.

It is based on the concept of 'an original position' in which a group of people come together to decide the basic principles on which they wish to order their society. In this 'original position', they are limited by certain clearly defined factors. They are rational beings with a coherent set of preferences — they will desire more 'social goods' rather than less, they will have enough knowledge to rank the possible alternatives, and they will try to protect their liberties. Their decisions will be made for perpetuity, and they can be relied on to implement whatever they decide.

The possibility that each will decide in his own vested interest is precluded by the concept of 'the veil of ignorance'. They do not know what their own position in the new society will be, so that they are able to judge with absolute rationality and fairness. The 'veil' cloaks such factors as their wealth, social position, colour, age, skills, training, intelligence and even personal psychology — thus an individual does not know whether he is an optimist or a pessimist, inclined to take risks or averse to them. Nor will each know his own particular value-system, so that they have no grounds for favouring, say, Buddhists over Ethical Humanists. There will be no basis for bargaining, and no addiction to envy (which might lead them to make non-maximising choices in order to hold each other down). In this state, it is Rawls's contention that the group would reach a 'reflective equilibrium' in which what was purely rational would coincide with what was intuitively felt to be fair and just.

The difficulties of this intricate theory are considerable. For example, one can theoretically exclude knowledge of an individual's psychological make-up, but hardly its effects on his decision-making. A gambling man of absolutely no moral standards even under the 'veil of ignorance' might well opt for an unjust situation in the hope that he would benefit from it. In terms of the theory, all 'social goods' or 'primary goods' are reduced to the same level — the term includes everything from the most altruistic and spiritual satisfaction to the grossest material satisfaction, without distinction. We have further to assume that the participants do not make any errors of calculation or reasoning, that they do not face any situations in which there are equal probabilities, and that there is only one strategy which will produce the right answer.[15] However, it has been the starting point for some fresh thinking about the problems of equality and liberty, and Rawls's principles — that is, the principles which he thinks would govern the new society — should be stated in full.[16]

1 The first principle is that

> each person is to have an equal right to the most extensive total system of equal basic liberties compatible with a similar system of liberty for all.

(1)

The second principle is that

> social and economic inequalities are to be arranged so that they are both a) to the greatest benefit of the least advantaged, consistent with the just savings principle, and b) attached to offices and positions open to all under conditions of equality of opportunity.

(2)

The 'just savings principle' is a complicated arrangement for allowing people a certain amount of savings during their lifetime, dependent on the state of the economy. In a wealthier society, people would be allowed to save more than in a poor one. No man may infringe another's liberty, but this is the sole constraint on basic equality. The first principle is to have absolute priority over the second — equality and liberty come before the arrangement of inequalities; and the second part of the second principle is to have a priority over the first part — that is, the maintenance of equality of opportunity takes precedence over the greatest benefit of the disadvantaged.

It can be seen that Rawls is really proposing three different concepts, ranked in this order:
 (i) equality in basic liberties;   (1)
 (ii) equality of opportunity for advancement;   (2)
 (iii) positive discrimination in favour of the underprivileged to ensure equity.   (3)

Rawls's argument (developed at a length of a quarter of a million words written over twelve years) starts from a Kantian concept of 'justice as fairness', which is basically an intuitive conviction, and curves back to the same conclusion in the light of a series of very stiff exercises in rational thinking. The concept of the 'rational equilibrium' predicates that the end product of the two processes must be identical. Like Tawney, he believes that injustice and inequality are basically wasteful and inefficient in terms of human resources. He is also much committed to the maintenance of liberty, and to a stable social order, and sees no conflict between the two — a fact which sharply distinguishes his thinking not only from the historical dynamism of Dahrendorf, but from that of Hegel or Marx or Marcuse.[17]

It is apparent that both equality and equity are second-order concepts — that is, they are means for the attainment of ends rather than ends in themselves; and the first-order concept — the primary principle which orders their relationship — is social justice.

Rawlsian theory and social justice

Two studies in the social policy field use Rawls's basic formulations to argue that the proper aim of social policy is the pursuit of social justice. These are Albert Weale's *Equality and Social Policy*[18] and W. G. Runciman's *Relative Deprivation and Social Justice*.[19] Weale stresses the importance of social policy studies as a testing ground for social justice. The major social services — income-maintenance, health, education, housing — account for about one quarter of the Gross National Product, and nearly half of all public expenditure, and are therefore to be regarded as 'social goods' in the Rawlsian sense. He holds that it is necessary to distinguish between substantive equality (the probably unattainable principle) and procedural equality (means for actually achieving equality) and argues, following Titmuss, that there are three basic positions which may be taken on the relationship between public and private provision:

  (i) the state provision of social services is seen as transitory — with greater affluence, we can expect to see a greater extension of market provision;
 (ii) the state provides a minimum range of social services which acts as a safety net, and is supplemented by private provision;
(iii) the state provides a full range of services freely available to all.

Of these, the third is the most 'egalitarian', but in practice we tend to reach a mixed solution depending on the nature of the service and the current circumstances. Most of our social policy is in fact incrementalist; we make marginal changes in existing situations rather than going back to first principles on ideological grounds. Thus we get a mix of private and public provision in each field.

Runciman, as the title of his book suggests, is more concerned with problems of practical equity than those of theoretical equality, and with attitudes rather than with policies. His basic question is 'what is the relationship between the inequalities in a society and the feelings of acquiescence or resentment to which they give rise?' As he points out, it is not a simple relationship. 'The reactionary peasantry, the affluent radicals, the respectful poor are all familiar from the histories of many places and times.' This inconvenient fact may be dismissed as 'false consciousness' but it is none the less a social reality. A detailed national field study (1962) is used to demonstrate in terms of reference group theory that there is still no clear correlation between feelings of relative deprivation in terms of class, status and power. As Dahrendorf points out in another context, such evidence destroys the Marxist contention that there is a direct and unfailing correlation between the extremity of class situation and the intensity of class conflict.[20] 'Of all its various determinants', Runciman concludes,[21]

> one of the least powerful is the abstract ideal of social justice. Yet the notion of social justice is somehow implicit in every account of how people feel about social equality.

He goes on to consider the problem of how far the views of his respondents may be said to be conditioned by personal interest rather than communal interest, and concludes that 'the relative deprivation of status felt by manual workers and their families was probably less often also less intensely fraternalistic in 1962 than in 1919.' After a discussion of the problems of assessing what are variously called 'social needs' or 'wants' or 'aspirations' or 'envy', he rejects the view that one can set a 'minimum need' or 'subsistence level' (though he admits that there may be absolute needs in the sense of what is required by human organisms for survival), and comes to the conclusion that only a theory of justice can solve these difficult questions. Rawls does not make an appearance until page 297, and the theory is very briefly summarised, but it is used to make a variety of new and extended points.

Runciman argues that the three basic criteria for the distribution of social goods are need, merit and contribution to the common good. It follows that the just society will not be a totally egalitarian society. People with special needs will require compensatory provision. Jobs which carry special responsibility or danger or long hours should carry salary differentials. That archetypal group who are still sitting in the original position under the veil of ignorance will want to build some incentives into their society, some reward for skill and achievement which is valuable to society as a whole. But with these limitations, the model of society implied by the contractual theory is one in which there will be no inequalities of wealth which cannot be justified on these grounds:[22]

> in a socially just society there will be a continuous transfer of wealth from the richest to the poorest except where those above the poorest

can vindicate their right to their greater wealth by reference to these principles. In the absence of special claims, there will be a constant regression towards the mean.

The theory is 'fairly radical in its implications' because the test of inequalities is whether they can be justified to the loser, not to the winner. This is because in 'the original position' any participant is a potential loser, and must make his decision with this knowledge in view.

When it comes to inequalities of status, Runciman contributes a formulation of his own: the distinction between praise and respect. There is no social injustice in applauding the individual excellence of great artists or statesmen or inventors or craftsmen. We may praise the professor and the garage hand equally if they do their job well, and praise the garage hand more if he does his job better. Respect is a different kind of concept, bound up with allocated social roles and institutionalised notions of class membership, a matter of in-built privilege which cannot be shown to be just. The only just maxim is to respect all men equally — 'free inequality of praise, no inequality of respect'. We do not praise a man for the colour of his skin. We should not respect him either more or less because of it.

In a society organised on these principles, inequalities of power would be considerably less than in the societies we know. Authority would only be legitimate if it were exercised for the common good, and by common consent. There would have to be safeguards against tyranny, and probably a fair degree of consumer/worker participation.

Runciman concludes that we do not know what a totally just society would be like, and we are unlikely to attain it. He is in agreement with Tawney that the search rather than the finding is the important element. Unlike Tawney and Rawls, he is not prepared to argue that an egalitarian or just society would necessarily be more efficient than an inegalitarian or unjust one. But he does end with a vision of 'a just society with the social and economic lineaments of twentieth century Britain which would neither be an inchoate and undisciplined rat-race nor an army of sullen and mediocre conformists.'[23] If Rawlsian theory can point us in that direction, it has something to offer.

The scope of social justice

Very few political thinkers up to the present century have been able to think about justice, political, economic or social, over the whole range of human diversity. Even in the Athens of Pericles, upheld for centuries as the ideal of political freedom, equality was confined to free adult males. There was no representation for women or children or slaves — who together made up something like 75 per cent of the population; and equality only extended to voting rights. There were considerable economic inequalities, and the social distinction between *hoi polloi* and *hoi oligoi* was very basic. The French Revolution did not extend the concept of liberty, equality and fraternity to the aristos, and sporting a tricolour in his cap did not save Louis XVI. Marx is not only able to think in terms of the dictatorship of the proletariat, but in terms of the dictatorship of the *industrial* proletariat — a very small part of the population of Germany in his day. Agricultural workers, independent artisans, people in small businesses, white-collar workers, members of the professions are dismissed contemptuously as members of the lumpenproletariat or petty bourgeoisie. Maoist thought is basically egalitarian — but not in regard to foreigners (for whom it retains some of the suspicion associated with the Middle Kingdom's traditionalist views. Luther believed in the power of princes. Rousseau was a patriarchalist. Many political philosophers do not seem to be clear whether their references to 'men' should be construed as *homines* (members of the human race) or *viri* (male members of the human race). Even the most recent edition of Sabine's standard *History of Political Theory*[24] does not contain a single indexed reference to the rights of women, and Rawls does not include in the detailed specifications for the 'veil of ignorance' that participants in the social contract should not know what sex they are — though it is noticeable that the earlier chapters of his twelve-year opus refer to 'men', while the later ones refer to 'people' or 'human beings'.

In much egalitarian thinking, some people have been distinctly more equal than others. The distinctive twentieth-century contribution seems to be the ability to think across categories, and to see common humanity as the starting point for theories of social justice.

We now have the basic equipment with which to look at the social policy of our own society, and to test its potential for increasing social justice. The requirements are:

 (i) that it must safeguard basic liberties;
 (ii) that it must provide for positive discrimination in favour of the underprivileged;
 (iii) that it must, given the priority of factors (i) and (ii) provide equality of opportunity;
 (iv) that it must cover all human beings without exception;

   (v) that it must include social services as 'social goods';

  (vi) that it must be impartial in the sense that such differentials as exist are as acceptable to the losers as to the winners and agreed to be fair;

 (vii) that it must cover economic, social and political aspects of life;

(viii) that it must (and indeed will) be socially cohesive.

Runciman makes the point that such a list of the attributes of social justice is not the exclusive property of any one political party, and Weale reaches a similar conclusion. Socialists will tend to collective solutions and Conservatives to individualist ones, but both favour a mixture of public and private provision, and both include appeals to social justice in their election speeches. There are probably few people in our society who would not assent to the requirements in principle. The difficulty comes in the working out.

One of the chief reasons for this is of course that human beings are not wholly rational creatures. Their practical decisions are conditioned by many emotional factors, including self-interest, in-built attitudes based on early experience, and a variety of sympathies and antipathies developed through the years. The philosophers' 'rational man' is as much an abstraction as the social contract. However, if Rawls is right, pure rationality and intuitive feeling ultimately coincide. Most people have some basic idea of fairness or social justice, and if this does not strongly motivate their actions, it is at least a common factor on which to build.

Measuring social justice

Tawney described the movement towards social justice as happening 'with almost melodramatic sedateness'. Dahrendorf concludes after a survey of shifts in economic structure and social class since the time of Marx, that the provision of a wide range of social services guarantees certain basic rights of citizenship — 'a reality that forcefully counteracts the remaining forms of inequality and differentiation'.

It is a matter of common observation that 'forms of inequality and differentiation' relating to race, sex, income and wealth do still exist in British society. What is new in the past few years is that these are now being documented, and in some cases adjudicated upon, by statutory bodies — the Commission for Racial Equality, the Equal Opportunities Commission, and the standing Royal Commission on Income and Wealth.[25] The three sets of interests are, for the most part, being pursued independently: a suggestion by Lady Seear that a combined Commission should be set up to cover the work of the EOC and CRE to cover all forms of social discrimination was rejected by a spokesman for the CRE on the grounds that 'the differences [between sex and race discrimination] far outweigh the similarities.'[26] Meanwhile, the supporters of the poverty lobby concentrate on issues of income and wealth in the belief that these are the basic elements in social injustice, and that the primary disadvantages of being black or female are economic disadvantages shared by other sections of the population. The Low Pay Unit is concerned with people who are poorly paid, irrespective of race or gender.

Measuring developments relating to social justice involves some sort of yardstick of time. Dahrendorf measured over more than a century, and was able to show major changes. If we make comparisons over thirty or forty years, it is still possible to demonstrate considerable advances on all fronts. For instance, C. G. Trinder has conflated figures from the first report of the Royal Commission on Income and Wealth with earlier figures for the ownership of wealth, and although these show very little change in the period 1967-72, they show very large changes in the spread of wealth since 1936-8, and even larger changes since 1911-12. A study of the PEP Reports on the Health Services (1936) and the Social Services (1937) show massive improvements since that time. The economic and social position of women has certainly improved since Sir Almroth Wright wrote *The Unexpurgated Case against Woman Suffrage* in 1913, or since (as late as the 1930s) married women in the Civil Service and some other occupations had to keep their single names in order to avoid losing their jobs.

But most commentators in the social services measure over much shorter time-spans, and confine their analyses to more recent periods. One reason for this is that much of their work is statistical, and it is seldom possible to get long runs of figures on comparable bases, since statistical techniques are constantly being refined. Another is the belief that we have now reached something of a plateau in the development of social justice, and that some of our assumptions about the inevitability of progress have been over-optimistic.

In the decade after the Second World War, it was generally assumed that publicly provided social services would necessarily lead to a vertical redistribution of resources in favour of under-privileged groups. There was a considerable complacency about the achievements of the welfare state, based on two assumptions — first, that the methods of raising revenue through direct income tax, national insurance contributions, and indirect taxes such as purchase tax (later VAT) and local rates or charges were progressive: that is, that they took a larger proportion of the income of higher income groups; and second, that the services and benefits provided with this revenue would benefit those with lower incomes most. The evidence suggests that rates, indirect taxation and National Insurance contributions are regressive in their incidence, and that income tax is proportional over the most common income ranges, and only progressive among tax-payers at the top rates. J. L. Nicholson has concluded that 'the progressive effects of some taxes is largely offset by the regressive effect of others, and all taxes combined have very little net effect on . . . inequality.'[27] For the second point, some publicly provided services appear to have benefited middle and upper income groups as much as, if not more than, the poor, and those services which have been provided for the poor only have been poor quality services. Evidence on the utilisation of health care is mixed and difficult to interpret because the less well off tend to have greater health needs; but the quality of services is often better in middle-class areas, the middle classes recognise symptoms more quickly, and because they are more articulate, they often secure a better quality of service.[28] In the field of education, the size of classes is smaller and the quality of schools higher in better-off areas, and children of middle and upper income group families are more likely to make full use of secondary education and go on to further or higher education.[29]

In housing policy, working-class families are more likely to occupy housing in the public sector, but under the existing system of housing finance, it is not at all certain that subsidies to public housing are any more financially advantageous to the recipients than are tax relief on mortgage interest payments and tax free capital gains to owner occupiers.[30] In income maintenance policy, the step away from flat rate contributions and flat rate benefits to earnings related contributions and earnings related benefits has reduced the equalising effect of insurance benefits. Mike Reddin, in a closely argued paper, demonstrates that the overall effect of social insurance and pensions policy is to skew resources towards the single, the long-lived, and women.[31] Even means-tested benefits or exemptions from charges have in practice been found to be less redistributive than was assumed. Some evidence on the mechanisms of the 'Poverty Trap' is given in Chapter 3.

These complex interactions of payments and benefits are difficult enough to assess, but in addition their overall redistributive impact has to be set against differences in need. Not all individuals, families and households can derive the same benefit from the same level of provision, because they have different needs. For instance, the disabled require additional help to maintain them at the same standard of living as the non-disabled, because of the extra costs of transport, food, clothing and attendance that arise from disability.[32] The Plowden Report provided the sharpest argument for positive discrimination, on the grounds that children living in the inner cities and other areas of social deprivation required not the same educational provision as other children, but better provision, to compensate for the disadvantages of their home environment.[33]

There is considerable disagreement about whether, and to what extent, there has been a redistributive shift in the ownership of wealth. Atkinson contended in 1972 that over a quarter of total personal wealth in Britain was in the hands of the richest 1 per cent of the population, and that as much as three quarters belonged to the top 10 per cent. He concluded that there had been 'no marked decline in the degree of inequality'.[34] Polanyi and Wood, two economists at the Institute of Economic Affairs, wrote a rejoinder claiming that the evidence could be interpreted differently. They argued that when allowances had been made for the inadequacies of the statistics, the growing proportion of social capital and other factors, the distribution of private wealth would approximate to the top 10 per cent owning 30 per cent, and that this was a reasonable figure if one allowed for private savings.[35]

The analysis of income inequalities by reference to Inland Revenue data has long been subject to criticism, and Nicholson and colleagues at the Central Statistical Office have attempted to overcome the principal weakness of the data — the narrowness of the definition of income — by building a model based on the Family Expenditure Survey of net living standards after the effects of taxes, benefits and services. This analysis is now published each year in *Economic Trends* and it takes account of the redistributive effects of direct and indirect tax, including National Insurance contributions, rates and income tax, as well as the benefits of food and housing subsidies and benefits in kind such as education, health care and welfare foods. The conclusion of this analysis is that 'the inequality of original money has been . . . largely offset by an increase in the extent of redistribution through all taxes and benefits.'[36] This attempt to assess the redistributive effects of social and fiscal policies has been criticised, notably by Webb and Sieve.[37] Field *et al.* suggest four ways in which the CSO analysis overstates redistribution: the Family Expenditure Survey sample underrepresents the poor and the rich, not all taxes are included, not all benefits are included, and it is assumed that all benefits are consumed equally.[38]

In order to make some sense of this torrent of claims and counter-

claims the Labour government in 1974 established the standing Royal
Commission to investigate the distribution of income and wealth in the
UK (the Diamond Commission). The Commission has already begun to
produce reports containing a mass of sophisticated research.[39]

Conclusion

Better methods of analysis make us more aware of the dimensions of
inequality and inequity. That is in itself a step forward, because the
first requisites for the solution of any social problem are its formulation
and documentation.

It is probable that many inequities and some inequalities remain
uncorrected not because of the absence of political agreement or lack
of resources, but because of widespread misunderstanding about the
impact of existing policies and the nature of current experience of underprivilege. There are no final solutions to the problems of inequity and
inequality, but the goals of a just society are becoming clearer. We still
have much to discover about the means to those ends.

References

1   R. Dahrendorf, 'The Nature and Types of Social Inequality', in
A. Beteille, *Social Inequality*, Penguin, 1969, p. 21.
2   For example, John Ball's
When Adam delved and Eve span
Who was then the gentleman?
which emerged during the Peasants' Revolt of 1381; or the four-
teenth century *Roman de la Rose:*
Naked and impotent are we all,
High-born or peasant, great or small,
That human nature is throughout
The whole world equal, there's no doubt.
(Trans. F. S. Ellis, lines 19,411-14, quoted by G. H. Sabine,
History of Political Theory, Harrap, 3rd edn, 1963, p. 315.)
3   R. Filmer, *Patriarcha, or, the Natural Power of Kings*, Walter Davis,
1680. G Winstanley, *The Law of Freedom*, a collection of pamphlets written between 1648 and 1650, Penguin edn, 1973, ed.
Christopher Hill. The Diggers, an off-shoot of the Levellers of the
Cromwellian period, tried to establish an agricultural commune on
common land at St George's Hill near Cobham in Surrey, but were
turned off by the dragoons on the order of Puritan landlords.
4   M. Friedman, *Capitalism and Freedom*, University of Chicago Press,
1962, p.2.

5   F. A. Hayek, *The Constitution of Liberty*, Routledge & Kegan Paul, 1960, p. 88.
6   R. Dahrendorf in Beteille, op cit., p. 42.
7   First draft of the American Constitution.
8   R. H. Tawney, *Equality*, Allen & Unwin, 1931, revised edn, 1952, p. 12.
9   Tawney, op. cit., p. 47.
10 R. M. Titmuss, *The Gift Relationship*, Allen & Unwin, 1970.
11 J. Rawls, *A Theory of Justice*, Clarendon Press, 1972.
12 J. Locke, 'The True End of Government', in *Of Civil Government*, Everyman edn, 1940, pp. 173-4.
13 J.-J. Rousseau, *The Social Contract and Discourses*, first published 1762, Everyman edn, 1913.
14 S. Freud, *Group Psychology and the Analysis of the Ego*, Hogarth edn, 1959.
15 B. Barry, *The Liberal Theory of Justice*, Oxford University Press, 1973, chapter 3 *passim*.
16 Rawls, op. cit. The principles are stated at several points in the exposition, but in their fullest and final form on pp. 302-3.
17 See Hegel's *Philosophy of History*, Marx's *Das Kapital*, and H. Marcuse, 'Repressive Tolerance', in R. P. Wolff, R. Moore and H. Marcuse, *A Critique of Pure Tolerance*, Beacon Press, Boston, 1975.
18 A. Weale, *Equality and Social Policy*, Routledge & Kegan Paul, 1978.
19 W. G. Runciman, *Relative Deprivation and Social Justice*, Penguin, 1972.
20 R. Dahrendorf in Beteille, op. cit., p. 117.
21 Runciman, op. cit., p. 291.
22 Runciman, op. cit., p. 316.
23 Runciman, op. cit., p. 343.
24 Sabine, op. cit.
25 See papers in *The Year Book of Social Policy in Britain* (Routledge & Kegan Paul): Eric Butterworth, 'Race Relations: the Next Step' (1973 edition); Alan Little, 'The Race Relations Act' (1976 edition); Nancy Seear, 'Equal Opportunities for Men and Women' (1973 edition); Christian Howard, 'Women and the Professions' (1973 edition); C. G. Trinder, 'Income and Wealth: first Reports from the Royal Commission' (1975 edition).
26 Little, op. cit., p.96.
27 J. L. Nicholson, 'Distribution and Redistribution of Income in the UK', in D. Wedderburn (ed.), *Poverty, Inequality and Class Structure*, Cambridge University Press, 1974, p. 81.
28 Le Grand, 'The Distribution of Public Expenditure in the National Health Service', evidence to the Royal Commission on the National Health Service, June 1976.
29 F. Field, *Unequal Britain*, Arrow Books, 1974.
30 C. Boyd, 'A Fair Share', *Roof*, September 1977.
31 M. Reddin, 'National Insurance and Private Pensions', in *The Year Book of Social Policy in Britain 1976*, Routledge & Kegan Paul, 1977.

24   Equality and Equity

32 J. R. Bradshaw, *The Financial Needs of Disabled Children,*
    Disability Alliance, 1976.
33 *Children and their Primary Schools,* report of the Central Advisory
    Council for Education (England), vol. 1 HMSO, 1967.
34 A. B. Atkinson, *Unequal Shares,* Allen Lane, 1972, p. 45.
35 G. Polanyi and J. B. Wood, *How Much Inequality?,* Institute of
    Economic Affairs, 1974.
36 Nicholson, op. cit., p. 81.
37 A. L. Webb and J. E. B. Sieve, *Income Redistribution and the*
    Welfare State, Bell, 1971.
38 F. Field, M. Meacher and C. Pond, *To Him Who Hath,* Penguin,
    1977, p. 185.
39 *Royal Commission on Income and Wealth,* Cmnd 6171, Cmnd,
    6172, Cmnd 6383, HMSO, 1975–6.

Chapter two

Needs and Resources

The gap between needs and the resources available to meet them has always been at the heart of debate about social policy. Up to the mid 1960s the conflict between need and resources was obscured because of a growth economy. From the mid 1960s to the mid 1970s there was at least the expectation of growth to sustain the hope that needs could continue to be met. Now for the immediate future there is little prospect of economic growth, and without growth and with dramatic rates of inflation there has been a hardening of attitudes about publicly provided social services. No longer are competing claims for resources dealt with on the basis of deferment — 'not this year but perhaps next year' has been replaced by 'if not already, then not at all'.

In the previous decade protagonists in the state v market controversy fought a fierce battle over the desirability of publicly provided social services and the limits of tax revenue. There are now few advocates of increased public expenditure on social services and most energy is being directed to a rearguard action to defend what exists. The British Association of Social Workers for instance launched a campaign against the cuts imposed in 1973 with the mild exhortation 'Care Costs'.[1] They had to follow it by backing the more emphatic statement 'Fight the Cuts', as local authorities and government departments vied with each other to reduce expenditure and curtail services.

Glennerster has identified four types of interpretation of public expenditure issues:

(a) an optimistic perspective which sees the problem as resulting from a medium term economic crisis, assuming that when income from development of the North Sea Oil becomes available it will be possible to finance public spending in the traditional manner;

(b) a perspective which sees social policy as detrimental to economic growth. The scale of public spending, level of taxation and increasing manpower requirements of the social services over the past fifteen years are viewed as at the root of Britain's economic problems. A decline in social services is seen as necessary for the country's economic recovery and success;

(c) an argument that the scale of government activity has grown to such an extent that the political system is no longer able to control it. This is a political argument. Social services are seen as having little opportunity to expand, indeed even a period of marking time is seen as contributing little to the economy's improvement; and

(d) a neo-Marxist interpretation where present difficulties reflect the basic contradiction of capitalism. A high level of public spending to maintain and increase productivity, essential to the capitalist system, is increasingly difficult to realise and therefore there is recourse to borrowing. In the end this becomes impossible and social services 'contribute to the collapse of the system and so of themselves'.[2]

None of these dominant schools of thought believes that there is now a case for higher levels of public expenditure and taxation. Even the 'North Sea oil optimists' believe that for the time being social ends must become subservient to economic means. Only when the economy is back on the rails will it be possible to begin a moderate expansion in the social services. Meanwhile we should mark time. The social services together with 1.6 million unemployed are now more clearly than ever before the handmaids of economic policy. In this chapter we rehearse some of the arguments for and against more resources for publicly provided social services. First we consider the concept of need.

Need

Some commentators have seen the recent debate about cuts in public expenditure as an ideal opportunity for government and local authorities to examine priorities:[3]

> To spend is to choose . . . expansion allows priorities to be blurred, or to be expressed in relative increases; retrenchment forces decisions between rival programmes battling for a steady or diminishing supply of resources.

The most often used criterion suggested for making such decisions is 'need'. Resources must be allocated to those individuals and groups most in need, it is argued. The ordering of need to determine priorities implies that there is a hierarchy of need. As with all evaluative concepts, however, the difficulty is in obtaining a consensus as to what constitute appropriate criteria by which needs can be ranked relative to one another in such a hierarchy. This difficulty is compounded by the different interpretations that can be placed on similar situations and the meaning that potential recipients of services place on their plight.

Technically, it is possible to identify 'absolute need' as it is to identify 'absolute poverty' — a state where survival of the human organism is threatened. Thus Seebohm Rowntree was able to identify those in absolute poverty by itemising the biological requirements in respect of food, fuel, shelter and clothing below which people would be unfit for work. It was therefore possible to state that those who were not obtaining these minimal requirements were in absolute poverty.

It is impossible, however, to divorce the plight of those in such a state from the wider social context which has contributed to that situation or to ignore the attitudes and values that are a reaction, and in some senses a compensation, to that situation. Often these attitudes and values of potential recipients may appear incomprehensible (and irresponsible) to those in authority. George Orwell is one commentator who has sought to convey how these differing expectations and meanings associated with the same situation may arise.

In *The Road to Wigan Pier* he argued that while adequate nutrition is necessary to maintain good health this did not mean that the miners, the group he was commenting upon, would necessarily allocate any of their limited resources to improving their diet:[4]

> The basis of their diet is white bread and margarine, corned beef, sugared tea, and potatoes — an appalling diet. Would it not be better if they [the miners] spent more money on wholesome things like oranges and wholemeal bread . . . . Yes, it would, but the point is that no human being is ever going to do such a thing. The ordinary human being would sooner starve than live on brown bread and raw carrots. And the peculiar evil is this, that the less money you have the less inclined you feel to spend it on wholesome food. A millionaire may enjoy breakfasting off orange juice and Ryvita biscuits; an unemployed man doesn't. . . . When you are unemployed, which is to say when you are underfed, harassed, bored and miserable, you don't want to eat dull wholesome food. You want something a little bit 'tasty'. . . . White bread-and-marg. and sugared tea don't nourish you to any extent, but they are *nicer* (at least most people think so) than brown bread-and-dripping and cold water. Unemployment is an endless misery that has got to be palliated and especially with tea, the Englishman's opium. A cup of tea or even an aspirin is much better as a temporary stimulant than a crust of brown bread.

Orwell's own values, with statements about 'ordinary human beings' are all too evident but they serve to emphasise that it is impossible to divorce values from an attempt fully to understand what is meant by the impact of 'absolute poverty' — how people interpret and respond to it. Similarly, with 'absolute need'. Different values and standards of behaviour mean that establishing a hierarchy of need is fraught with difficulty as, indeed, is the attempt to identify need where no attempt is made to rank items in terms of relative importance. David Harvey,[5] for example, identifies nine areas where there could be possible need:

    (i) food;
    (ii) housing;
    (iii) medical care,
    (iv) education;
    (v) social and environmental service;
    (vi) consumer goods;
    (vii) recreational opportunities;
  (viii) neighbourhood amenities;
    (ix) transport facilities.

This is more specific than Kathleen Slack's categories of preventing suffering, protecting the weak, and promoting individual and social good.[6] But the result, while of interest, is of little use to the policy maker. The categories are so broad that they can encompass many different interpretations rather than clarifying the relationship between such interpretations. The list was published in 1973, and only four years later the omission of 'employment opportunities' is conspicuous by its absence — indicating that need is relative not only between different sectors of society at the same point in time but also over time as experience and expectations change. It is interesting to note that those writers who criticise the welfare state for failing to meet needs, no matter how defined, do not advocate that any alternative system will eliminate need.[7] As need is evaluative and relative no society can eliminate need. Attempts can be made to meet and minimise the impact of need — but all need cannot be eliminated.

The response to such difficulties among some commentators has been to see the concept of need as only having conceptual use and value if applied to demand. Others have emphasised that the question that should be asked is not 'what is need?' and how is it defined but 'who defines need?', for if need is relative it is relative to standards established by certain groups in society.

NB

Need as demand

Need is not solely demand. Demand refers to need that is backed by the money to pay and is therefore an important component of any definition. The difficulties associated with how demand is articulated, and the social processes behind these difficulties, means that it is misleading to restrict need to demand. An example can be taken from the market versus the state controversy conducted between the Institute of Economic Affairs and the late Richard Titmuss. This debate has been criticised by Culyer as being too polemical and divorcing demand from supply.[8] Both points are valid, but the fact that the debate was polemical and conducted on a narrow front meant that the issues emerged in a particularly clear manner.

In one of the early rounds of the debate Jewkes and Jewkes stated:[9]

> Does not equality become a very odd thing in a system such as the NHS where, in effect, people with small incomes *who are rarely sick* subsidise people with large incomes who *frequently fall ill and* make large demands on the Health Service? (emphasis added)

If the parts of the statement that have been italicised are deleted then it reads in a much less contentious manner. In fact the working class, as defined in terms of occupation, make less use of the facilities than do the middle class. No one knows why this is, for various statistical measures indicate that the working class are not healthier than other groups, indeed they often suffer from poorer health than other groups.[10] Factors such as different concepts of what is 'good' or 'bad' health, knowledge of facilities, a mother feeling that it is necessary to 'carry on' as someone has to look after the family, have all been advanced. Although largely based on stereotypes such explanations probably contain an element of truth as to why the working class under-utilise the NHS. They also indicate that the statistics of treatment cannot be accepted at face-value in the way that the Jewkeses did.

The manner in which they interpret the statistics indicates the swingeing nature in which the market v state controversy was conducted rather than shedding light on need and how it relates to the health care that is received. Similarly, waiting lists are not reliable indicators of unmet need unless it is clear how the list is constructed — after a certain point many such lists are closed even if there are potential recipients who could be placed on them.[11]

Demand is therefore part of need but it does not reflect the complete picture. In spite of this difficulty it is felt that 'need as a demand concept' is the only way that a theoretical advance can be made in providing an answer to that deceptively simple question 'what is need?' Thus

Nevitt has recently argued that:[12]

> I have emphasised that 'need' can only be a useful concept if it is
> equated to a demand by governments or individuals for goods and
> services. So long as prices and quantities are omitted from estima-
> tions of 'need', the concept can have neither theoretical nor empir-
> ical value, and it properly belongs not to the social sciences but to
> the vocabulary of political rhetoric.

Nevitt feels that students of needology (a term forwarded by A.
Williams[13]) are suspicious of the market model. This is probably true,
but they are suspicious of a situation where it is assumed that to inter-
ject prices and quantities necessarily makes the concept of 'need' more
scientific. Difficulties associated with compensating victims of industrial
accidents indicate the complex issues of value-judgments associated
with assessing 'the quality of life' experienced by an individual. Such
difficulties should not act as a deterrent to measurement, although the
basic problem will always remain — it is only one variable in decision-
making. Measurement may be a necessary step but it is not sufficient
in itself — it cannot be divorced from interpretation, interpretation
which inevitably involves 'the vocabulary of political rhetoric' as the
Jewkeses' quotation clearly indicates.

Nevitt argues that 'need as demand' avoids the difficulty of confusing
personal want with personal need. I may want a Porsche sports car but
unless this becomes a demand in the market, either through my efforts
or a sponsoring authority, it is not a need. Need is therefore a personal
want that is recognised as legitimate through the process of demand in
the market. This applies also to situations where others may advocate
a need on my behalf although I do not experience the situation as leading to a personal want. Unless the process of demand occurs, I am not
in a state of need. But to exclude from systematic analysis factors relating to how demand becomes articulated, no matter how qualified the
argument, imposes an artificial theoretical clarity on the world where
decisions are made on the basis of value judgments which may be far
from clear. It is these value-judgments that have to be incorporated
into a definition of need. As Culyer states about the National Health
Service:[14]

> The making of value judgements lies at the heart of medical care
> delivery in general, is crucial in the concept of the NHS and is
> the very essence of establishing the meaning of the word 'need'.

He further goes on to state when attempting to construct an index by which to ration health care resources[15]

> the selection of variables for inclusion in the index and the weights attached to them are *policy* decisions embodying particular value judgements. They are not matters that can be decided by social science (or any other kind), nor are they matters, in a *national* health service, that should be decided by persons without public accountability.

Need and the 'gatekeeper'

In this extract Culyer is concerned with the role of the medical profession in limiting access to scarce resources. The role of professional practice and autonomy is crucial as is the role of the citizen in the decision making process: the chapters on 'Professionalisation' and 'Citizen Participation' clarify these issues which have a direct bearing on the definition and meeting of need.[16] It is important, however, to be clear that it is not just those occupations traditionally defined as 'professions' that are solely involved in defining 'need'. All occupational groups that are involved in the process of deciding access to scarce resources have recourse to the concept of 'need', either explicitly or implicitly. Such occupational groups may not enjoy the status of 'expert' or 'professional' but, none the lesss, influence access to scarce resources by acting as advocates for those who meet certain criteria and defenders against those who do not. One example is the housing visitor who has to assess the housing need of a family as well as passing judgment on the living standards of that family. Problems of varying definitions of hygiene and cleanliness in different sectors of the society inevitably impinge upon the subjective evaluation that the housing visitor makes — an evaluation with crucial importance in deciding the quality of future housing for that family. Such problems are especially acute when the evaluation is of an immigrant group with different customs and values. A recent Political and Economic Planning report illustrates the problem:[17]

> Housing visitors are generally instructed to assess how hard the applicant is trying, regardless of the physical circumstances imposed on him or her; this is a genuine attempt at objectivity, but the ratings are still bound to be subjective. If, therefore, minorities are given lower ratings, to say that this is wrong is only to oppose one subjective assessment by another. As long as the system of subjective assessments of standards continues — and none of the authorities

show the slightest sign of abandoning it — it will be possible for one person, or one group of people, to be favoured at the expense of another, purely because of the housing visitor's way of looking at things.

In such a situation it is perhaps appropriate to use the term 'gatekeeper', originally forwarded by Pahl,[18] to describe the person or occupational group who acts as a defender of their agency's resources. The health and social services contain many such gatekeepers — not all of whom are accorded full approval for their decisions by many commentators who, acting as advocates for those they feel are 'in need', find their activities thwarted by such persons.[19] The desk clerk at the local Department of Health and Social Security office has a reputation of considerable notoriety as an obstructive, some would say vigilant, gatekeeper. It is doubtful whether there is any adult in the country who has not encountered the hurdle of the receptionist in gaining access to the doctor; and one study of a social services department has concentrated specifically on what it called 'The Point of Entry'.[20]

Such gatekeepers not only decide access to resources; they may also decide the allocation of certain types of resources. There is, therefore, a decision on whether need exists and the most appropriate manner in which that need can be met. To define need theoretically does not necessarily tell you how to meet that need either effectively or efficiently. In practice, however, the two are inextricably linked. Need as a criterion upon which to decide the ordering of priorities is therefore applied to two types of decision:

(i) whether to allocate resources;
(ii) what type of resources to allocate.

In such decisions the focus of concern can be the individual as a member of a group, for example single-parent families, or the individual as resident of a certain geographical area, for example the inner-city zone. Both approaches have their difficulties.

The chapter on 'Universality and Selectivity' indicates the difficulties associated with take-up of selectively based services and benefits for those with certain types of need. There are the twin problems of lack of information and stigma that operate to keep the number of recipients down. Here the role of the gatekeeper is crucial in possibly reinforcing feelings of social opprobrium in those who initiate contact. They may also be reluctant to identify possible recipients. So, for example, social services departments were accused of 'dragging their feet' in establishing 'At Risk' registers under the terms of 1970 Chronically Sick and

Disabled Persons Act as they did not want the additional financial burden of statutorily having to provide services for those that they did not already have on file.[21]

At first glance the 'blanket approach' of providing resources for a geographical area appears to avoid the problem of the individual failing to come forward. It is possible by using various indicators to isolate certain geographical areas of need — the inner city, regions of industrial decline and stagnation and the like. Statistical criteria can be used to advance an argument of 'territorial justice' — areas with like populations should have like services and facilities. If one such area is lacking a certain facility that the other possesses then it can be argued that the former is in 'need' and this can be corrected on the basis of arguing for territorial justice.[22]

There is the danger, however, of falling victim to 'the ecological fallacy'. To classify an area as a multi-problem and deprived zone does not mean that an individual living in that zone will necessarily suffer from multiple problems and deprivation. All the individuals in an area with a high rate of delinquency are not necessarily delinquent.[23] It was discovered on the Educational Priority Areas programme that to provide resources for a geographical area means missing a considerable number of individuals for whom there ought to be concern while including many to whom the criteria do not apply with the same urgency.[24]

In 1972 Bradshaw published 'A Taxonomy of Social Need'[25] which distinguished between four categories of need:

normative need:	the way the expert or professional defines need in a given situation;
felt need:	need felt by the individual in terms of want;
expressed need:	need that becomes a demand; and
comparative need:	the principle on which 'territorial justice' is based. If X and Y have similar characteristics and Y is in receipt of a service not received by X then X is said to be in need.

Such a taxonomy does not seek to define what is meant by 'need' but to indicate the elements that are included in the attempts of others to define need. The responsibility for using the taxonomy and in defining need is left to the policy-maker.[26] The values of the policy maker and the constraints within which he operates are, therefore, of crucial importance. Foremost among such constraints, and the focus of much controversy, is the raising and distribution of resources. In the following section on resources, consideration is given to the raising of revenue and the role of public expenditure. This is not meant, however, to imply that money is the only resource available to the community.

'Resources' refers to more than just revenue — it includes manpower, skills and plant and a more comprehensive and critical approach to their use and effectiveness. The role and deployment of staff in post is undergoing a re-appraisal as is the contribution that the volunteer and voluntary organisations can make — see the chapter on 'Voluntary Organisations'. Critical evaluation of proposed capital projects has led to cheaper alteratives such as sheltered housing being adopted — on the grounds that it is both cheaper and more effective in maintaining the independence of the residents.[27] Further, a more integrated approach to the use of existing buildings is being sought — for example, social services may use the building that education has as a youth club for a day-centre. To talk of resources refers therefore to the complex interplay of money, staff and buildings. In the following discussion 'resources' refers to revenue — however raised — to highlight the importance of different approaches to expenditure and how such political considerations reflect important conceptions of what is need and how it can be adequately met.

Resources

What are resources needed for social services required to do?

First, they are required to maintain the *level* of benefits and services that are already being provided by public agencies.

Second, they are required to maintain the *value* of benefits and services in the face of inflation in prices and wages.

Third, they are required to maintain the *quality* of the benefits and services in the face of increases in the population in need. For example, the increase in the proportion of elderly in the population requires more resources (and the reduction in the birth rate may release resources for other purposes).[28]

Fourth, resources are needed to meet needs not being met now. These may be either new or improved benefits or services, or increased demand for existing benefits and services.

A good deal of the increase in resources needed for the social services is automatic or semi-automatic. That is the demand for more resources is not the direct result of the provision of new services by government. Most of the demand comes from changes which are more or less outside government control — changes in the rate of unemployment or inflation,

the increased take-up of services for which there is a legal entitlement —
more children staying on at school or going to university, an increase in
prescribing by doctors. Higher standards of provision create their own
demand — better housing conditions have been one factor responsible
for the dramatic increase in the proportion of old people living alone
and the increase in the proportion living alone will itself lead to greater
demands on the health and welfare services.

What then are the sources of revenue for publicly provided social
services? Note that not all social policy is financed from public expenditure. To provide a complete assessment of the total amount of resources
spent on social welfare provision it is necessary to take account of four
other types of expenditure in addition to public expenditure.

1 Private purchases of social services such as contributions to BUPA
for private health care, education purchased in the private school system
and private insurance schemes. These private purchases can be either
purchases from a public service, such as charges for dental treatment
or spectacles, or purchases from the private sector in the form of
insurance contributions or fees.

2 Social fringe benefits provided by employers such as non-contributory pension schemes, sickness cover, free or subsidised housing or
transport.

3 Net expenditure by voluntary bodies using funds raised from the
population.

4 The most important source of social expenditure other than what
is technically regarded as public expenditure comes in the form of
tax concessions — tax relief on occupational pension contributions, on
mortgage interest payments and allowances for elderly people, children
and single parents. These concessions and allowances are a crucial part
of social welfare payments, but because of public accounting conventions they do not appear as public expenditure. There has always been
something of an argument about whether tax allowances should be
treated as public expenditure and it has been argued that revenue fore-
gone by the exchequer is not the same as revenue collected and redistri-
buted. However, they both have the same impact on the public sector
borrowing requirement and the fact that for instance child tax allowances have exactly similar effects to child benefits and yet do not count
as public expenditure is a considerable anomaly.

The sources of revenue for public expenditure come from:
Taxes on income;
Taxes on expenditure;
National Insurance contributions;

Rates;

Other receipts and borrowing.

The proportion of revenue derived from the different sources varies from year to year and the proportion derived from borrowing, particularly borrowing abroad, led to concern in 1975 and 1976 about the size of the public sector borrowing requirement, a loan from the International Monetary Fund and an agreement with them that led to further cuts in public expenditure.

The best method of raising revenue is a matter of dispute but so is the amount of domestic expenditure devoted to public expenditure. The 1976 White Paper on public expenditure states that 60 per cent of Gross Domestic Product is devoted to public expenditure.[29] As Glennerster[30] comments:

> The implication is that only 40% of the economy remains in private hands. That is, of course, rubbish. . . . The figure for total expenditure that is so often quoted includes both expenditure on goods and services which do form part of the gross national product *and* transfer items like pensions and other kinds of income support which do not.

The role of transfers in public expenditure is too often misunderstood. In the case of transfers money is taken out of consumer expenditure by taxes and contributions but transferred back to it in the form of pensions and benefits — it is a redistribution from one consumer to another. While transfers are not a withdrawal from consumer expenditure they may effect a reduction in capital formation because it is argued that pensioners and other social security beneficiaries are likely to spend their money whilst those from whom it was taxed would have been more likely to save it.

An increasing proportion of revenue taken out of consumers' expenditure through taxation goes not to current public expenditure or to public capital formation but back to the private sector as capital grants to private industry through agencies such as the Public Enterprise Board.

If allowances are made for this 'double counting' only about a third of GNP goes on public expenditure on goods and services. There has been a long wrangle about the merits of private and public consumption. J. K. Galbraith[31] in a book which greatly influenced the aspirations of the 1964-70 Labour government (if not their achievements) drew a contrast between 'private affluence and public squalor'. He described how in the USA the priority given to private consumption had led the economy to extravagant over-production of more and better consumer goods at the expense of the quality of publicly provided services and the environment. One of the keynotes of the Labour Party election campaign in 1964 was the need to alter the balance between 'starved community services and extravagant consumption'.[32] Labour's plans depended on a growth in the economy that was never achieved, and plans for 1964-70 were scrapped.[33] Since 1969 a series of White Papers have been published setting out public expenditure proposals over a five year period. As predictors of what will actually happen they have been of limited use. They have been revised and re-revised with changes of government and with one economic crisis after another, and until the Treasury succeeded in imposing cash limits on the spending departments in 1976 they invariably overspent the budget allowed for them. It is worth describing parts of some of these White Papers to illustrate how governments have in practice been vying with each other to control public expenditure. In the first White Paper (1968-9 to 1971-2)[34] the Labour government proposed an increase in the Health and Welfare budget of 3.8 per cent per annum but much of this was needed to meet the needs of an increasing population. It was suggested that real improvements could only come from increases in efficiency. Expenditure on social security benefits would arise from increases in the dependent population and inflation. In a most revealing sentence the White Paper said:[35]

> Increased expenditure on social security benefits has to be met by
> higher insurance contributions and taxation raised from the
> nation as a whole. The extent to which it will be possible to make
> further real improvements in the level of benefits over and above
> expenditure required to take account of price movements therefore
> depends on the rate of growth of national wealth.

Thus the Labour government had decided that taxes and contributions were high enough and any improvements must come from growth.

When the Conservatives came to power in 1970 they published their own expenditure White Paper. This aimed to reduce public spending and taxation and lop £1,600 millions off spending plans by 1974-5.[36] This process was begun with the famous Barber budget in 1971 when income tax was cut by a 'jolly, jolly sixpence' and free school milk was abolished and school meals prices raised. The Conservatives' second White Paper[37] restored most of the cuts in response to rising unemployment. The pattern of revision and reduction continued after Labour returned to power in 1974. The anti-public expenditure ideology is in the ascendant in all the main political parties and in much of the academic and media commentary on public affairs. The composite anti-public expenditure ideology was well put in a paper by R.G. Smethurst.[38]

> The public sector in the U.K. is particularly large. This not only means that there is a large sector which is unresponsive to public demand and the forces and discipline of the market, and therefore with a tendency to inefficiency; it also means a particularly heavy tax burden. In addition because despite this tax imposition the government cannot wholly cover its expenditure, we have a very large national debt, the management of which inhibits the effective use of monetary policy and an expansion in the money supply which has direct inflationary effects. Demographic trends make it inevitable that if present policies continue public sector demands will rise, producing higher tax burdens or more inflation, or both. Yet already taxation has had an adverse effect upon incentives to innovate and restructure British industry and upon the work effort of the labour force. High taxes also discourage saving. What this means is a high level of consumption which sucks in imports; a low level of growth and rate of productivity, less incentive to invest high and growing wage costs per unit of output — all of which make British exports less competitive. Hence recurrent balance of payments crises which force the government further to curtail demand by raising taxation — a self defeating process. Hence devaluation and hence Britian's low rate of growth and relatively declining standard of living.

Not all those who would believe that the limits of public expenditure have been reached would support all the arguments in this paragraph. However, it contains most of the most often expressed criticisms of public expenditure. Those who seek to defend public expenditure are drawn into replying to economic criticisms with an economic defence. Thus they argue that social services are a productive investment. Expenditure on health care increases the productivity of the labour force; education improves their efficiency and skill; housing is good for health and morale; cash transfers act as an economic stabiliser providing purchasing power in depressions and reducing insecurity. Pensions ease the burden on the children of the aged and release money for investment.

These claims may be correct. The economic value of social expenditure may be under-valued but there is a more fundamental objection to these arguments. Why should either economic or social programmes be geared to production per se? What is the intrinsic value of producing one more motor car more cheaply than the Japanese? If they are, human betterment becomes a means to an end instead of an end in itself. In defending social expenditure as a productive investment we may be ignoring the more fundamental question — production for what? If we pursue economic growth at the expense of social justice then we have got all our values mixed up.

Apart from these arguments the main thrust of the opposition to the economists' case against public expenditure is that important parts of their case are just not true. In particular, is it true that

1 Public expenditure is *too high* in the UK — or
2 that taxation is *too high*; or
3 that increased taxation would have an adverse effect upon incentives?

Current government expenditure in Britain is not dramatically different from that of other industrialised countries. These types of comparisons are notoriously difficult to make but those who have compared the proportion of GNP going on goods and services have found the UK in the middle of the league table despite the fact that our defence expenditure and debt interest take up a larger proportion of expenditure than in most other countries.[39]

Nevertheless over recent years our expenditure has been greater than revenue resulting in a large public sector borrowing requirement. This imbalance was the result of a number of factors including very rapid rates of inflation, increased expenditure on unemployment benefit and direct and indirect subsidies to the private sector in the form of direct grants or the waiving of revenue from Corporation Tax. So it was hardly the result of overspending on social services and could have been dealt with by increases in taxation or reductions in public expenditure. Thanks partly to the terms laid down by the IMF and thanks also to the belief that we are already too highly taxed — the cuts came in public expenditure.

Are taxes too high? Again international comparisons of taxation as a percentage of GNP tend to show the UK in the middle of an international league table.[40] To compare tax systems it is really necessary to look not just at the overall GNP taken in revenue but at the structure level and transfer of taxes. Brown and Dawson[41] who did this found that a relatively larger proportion of our tax revenue was raised by indirect taxes than by direct taxes and social security contributions and though our rates of income tax might appear high on a simple comparison, if 'equivalent purchasing power exchange rates' are used for the comparison, only at the very highest income does the UK have higher tax rates.

Nevertheless as Brown and Dawson argue, the UK could have the lowest taxes in the world and still be over taxed if the public provision of goods and services is at the expense of work effort.

This leads to the question, what evidence is there that high taxes have an adverse effect on incentives? The general conclusions of Brown and Dawson are that there is a considerable misunderstanding about how much income is paid in tax in the UK; if there is an effect on incentives then in theory direct tax would have no greater effect than a diminution in purchasing power brought about by indirect taxes; only the minority of the workforce have the opportunity to work more or less — overtime where it is available is often compulsory; those who might be expected to have most freedom to work more or less and whose decision may be expected to affect the economy — the entrepreneur — appears to be motivated by power, status and prestige rather than money; and finally there may be as many who work harder to make up for taxation as are driven to emigrate, retire early or choose careers in the Civil Service rather than business because of the marginal rate of taxation in the UK.

Richard Crossman[42] towards the end of his period as Secretary of State for Social Services suggested that, because income tax is so unpopular, revenue could more easily be raised by progressive national insurance contributions.

Local authority revenue

Traditionally there has been the assumption that the rates provide the backbone of local authority revenue. In reality this has only been one of many varied sources — in the early 1960s, for example, the rates accounted for just under a third of local authority revenue, the rest consisting of loans and government grants. The effect of inflation has meant that existing services cost more to provide at a time when the statutory requirements placed on the local authorities have increased. The result has been that it has proved impossible for the rates, always a sensitive issue in local politics, to keep abreast of increasing costs and commitments. By the mid-1970s the rates only accounted for approximately a fifth of local authority revenue,[43] central government playing an important role in providing revenue through the rate support grant.

This increasing dependence on central government, and the control this implies on spending through the level of the rate support grant, has led to concern about the relationship between local authority autonomy and central government direction. The nature of this relationship raises the question of who is responsible for deciding the allocation of scarce resources. The Layfield Committee on Local Government Finance,[44] reporting in 1976 stated:

> We need a system that makes it unambiguously clear who is responsible for spending public money so that they can be held accountable through the ballot box for the decisions to spend and for the taxes raised to finance that expenditure.

The Layfield Committee decided in favour of local autonomy and advocated a local income tax. One year later in 1977 the Labour government rejected such a decision, reaffirming the dependence of local authorities on central government as essential to maintain overall control of the economy.[45] Although adopting one of the Layfield recommendations, to base rating valuation on capital rather than rental values, such a reaffirmation has done little to quell local authority anxiety about the source of adequate funding of services for which it is responsible.

At present only a small part of the rate support grant is earmarked for specific services and projects. The fear of the local authorities is that this will increase. Arguments for and against local authority autonomy reflect issues as basic as those relating to the size of public expenditure. Such issues are concerned with value judgments and assumptions as to the nature and meaning of the welfare state — the same value judgments and assumptions used by policy makers in deciding the answer to the question 'what is need and how is it to be met?'

The era of constraint

The 1970s were to be the era of reorganisation. Social services departments were created and local government and the National Health Service were reorganised. Ironically, such developments were overtaken by the era of constraints in which it was necessary to question priorities, an exercise such developments were supposed to facilitate. In the process many felt that the new structures were ineffective and that they may have contributed to, and exacerbated, the difficulties. It became clear that decisions about balancing needs and resources are:[46]

> the product of a dialectic between the demands generated by ongoing programmes, economic expediency, social values, administrative convenience and political pressures, constraints and opportunities.

In such a context it is still possible for the academic commentator to argue whether 'need' is a useful or useless concept; but for the decision-maker consideration of the question 'what is need?' becomes unavoidable.

References

1   British Association of Social Workers, 'Care Costs', *Social Work Today*, 29 May 1975, pp. 153–4.
2   H. Glennerster, 'The Year of the Cuts' in K. Jones, M. Brown and S. Baldwin (eds), *The Year Book of Social Policy in Britain 1976*, Routledge & Kegan Paul, 1977, pp. 14–15.
3   R. Klein *et al.*, *Social Policy and Public Expenditure, 1974*, Centre for Studies in Social Policy, 1974, p. 81.
4   G. Orwell, *The Road to Wigan Pier*, Penguin edn, 1970, pp. 85–6.
5   D. Harvey, *Social Justice and the City*, Edward Arnold, 1973, p. 102.
6   K. Slack, *Social Administration and the Citizen*, Michael Joseph, 1966, p. 93.
7   V. George and P. Wilding, *Ideology and Social Welfare*, Routledge & Kegan Paul, 1976, pp. 133–5.
8   A. Culyer, *Need and the National Health Service*, Martin Robertson, 1976, pp. 88–93. The issue is further considered in Chapter 3.
9   J. Jewkes and S. Jewkes in D. Lees, *Monopoly or Choice in Health Services*, Occasional Paper 3, Institute of Economic Affairs, 1964, p. 36.
10 D. Reid, *Social Class Differences in Britain*, Open Books, 1977, p. 123.
11 On the operation of waiting lists and the relationship to waiting for appointment see G. Forsyth and R. Logan, *Gateway or Dividing Line*, Oxford University Press, 1968.
12 D. Nevitt, 'Demand and Need', in H. Heisler (ed.), *Foundations of Social Administration*, Macmillan, 1977, pp. 125–6.
13 A. Williams in A. Culyer (ed.), *Economic Policies and Social Goals: Aspects of Public Choice*, Martin Robertson, 1974.
14 Culyer, op. cit., p. 44.
15 Culyer, op. cit., p. 104.
16 It is worth noting that commentators such as Ivan Illich argue that professional groups help perpetuate the situation that they are supposed to alleviate — hence he refers to 'the disabling professions'.
17 D. J. Smith, *Racial Disadvantage in Britain: The PEP Report*, Penguin, 1977, p. 276.
18 R. Pahl, *Whose City?* Longmans, 1970, p. 215.
19 B. Jordan, *Poor Parents*, Routledge & Kegan Paul, 1974.
20 A. S. Hall, *The Point of Entry*, Allen & Unwin, 1974.
21 D. Guthrie, 'Who are the disabled?', *The Times*, 23 February 1970.

22 B. Davies, *Social Needs and Resources in Local Services*, Michael Joseph, 1968.
23 A. Bottoms *et al., The Urban Criminal*, Tavistock, 1976, pp. 37-8.
24 A. H. Halsey (ed.), *Educational Priority Areas*, vol. 1, HMSO, 1972.
25 J. Bradshaw, 'A Taxonomy of Social Need', in G. McLachlan (ed.), *Problems and Progress in Medical Care, Seventh Series*, Oxford University Press, 1972, pp. 69-82.
26 Bradshaw, op. cit., p. 74.
27 N. Bosanquet, *New Deal for the Elderly*, Fabian Tract 435, 1975.
28 Central Policy Review Staff, *Population and the Social Services*, HMSO, 1977.
29 *Public Expenditure to 1979-80*, Cmnd 6393, HMSO, 1976, p.1.
30 H. Glennerster, 'In praise of public expenditure', *New Statesman*, 27 February 1976, p. 252.
31 J. K. Galbraith, *The Affluent Society*, Penguin, 1972.
32 Labour Party, *Signposts for the Sixties*, 1961.
33 B. Abel-Smith, *Labour's Social Plans*, Fabian Tract 369, 1966.
34 *Public Expenditure 1968/69-1973/74*, Cmnd 4234, HMSO, 1969.
35 Op. cit., p. 55.
36 *Public Expenditure 1969/70-1974/75*, Cmnd 4578, HMSO, 1971.
37 *Public Expenditure to 1975/76*, Cmnd 4829, HMSO, 1971.
38 R. G. Smethurst, 'Welfare Economics and the Economics of Welfare' in *New Thinking About Welfare*, Association of Social Workers, 1969.
39 T. P Hill, 'Too much consumption', *National Westminster Bank Review*, February 1969.
40 Hansard, vol. 938, cols 127, 128.
41 C. V. Brown and D. A. Dawson, *Personal Taxation Incentives and Tax Reforms*, PEP Broadsheet 506, 1969.
42 R. Crossman, *Paying for the Social Services*, Fabian Tract 399, 1969.
43 In 1963 the rates provided 31.0 per cent of local authority income, by 1974 this had fallen to 22.6 per cent. Source: *Social Trends No. 6*, 1975, p. 199, Table 13.5.
44 The Layfield Report, *Local Government Finance: Report of the Committee of Inquiry*, Cmnd 6453, HMSO, 1976.
45 Green Paper on Local Government Finance, Cmnd 6813, HMSO, 1977.
46 Klein, op. cit., p. 17.

Universality and Selectivity

A universal social service is, in the strict sense of the term, one to which all citizens contribute equally, and from which all are entitled to draw equal benefits. A selective social service is one which is paid for out of public funds, and available only to certain applicants on externally imposed conditions.

In fact, there are no totally universal social services in Britain. We contribute unequally through rates, taxes and wage-related social insurance contributions. Dependent groups in the population may be said to make their contributions over time (children will contribute in the future, the retired and the unemployed have mostly contributed in the past) but the value of the contributions will vary with income, and with the period in which those same contributions were made. There are very few services which we all receive equally, though one can find examples in the public health field. The control of epidemics, refuse collection, and measures against air pollution and food contamination may be said to provide equality of benefit, because we are all equally capable of contracting cholera and typhus, we all breathe, and we could all suffer from food poisoning; but other social services are only provided, or only provided free, on some test of need.

For example, Family Allowances, which have often been quoted as a 'universalist' benefit, are only paid to families with dependent children. Consultation with a general practitioner is free, but prescriptions must be paid for except by families with low incomes, children, expectant and nursing mothers, pensioners and people with certain specified chronic conditions, such as diabetes and endocrine disorders. Supplementary benefit — now the passport to some other free services — is subject to a means test. Services for special client groups — the old, the blind, handicapped children and so on— are only available to people deemed by some public authority — usually a doctor or a social worker — to fall within the specified group.

There are good grounds, therefore, for Mike Reddin's verdict that 'the debate on universal versus selective benefits cannot be a discussion of absolute or diametrically opposed systems' because what we have in fact are 'selectively financed universal services selectively used'.[1]

So what has the debate been about?

First it has been about *ideology* — about the goals of social policy. On the one hand those disciples of the visionary collectivism which led to the welfare state legislation of 1945-8 who in the Fabian Society and elsewhere continue to advocate an institutional model of social welfare have tended to advocate universalist policies. On the other, the major advocates of the residual model of welfare — Milton Friedman and the Chicago economic school in the USA and the Institute of Economic Affairs in the UK — have been the main advocates of selective social provision.

It is not inevitable that believers in the institutional model of welfare should necessarily have an unqualified commitment to universal services, nor that residualists should necessarily support selectivity, but because at least at the academic level, the discussions have been carried on between these different schools of thought, it has tended to be an ideological debate.

The debate has also become involved with disputes about *the efficacy of the market and consumer choice*. Again it is not inevitable that this should be so. There is no reason why universal services should not be supplied through private agencies and there are many selective services provided by public agencies. But it has been those who believe in the principles of private enterprise and a *laissez-faire* economy who have led the call for more selective services.

The debate has been about the practical realities of *public expenditure* — about what we can afford in the way of social services and about whether the levels of taxation needed to finance public expenditure are or are not destroying the incentives of the working population to earn and save and create wealth. Those proposing selective measures have also tended to believe that we have reached the limits of public expenditure and taxation, and that if we want to help those in need, the money must come from concentrating existing resources through selective measures. Those who have advocated or defended universalist measures have argued that we are not over-taxed, that taxation does not affect incentive, and that there should be further redistribution from private consumption to public provision.

Again this is a description of the way the debate has developed rather than of a principle inherent in it. A generous selective policy may involve as much public expenditure as a limited universal policy.

The debate has also been about *administrative feasibility and effectiveness* - the right of the general public to know about and understand the entitlements; about the difficulties and frustrations of applying for selective benefits; about the discretionary powers of officials, and about the costs of administration. Most of this debate has centred on means-tested benefits and exemptions and non-take-up, and because stigma has been thought to be a reason for non-take-up, stigma became associated with selectivity. Universal services are good, it is argued, because everyone benefits from them. There is no inequality built into the exchange and thus stigma is avoided. On the other hand selective services are based on an unequal exchange relationship — some are givers, others receivers and those receiving are stigmatised.

Stigma is crucial in determining the acceptability of social policies. Not enough is known about how exchange theory does operate in social policy — why some people claim benefits and others do not or even whether people do feel stigma through dependency and how it can be avoided. However universal policies do not necessarily provide status and selectivist policies do not necessarily stigmatise. The selective benefits for the disabled do not appear to be associated with stigma and the universal health service in many instances stigmatises in the way people are treated.

All the arguments about universality and selectivity tend to flow into each other and to be used to reinforce each other. The debate has been carried on at two levels; at one level the ideas of principle have been fought out by supporters of different normative theories. At the other level policy makers are striving to distribute scarce resources to large numbers of people in need. At the first level the debate is an ideological one and at the other level it is about the most effective way of allocating services. The academic debates have tended to lose sight of the realities of power. Whatever the government's ideological perspective, when faced with the context of policy making, the administrative constraints and the scarcity of resources, policy innovations have been selective.

As Richard Titmuss said:[2]

The challenge that faces us is not the choice between universal and selective service. The real challenge resides in the question: what particular infrastructure is needed to provide a framework of values and opportunity bases within and around which can be developed socially acceptable selective services able to discriminate positively with the mimimum risk of stigma in favour of those whose needs are greatest.

In order to evaluate the components of the universalist and selective argument, it is useful to know something of their historical development since the early post-war period.

The Labour government, 1945-51

Hugh Dalton called this period 'The Five Shining Years', and wrote in his memoirs: 'There was exhilaration among us, joy and hope, determination and confidence. We felt exalted, dedicated, walking on air, walking with destiny.'[3] Such hyperbole was not unusual among the members of the new Labour administration. Perhaps it derived partly from the crude propaganda and polemic of war-time — the closing paragraphs of the Beveridge Report[4] with their resounding appeal to the British people to fight for the 'twin victories' — against Nazi Germany and against social injustice — seem somewhat overwritten today; but the social injustice of the 1930s was real enough, and the overwhelming Labour victory at the polls was seen as the beginning of a new era.

Such a mood of exaltation lends itself to sweeping statements, and to a certain impatience with administrative detail. The Beveridge Plan of 1942 had been hailed by the Left with the slogan 'social security from the cradle to the grave', and this was partly Lord Beveridge's doing, for the principles of his plan included, *inter alia*, comprehensive social insurance coverage, flat-rate contributions and flat-rate benefits, which sounded like pure universalism; but in fact the details of the scheme were not universalistic. It was not financially watertight — there was provision for Exchequer contributions, which meant that some people would in fact be contributing more than others through rates and taxes, in spite of the flat-rate insurance contributions. Though the scheme ironed out many anomalies in the payment of benefit, such as the differential rates of benefit for the unemployed, the sick and the retired, it was not fully comprehensive. It did not give full coverage to housewives, single parents other than widows, the civilian disabled, the self-employed, or to those without contribution rights. The proposal for a National Assistance scheme for those who 'fell through the net' of insurance testified to the fact that the net had holes in it.

Nevertheless, Lord Beveridge's scheme was widely spoken of as universalist, and the principles rather than the details caught the public imagination. The same was true of the National Health Service — Aneurin Bevan wrote of a Health Service which could give all citizens access to 'the best that medical skill can provide' with apparently little understanding of the problems of scarce resources, maldistribution, and spiralling demand. The idea that health care, like roads and tap water, should be provided to all who cared to use it, was to prove a considerable over-simplification.[5]

The exaltation clearly could not last; for the five years of intensive legislative activity which put the outlines of a modern welfare state on the Statute Book were also years of readjustment to peace-time conditions — of demobilisation, of dislocation in industry, of rationing, of black market activities. Money was scarce, for though we had a framework of administrative machinery for the welfare of the people, we only slowly began to understand the problems of running it.

The right-wing back-lash

When Winston Churchill first read the draft of the Beveridge Report in 1942, he sent a sharp note to the Cabinet (which then included members of the Labour Party) warning them about 'false hopes and visions of Utopia and Eldorado'.[6] He resigned immediately on the announcement of the election results in 1945, saying that the verdict of the electorate was so clear that he did not wish 'even for an hour to be responsible for their affairs'. This bitterness was carried through into party politics. Conservatives tended to treat the Labour government, the first with a clear majority in the House of Commons, as an aberration from which the British people would eventually recover.

The attack on the welfare state came from several directions: from the British Medical Association, which fought Aneurin Bevan in the creation of the Health Service; from jeers in the right-wing press about patients who 'queued for wigs and aspirins'; from the publications of the Bow Group and the Institute of Economic Affairs. As early as February 1952, *The Times* published two articles on 'Crisis in the Welfare State', advocating retrenchment on the grounds of economic expediency. Enoch Powell and Iain Macleod, then Conservative back-benchers, produced a pamphlet on 'The Social Services — Needs and Means' which attacked the principle of universality on the grounds that the country could not afford it and was not in fact achieving it.

The focus of the attack concentrated on the national insurance scheme. The Right argued that because insurance benefits were below subsistence level the system had failed and that the solution should be to further encourage the growth of occupational pension schemes. The Left called for a universal earnings related scheme. Means tested benefits were already growing in importance; large numbers of insurance beneficiaries were having to supplement their incomes with means tested assistance, school meals which it had been proposed should be free, were charged for and a prescription charge was introduced.

By 1960, a buoyant economy led to a different kind of attack. T. H. Marshall describes the development of the argument that 'the time had come to give the Austerity Society a decent burial, and to welcome an Affluent Society in its place . . . an Affluent Society should not need to maintain a complicated and expensive apparatus for waging war on poverty.'[7] The grounds of attack shifted from the contention that the welfare state was an impossibility because we could not afford it to the contention that it was out-dated because we did not need it. A Conservative MP wrote in *Crossbow:*[8]

> To apply the Beveridge principle in 1960 is to swallow the drug after the disease is gone. For primary poverty has now almost disappeared. Full employment has lifted the mass of our working population to a level of affluence unprecedented in our social history.

Proposals for diminishing the public sector of the social services and expanding the private sector were widely canvassed by members of the Institute of Economic Affairs.[9] Much of the argument was concentrated on the National Health Service, where Jewkes and Jewkes opened the battle in 1961 with a book[10] in which they argued that a free optimal service of the kind envisaged by Bevan was unrealistic, because health needs were self-expanding. They recommended a scheme of voluntary insurance and private payments backed by a free (minimal?) scheme for those with low incomes. This was followed by a series of articles in which D. S. Lees, the Reader in Economics at the University of Keele, and other writers supported the Jewkes' view against Professor Titmuss and his colleagues at the London School of Economics.[11] The IEA and its supporters argued that freedom of choice was fundamental in a free society, and that this could only be obtained through a free market. Medical care was like any other commodity, and should be bought and sold. Professor Titmuss and his colleagues argued that the market system was inappropriate, and could be demonstrated to have failed in the USA where the sick, the poor and the aged were unable to obtain adequate care through voluntary insurance. They held that a free service was ethically superior. The cash nexus was not an appropriate mechanism for times of personal misfortune, which should be met by collective provision, the well paying for the sick. Richard Titmuss wrote:[12]

Dr. Lees . . . devotes his study to the economics of medical supply and demand. This is what divides us. I do not believe — either as a method of study or as a value judgement — that the economics of medical care can be considered apart from the ethical and social values.

The debate spread to other areas of social policy, such as education and pensions, the IEA widely canvassing the idea that a voucher system should replace free entitlements. In 1968, Mark Blaug supported such a system on the grounds that it would 'stimulate the growth of private schools, private hospitals, private medical insurance, private housing, private pension schemes' and that it might be 'the selective pattern carried to its logical conclusion'.[13] It was the Fabians who suggested to him that it would be 'selectivity gone mad'.

◁ Labour's re-thinking ▷

There were two distinct strands in Labour's reappraisal of the situation. The first was the 'rediscovery of poverty' by the 'high priests of universalism', Professor Titmuss, Professor Abel-Smith and Professor Townsend[14] in 1965. In reply to the Conservative attack, Abel-Smith and Townsend's Occasional Paper in Social Administration, *The Poor and the Poorest,* hammered home the message that poverty had not been conquered, and that there were pockets of acute poverty in a supposedly affluent society. The title of Brian Rodgers' book was changed from 'The Conquest of Poverty' to *The Battle Against Poverty* shortly before publication in the light of these findings.

The Child Poverty Action Group was founded in 1965 to campaign against poverty. It was concerned about adequacy — the adequacy of family allowances and insurance benefits, but it also began to pioneer the welfare rights movement in Britain as means tested benefits became more important and new ones were introduced. Peter Townsend invoked the spirit of 1948, recalling the 'theme of equal rights or social equality', and attributing the waning support for universality within the Labour Party itself to the subordination of social objectives to economic objectives. Labour ministers, he argued, were no longer interested in large-scale planning, but only in piecemeal improvisation. Pressures from the City, from the USA and from the financial centres of Europe had led to the predominance of Treasury thinking over political and social initiative.[15] He had earlier expressed the view that 'subscription to the values of expanding output has sapped the moral values of the Left' — a view which drew a reply from Harold Wilson.[16]

Second, by 1967, the brief period of affluence was over, and the talk was again of retrenchment and expenditure cuts. Britain was forced into devaluation on 18 November, and a fortnight later, a major conference on the social services was initiated by the government at Lancaster House. The First Secretary of State, Michael Stewart, who at that time held responsibility for the social services, started with a statement to the effect that

> The flat rate benefits characteristic of Beveridge's system were no longer entirely suited to present conditions, and had not eradicated poverty from certain groups . . . the task of operating the social services was limitless, but the nation's economic resources were limited . . . in the particular circumstances of the present, the Government had a further special duty to protect the most vulnerable sections of the community from the effects of the devaluation of the pound.

The government message in what was primarily a public relations exercise was that increased selectivity was inevitable, for two reasons: devaluation meant a poorer Britain, with less to spend on the social services; and the dependency ratio was increasing: a rise in the birthrate accompanied by increased longevity meant that more limited resources had to meet greater needs in the care of the young and the old.

The Labour Cabinet was split on the issue of selectivity. A powerful group, led by Ray Gunter and Douglas Houghton[17] argued for selectivity on the grounds of economic necessity. Against them were ranged Richard Crossman, Kenneth Robinson (then Minister for Health), Judith Hart and Peggy Herbison, backed by the Fabians, and arguing on grounds of social justice. The issue came to a head over the question of prescription charges, and in January 1968, the selectivists won. A charge of 2s.6d. per prescribed item was introduced, except for the exempted classes. The saving in the financial year 1968-9 was estimated at £25 million. There seems to have been some hope at the time that Britain's economic problems would be short-term, and that the charges would be no more than a temporary expedient.

The Fabian defence

The debate continued within the Labour Party and was articulated in two collections of Fabian Society papers — *Social Services for All?*[18]

and *Labour and Inequality*.[19] These papers provide an excellent introduction to both the complexities of the issue and the outraged feelings of the universalist Left at the performance of the Labour government in office.

Peter Townsend wrote:

> What is at stake is not just the most technically efficient or cheapest means of reaching an agreed end. It is the kind and quality of society we wish to achieve in Britain.

The debate covered the areas of social insurance and assistance, health, housing, family allowances and education. There was a good deal of discussion about 'what it is we are arguing about', and most of the writers were clearly prepared to accept some degree of selectivity. They did not object to unequal financing — it was agreed that the rich should pay more than the poor. They did not object to selective benefits — provided that the selectivity was by area or by client group and not by the delineation of a separate group of 'the poor'. Brian Abel-Smith, in a thoughtful paper, pointed out that there was in fact a substantial measure of agreement between the universalists and the selectivists. Both sides were agreed that total universality was a mirage:[20]

> For far too long, people on the left as well as on the right have believed that the slogans of the Beveridge era were descriptions of facts. But there never has been 'cradle to the grave' security in Britain. There never has been a 'safety net' beneath which none can fall.

Both sides were agreed that there was still poverty in Britain, and that it ought to be reduced if not abolished. The main source of argument was that the 'extremist Institute of Economic Affairs selectivists' wrote as though universal services were the rule, and selective services the exception, whereas in fact the reverse was the case. Poor families were 'already caged in a veritable labyrinth of means tests' which involved problems of how, when and where to apply, required the repeated filling in of obscurely worded forms with different formulations and different standards, and led to the maximum disclosure of the applicant's private affairs in return for the minimum disclosure by officialdom of his entitlements.

Mike Reddin, in a paper on Local Authority Means Tested Benefits, notes that 'the middle class versions of the means test, such as that for university grants, tend to be more civilised and socially acceptable devices' but that among the lower income groups, a study of means testing involved a 'voyage into the underworld'. He added up schemes for means tests administered by local authorities for rate and rent rebates, home help, day nurseries, children in care, educational maintenance, uniform grants, school meals, welfare foods for expectant and nursing mothers, contraceptive appliances (now free — perhaps Sir Keith Joseph's one gesture to universality), residential accommodation for the aged and infirm, and a variety of lesser-known benefits, and found that there were in all at least 3,000 means tests in operation, of which 1,500 were unique — i.e. they were specific to one particular authority which set its own conditions.

He pointed out that each of these involved verification of income for every applicant (this is particularly difficult for lower income families, whose income often varies from week to week). It also involved assessment by a relevant official; reassessment at stated intervals; the periodic revision of scales to meet changing circumstances; and the cost of publicity to claimants to inform them of changes in entitlement.

The tangle of means-testing created illogicalities, and hence injustice. A family might be refused a grant in one local authority when it would be entitled to one a few miles away, because of varying conditions and standards. There was a lack of relationship between means tests, even in the same authority — 'virtually all of these means tests "ignore each other".' There was no understanding of or concern for the cumulative effects on the recipient. He concludes 'each means test is, in the final analysis, a secondary tax system'.[21]

Positive discrimination and territorial justice

The position of the Fabian Left was further complicated by new ideas which were beginning to point to the need for the selective treatment of areas in special need. In 1967, the Report of the Plowden Committee made a powerful plea for positive discrimination for primary schools in decaying city areas,[22] and this led to the setting up of special action research schemes in what became known as Educational Priority Areas. The positive discrimination philosophy was futher expressed in the development of broader schemes for Community Development Projects and Urban Aid Programmes, which were to develop their own momentum in the 1970s.

Meanwhile, Bleddyn Davies published in 1968 his massive *Social Needs and Resources in Local Services,* which argued for 'territorial justice' between local authorities. The complexity of his systems of measurement and evaluation, and the comparative crudity of some of his basic assumptions (perhaps inevitable in a novel methodology), did not obscure the basic message: local authorities differed radically in terms of the resources they had at their command, the ways in which they were allocated, and the quality of service they provided. For the citizen in need, this often meant territorial injustice, since provision depended on where he lived rather than on what his needs were. Professor Pinker comments:[23]

> The difference between these two approaches is less than at first seems to be the case. Plowden's key point was that all local authorities — even the richest ones — should adopt positive discrimination programmes favouring their most deprived schools. Ideally, such programmes would involve other services, such as housing, social work and welfare provision. Those local authorities with the largest proportion of deprived schools would receive priority aid from central government. Plowden's concern was focused on the distribution of resources within local authorities, while Davies seems to concentrate on the overall distribution of services between local authorities.

> The argument on the Left moved from an ideological one to a technical one. Selectivity was acceptable to much of the Left if it did not involve a means test. Selective policies could be more egalitarian than universal, for to offer equal benefits to persons in unequal situations is not to offer equality but merely to underwrite existing inequality.

Selectivity and the Conservatives 1970-4

While Labour in office had adopted means tested benefits unwillingly (prescription charges) or as a temporary expedient (rate rebates) the Tories adopted selective benefits with a new ideological fervour. They came to power determined to cut taxation by 'cutting out unnecessary state spending'[24] and to 'confine the scope of free or subsidised provision more closely to what is necessary on social grounds'.[25] Charges for school meals were raised, free milk abolished for children over seven. A new means-tested benefit, the Family Income Supplement, was introduced for the low paid. Subsequently rents were raised and a new rent rebate scheme introduced. Rate rebates were also upgraded. The Tories also made valiant attempts to make selectivity work with massive publicity campaigns advertising benefits 'as of right'.

In other areas of policy they also made selective changes in social policy. The Crossman universal earning-related pension scheme was dropped in favour of a universal flat-rate scheme topped off with selective state or private provision. The government also introduced a number of new non-means tested selective benefits for the civilian disabled. The Attendance Allowance was a great success and was soon being claimed by more than those who it had initially been thought would be eligible. As well as the Attendance Allowance the Conservatives also established the Family Fund for severely disabled children and gave the responsibility for the Fund to a charitable trust.[26] This highly selective provision for the disabled has since been developed and extended by the Labour government in benefits such as the Invalid Car Allowance, the Mobility Allowance and the Non-contributory Invalidity Benefit. The policy is not without its critics: both the Disablement Income Group and the Disability Alliance[27] have called for a universal disability income to replace the growing hotch potch of benefits but it appears that the test of disability described by one writer as a 'physiological and psychological means test'[28] is more acceptable to claimants than an incomes test.

By 1972 the Conservatives had changed direction as the evidence of the failure of their means-tested strategy was produced.[29] The take-up of means-tested benefits was still universally low despite attempts to improve publicity,[30] they were cumbersome and expensive to administer, and efforts to streamline the multiplicity of benefits by 'passporting' eligibility from supplementary benefits or the family income supplement only had the effect of increasing the numbers of families subject to the 'Poverty Trap', the range of income where a loss of benefits and payments of tax would be in excess of an increase in income.[31] Means testing was unpopular, ineffective and creating a wide band of earnings over which there was no incentive at all, and when the Conservative government produced its proposals for a Tax Credit Scheme one of its principal aims was to reduce reliance on means tested benefits. The Tax Credit proposals were evidence that the Conservative adherence to means tests was diminished — it was a comprehensive and integrating measure, and if not in the strict sense universal, everyone was to receive the same credits. Like all universal schemes it was very expensive, calling for £1,300 million extra in public expenditure.

The present position

The incoming Labour government in 1974 was committed to reduce reliance on means tests. They turned their backs on the tax credit proposals because they could obtain better value for money by uprating existing patterns of benefits. But faced with record inflation, a crippling public sector borrowing requirement and the International Monetary Fund making a condition of a loan that Britain should reduce its public expenditure, what innovations they made have tended to be selectivist. There has been no diminution in the numbers of dependent on means-tested benefits. The principal universal benefit and the core of the government's policy — child benefit — was only saved by Cabinet indiscretion and a rearguard action within the Labour Party, and has been introduced at a level which improves the financial position of only a restricted number of families. With rising unemployment the numbers receiving supplementary benefit and other means-tested benefits have greatly increased.

In other areas of policy there have been small gains for the universalists: comprehensive schools were extended by central government mandate despite the setback of the Thameside judgment of July 1976 (a notable victory for selectivists and for the local authorities); pay beds are to be phased out and the National Health Service hospital services will become universal for the first time; a basically universal pension scheme has at last reached the statute book and will begin to operate from 1978.

Conclusions

Neither Conservative nor Labour governments are now prepared to advocate means-tested selectivity in the provision of social services. Conservative administrations still believe that poverty and problems of distribution are residual problems but their solutions are not those advocated by the Institute of Economic Affairs. They are prepared to maintain the basic universal structure, but innovations will be selective. Labour administrations, confused by economic pressures and the strong arguments for positive discrimination, make progress by selective incrementalism.

To a great extent the future of social benefits will depend on the spin of the economic coin. A prosperous Britain under a Labour administration might travel further along the road to universalism. But they would always be inhibited by the economic and electoral consequences of increasing public expenditure and taxation. An economically stagnant Britain with a Conservative administration might move to the Right, embracing the philosophy of the IEA, and dismantle what is left of the welfare state in the interests of consumer sovereignty.

Professor Pinker takes the view that the debate is dead — or as nearly dead as makes no difference:[32]

> In the context of democratic policies, the related concepts of relativism and proportionate justice act as a kind of catalyst, inexorably transforming universalists. Universalism and selectivism may therefore be seen to be alive in principle but dead in practice . . . the conflict that breaks out from time to time is largely a battle between ideological ghosts, but the echoes of their gunfire serve as necessary reminders to policy makers that issues of principle are involved. In different metaphorical terms, the ideological skeletons may hang in separate cupboards, but the same political wind rattles both sets of bones.

In pragmatic terms, he may well be right; but the 'ideological ghosts' may still fire real political bullets.

References

1   M. Reddin, 'Universality versus Selectivity', in W. A. Robson and B. Crick (eds), *The Future of the Social Services,* Penguin, 1970, p. 25.
2   R. Titmuss, *Commitment to Welfare,* Allen & Unwin, 1968, p. 135.
3   H. Dalton, *High Tide and After,* quoted by Pauline Gregg, *The Welfare State,* Harrap, 1967, pp. 1 and 36.
4   *Social Insurance and Allied Services,* Cmnd 6404, HMSO November 1942.
5   A. Bevan, *In Place of Fear,* Heinemann, 1952, p. 100.
6   W. Churchill, *The Second World War,* vol IV, Cassell, 1950, appendix F. p. 861.
7   T. H. Marshall, *Social Policy,* Hutchinson, 1965, 2nd edn 1962, p. 94.
8   Article from *Crossbow,* Autumn 1960, quoted by Marshall, op. cit., p. 93.
9   E. g. A. Seldon and H. Gray, *Taxation and Welfare,* Institute of Economic Affairs, 1967; A. Seldon, *Universal or Selective Social Benefits,* IEA, 1967, A. Seldon, *After the National Health Service,* IEA, 1968.
10 J. Jewkes and S. Jewkes, *The Genesis of the National Health Service,* Oxford University Press, 1961.
11 *Monopoly or Choice in the Health Service,* Hobart Paper, IEA, 1961.
12 R. M. Titmuss, 'The ethics and economics of medical care' in *Medical Care,* vol. 1, no. 1, 1963 (reprinted as chapter XXI of *Commitment to Welfare,* op. cit.).
13 *Social Services for All?,* Fabian Society, 1968, p. 39.

14 *Social Services for All?,* p. 30.
15 *Social Services for All?,* chapter 1, passim.
16 P. Townsend, *Sociology and Social Policy,* Allen Lane, 1975, p. 256 (reprinted from the *New Statesman,* 26 September 1959).
17 *Social Services for All?,* p. 1.
18 Ibid.
19 *Labour and Inequality,* Fabian Society, 1972.
20 *Social Services for All?,* p. 112.
21 *Social Services for All?,* p. 104.
22 Central Advisory Council for Education, *Children and their Primary Schools,* HMSO, 1967.
23 R. A. Pinker, *Social Theory and Social Policy,* Heinemann, 1971, p. 194.
24 The Conservative programme for the next five years: *A Better Tomorrow,* 1970.
25 Hansard 1970/1, vol. 806, col. 217.
26 L. Waddilove, 'The Family Fund', in K. Jones (ed.), *The Year Book of Social Policy in Britain 1973,* Routledge & Kegan Paul, 1974.
27 *Poverty and Disability,* Disability Alliance, 1975.
28 Helen Bolderson, 'Compensation for disability', *Journal of Social Policy,* 3, pp. 193–211.
29 Ruth Lister, *Take-up of Means Tested Benefits,* CPAG, 1974.
30 Peter Townsend, 'The Scope and Limitations of Means Tested Social Services in Britain', Manchester Statistical Society, 1972. Reported in *Sociology and Social Policy,* 1975.
31 D. Piachaud, 'Poverty and taxation', *Political Quarterly,* January–March 1971, pp. 31–44. J. Bradshaw and I. Wakeman, 'The poverty trap updated', *Political Quarterly,* October–December 1972.
32 Pinker, op. cit., p. 108.

Chapter four

Professionalisation

When the reorganisation of the health and social services took place in the early 1970s one of its notable features was the anxiety displayed by different occupational groups about the question of professional status. Social workers, liberated from their previous narrow occupational groupings by the formation of the British Association of Social Workers (BASW) and from functionally restricted tasks by the wide scope of the new social services departments, might be forgiven for feeling that they were no longer professionally *arriviste*: they had arrived. Probation officers discussed at stormy meetings whether they were primarily social workers or servants of the courts. In the end, they did not join BASW as a group, though many joined as individuals; and they stayed outside the social services departments, though their colleagues in Scotland were already part of the comparable social work departments.[1] Community workers debated long and earnestly whether they represented a separate profession, a profession which was part of social work, or whether they were ideologically opposed to professionalism anyway.[2] The Central Council for Education and Training in Social Work, formed in 1971, spread its wings to cover residential staff (in a document flatly entitled *Residential Work is Part of Social Work*[3]), day care staff[4] and those working with the handicapped.[5] The medical profession fought a losing battle for the control of social services departments, saw the demise of the Medical Officer of Health in the National Health Service Reorganisation Act of 1973, and turned round to face within the Health Service the competing claims of nurses and administrators for managerial roles.[6]

The issues concerned in these and other debates of the period were about several things: responsibility, competence, expertise, pay, status. They owed something to the heightened trade union activity of the time — more, perhaps, to the fact that the prospect of reorganisation created a temporary vacuum in which long-standing assumptions could be queried, and new claims asserted.

As Smith and Levinson note, 'There is always an unstable margin of competition for specific functions between occupational groups',[7] and reorganisation brought this to the surface. Out of reorganisation were to come new working relationships, new power structures, and new alignments. It was not surprising that the terms 'profession' and 'professional' were employed as touchstones of power and prestige.

What is a profession?

In popular speech, a profession is an occupation which requires a higher educational qualification — a degree, diploma or certificate. (At one time the converse was also true — a degree, diploma or certificate was expected to lead to professional status; but this assumption has been somewhat eroded by the problems of graduate unemployment.) Sometimes it is thought of as an occupation involving a degree of ethical responsibility — the medical and legal professions have concepts of 'unprofessional conduct' which can lead to members being struck off the register or disbarred. Clergymen may be unfrocked, officers in the armed forces cashiered. The comment 'that's a professional job' means that the job has been done well, and 'amateurish' usually means that it is less than professionally expert; yet in the sporting context, an amateur plays for the love of the game, and a professional gets paid for it. It is not many years since the world of cricket abandoned the distinction between 'Gentlemen' and 'Players'; and it is notable that some experienced voluntary workers in the social services, perhaps in reaction against the over-professionalism of the professionals, have begun to invoke a similar distinction.

The longer established professions had a recognisable uniform — the doctor's white coat and stethoscope, the lawyer's wig, the parson's collar, the academic's cap and gown; and though these are now being abandoned for all but ritual situations by a generation which does not care for uniforms, they may have played their part in creating an aura of expertise and a recognisable public image. Even today, individual professions tend to create their own conventions about dress — it would be difficult, for example, to mistake a gathering of health service administrators for community workers.

The considerable literature which has grown up on the professions reflects both the ambiguities and the stereotypes. Cogan[8] in an attempt to categorise the concept of a profession, distinguishes three main approaches to definition: *persuasive definition,* used to argue the case for or against the inclusion of a specified occupation in the ranks of the professions; *operational definition*, used when looking at the organisation or practice of a particular occupational group or groups; and *logistic definition,* which draws verbal boundaries round historical material and customary usage.

Such definitions will not necessarily include common elements, but many writers have concerned themselves with the construction of lists of what are thought to be the essential elements in a profession. Millerson, in a survey of twenty-one such writers,[9] points out that they list twenty-three different elements between them. No one item appears on all lists, and nine items receive only one mention. Among the most frequently mentioned traits are:

  (i) skill based on theoretical knowledge;
  (ii) the provision of training and occupation;
  (iii) tests of the competence of members;
  (iv) organisation;
  (v) adherence to a professional code of conduct;
  (vi) altruistic service.

The problem with this list is that it does not only apply to the recognised professions. Edwin Sutherland points out that it could equally well apply to professional burglars.[10]

> The one characteristic . . . which they lack is the ethical standards which minimise the pecuniary motive. When this point was mentioned to a professional thief, he admitted that his profession did not have this characteristic, but he added that the medical and legal professions would have very few members if that were used as a criterion of membership.

While a small number of occupations have traditionally been regarded as professions, and this recognition has carried some public trust and esteem, many other occupations have started to professionalise rapidly in the last twenty of thirty years under the impact of developing knowledge and technology. There is no longer (if there ever was) a sharp dividing line between professions and non-professions. Sociologists have therefore tended to concentrate on the process of professionalisation and on professionalism rather than on the question of whether a given occupation is or is not a profession.

'Professionalisation' applied to individuals and groups

'Professionalisation' may be viewed as the socialisation process by which individuals are drawn into the institutional context of particular occupations — what does it mean to become a doctor, a nurse, a monk or a policeman? How are knowledge and expectations about behaviour conveyed and internalised? Is the same sort of process at work in the preparation for practice of a social worker – or a banker – or a bus conductor, and if not, why not? Why do some occupations demand more in the way of personal commitment and/or social conformity than others – and where can the boundaries legitimately be drawn between 'education' (which ought to be liberating) and 'training' (which is necessarily restrictive)? Such arguments lay behind the rather cumbersome title of the Central Council for Education and Training in Social Work – the original Local Authority Social Services Bill mentioned only 'training', and 'education' was inserted during its passage through parliament at the insistence of a group of social administration and social work teachers.

But the concept of professionalisation can also be applied to whole occupational groups, and to their competing aspirations for status. Each successful claim necessarily diminishes the sphere of action of an existing group: thus medical practitioners may feel the scope of their work narrowed by the development of social work, and the growth in the management role of nurses and health service administrators; the clergy find some of their traditional pastoral work taken over by social workers, community workers and psychiatrists; solicitors view with some distrust the extension of executor's work and trust work by the banks; judges and barristers may be heard to speak with less than favour about administrative tribunals, which take work away from the courts.

Again, sociologists have tried to formulate lists of the elements in the process of professionalisation in particular occupations. Wilensky,[11] for example, proposes the following steps:

   (i) full-time activity at the task;
   (ii) the establishment of university training;
   (iii) the formation of a national professional organisation;
   (iv) redefinition of the core task, so as to give the 'dirty work' to subordinates;
   (v) conflict between the old timers and the new men who seek to upgrade the job;
   (vi) competition between the new occupation and related ones;
   (vii) political pressure to gain legal protection;
   (viii) a code of ethics.

We can test this list out against the historical facts of the development of medicine, nursing and social work in England.

The medical profession had centuries of 'full-time activity at the task' before it was recognised in the Medical Qualifications Act of 1858. Its relation to university training has gone through two contradictory phases. In the late eighteenth century, it was still possible for a Master of Arts of the Universities of Oxford or Cambridge to become a Doctor of Medicine by expounding a work of Galen in three written or six spoken lectures[12] without ever attending a patient. The great revolution of the period lay in getting the medical men out of the universities and on to the hospital wards. Today, in a very different educational context, this movement has gone into reverse. The Todd Report of 1968 stated:[13]

> Until the rise of scientific medicine, the apprenticeship system was on the whole an adequate basis for medical education. Medical knowledge was limited in extent, and general in nature; after a few years of apprenticeship, a young man could reasonably set himself up as an independent practitioner, capable of treating, within the limits of current medical knowledge, most patients who might come his way. . . . The assumption may well have been valid in the mid-nineteenth century, but advances in medical knowledge as well as the growth of specialisation were soon to make it quite unrealistic. Yet it remained to dominate medical education for nearly a hundred years. . . . We are convinced that undergraduate medical education should be firmly in the hand of a university.

The national professional organisation, the British Medical Association, was formed in three stages. Rosemary Stevens recounts the story[14] of how the Provincial Medical Association was set up in 1832 and how, in reaction against the dominance of London in the medical world, London members were not invited to join it until 1853. It took its present title in 1856. Nursing developed soon after to do the 'dirty work'. Brian Abel-Smith makes it clear[15] that the original status of nurses was not much above the domestic level, and that Miss Nightingale sought 'mature and respectable women used to hard work' rather than the ladies who 'rushed in to take brief and privileged courses of instruction as a prelude to appointment in their mid-20s to the key positions of the nursing world'.

The conflict between the old men and the new was less a matter of upgrading the profession as a whole than of including, with some reluctance, members of the Society of Apothecaries, 'relentlessly rising in status' to join the more prestigious members of the Royal Colleges of Surgeons and Physicians.[16] There was evidence of competition with other occupational groups — the long battle with the sanitary engineers ended with the dismissal of the members of the General Board of Health, including Edwin Chadwick and Lord Shaftesbury, in 1854. The Medical Act of 1858 set up Qualifications council, now the General Medical Council, with responsibility for accrediting medical courses, setting standards, and keeping a professional register.

Nurses had some sort of training and organisation from the time of the Crimean War, but it was not until 1919 that the College of Nursing Ltd (later the Royal College of Nursing) was set up.[17] Three years later, the Nurses' Registration Act set up a statutory body, now the General Nursing Council, on the model of the GMC, but under medical supervision. There was an embarrassing problem of what to do about 'existing nurses' — women who were experienced but unqualified — and the process of deciding in individual cases whether they could join the register or not took so long that the Minister of Health declared that 'many of the nurses would be dead and buried before they got on the register'.[18]

The 1919 Act gave the nurses a recognised legal position, and the task of shedding the 'dirty work' does not seem to have been long delayed. By the 1930s, many hospitals were appointing orderlies to do domestic work.[19] The code of ethics had existed — and been transmitted — since the days of Miss Nightingale. It is only in recent years that degrees in nursing have developed within the universities.[20]

Social work has a much more recent history. It developed as a separate occupation under the aegis of the Charity Organisation Society, founded in 1869, and training in association with the universities was started in the 1890s. BASW was not founded until 1970. The 're-definition of the core task' was undertaken by the Younghusband Report of 1959 which also introduced a lower grade of worker called a welfare assistant to carry out routine tasks.[21] The conflict between the 'old-timers' and 'new men' is only just beginning, but in a rapidly expanding service, many senior posts went to workers considerably less well trained than those who now work under them at field level. The National Institute for Social Work has run a series of senior courses to redress the balance. Political pressure built up through the 1960s to the Local Authority Social Services Act of 1970, which set up CCETSW to accredit courses, set standards and keep a register. Like nurses, social workers tend to have highly internalised values, but BASW has for some time been debating a code of ethics.

It seems clear that the steps in Wilensky's list are not progressive — several of them may occur concurrently, and they may occur in almost any order, but the formulation generally fits the facts. By these criteria, social work has arrived at the status of a profession.

'Semi-professions'

A more complex and interesting sociological approach is to view the acknowledged and established professions as representing one end of a continuum, and routine tasks which are generally acknowledged to be non-professional in character as the other. This approach is more useful than the simple dichotomy between professions and non-professions, because it allows for graduations of professionalism, and changes over time. In Elliott's formulation, it involves nine separate continua, and an occupation might be located at a different point on each of them:[22]

Non-professional		*Professional*
Technical, craft skill	Knowledge ←——————→	Broad, theoretical knowledge used in ↓
Routine	Tasks ←——————→	Non-routine situations to reach ↓
Programmed	Decision-making ←——————→	Unprogrammed decisions according to ↓
Ends decided by society (or other institution)	Authority ←——————→	Ends (derived from knowledge) decided for society (or institution within it) and supported by ↓
Other or non-work	Identity ←——————→	Occupational group because work and occupation are ↓
Means to non-work ends	Work ←——————→	Central life interest and are also the basis for ↓
Occupational/ class advancement	Career ←——————→	Individual achievement which involves meeting initial entry qualifications through ↓
Limited	Education ←——————→	Extensive education, showing skill and meeting other latent status requirements involved in the ↓
Specific	Role ←——————→	Total role (that is expectations extend beyond expertise and work situation)

This kind of analysis makes it possible to develop the notion of 'semi-professions' — occupations whose members make a claim to comparable status with the traditional professions, but whose 'training is shorter, their status less legitimated, their right to privileged communication less established, there is less of a specialised body of knowledge, and they have less autonomy from supervision or societal control.'[23] The semi-professions are usually to be found employed in organisations rather than themselves acting as employers or being self-employed (the 'self-employed' status of lawyers and most medical men has played a considerable part in their acquisition and maintenance of status, and considerable anxiety was expressed by the medical profession in 1948 lest the National Health Service should reduce them, as they saw it, to the level of salaried civil servants.[24]

In addition, many of the semi-professions are occupations where a large part of the labour force has traditionally been female and middle-class. Studies of social work[25] and nursing[26] suggest that male entrants and entrants with working-class backgrounds may press harder for status. Rosen and Jones write of male nurses, in contrast to female nurses:

> The man who comes into nursing usually comes in later, and with some reluctance. It is not part of his adolescent image of himself, but a mature decision made after considerable employment experience. His family probably had no contact with hospital work, and did not suggest it to him; his secondary modern school probably considered it a career for girls. After some years as an unskilled worker without qualifications, he saw nursing as a means of obtaining the education he missed, the qualifications he needed, and a job which he felt was worthwhile in human terms. Once in his profession, his enthusiasm is no less great, his devotion no less marked.

From 'status professionalism' to 'occupational professionalism'

'Status professionalism', in Elliott's analysis, relates to the days when the younger sons of the nobility and the gentry became doctors, lawyers or clergymen (or possibly officers in the navy or the more prestigious army regiments), continuing the way of life in which they had been brought up, often with relatively little impact on the organisation of work or contribution in the way of community services. 'Occupational professionalism' relates to a more modern concept of specialisation of knowledge and tasks, and is directly linked to the increasing division of labour in society brought about by industrialisation.

Discussion about these issues has been pursued on a variety of levels. At one end of the spectrum, there is a remarkable piece of evidence submitted to a Royal Commission by the Royal College of Surgeons[27] as late as 1958:

> There has always been a nucleus in medical schools of students from cultured homes . . . this nucleus has been responsible for the continued high prestige of the profession as a whole, and for the maintenance of medicine as a learned profession. Medicine would lose immeasurably if the proportion of such students in the future were to be reduced in favour of precocious children who qualify for subsidies from the local authority and the state purely on examination results.

Yet apart from such references to a mythical golden age, there are more realistic worries about the increase of 'occupational professionalism'. C. Wright Mills, for example, saw it as an unwelcome increase in technocracy where 'intensive and narrow specialisation has replaced self-cultivation and wide knowledge',[28] and more recently Ivan Illich has contributed his own astringent view of the disadvantages of medical specialisation.[29]

Several commentators have wondered whether the increasingly impermeable boundaries of professional organisation work in the best interests of the public the professionals exist to serve. Herman and Ann Somers have described the multiplication of scientific and technological developments in medicine and the way in which 'the traditional symbol of medical care − the kindly old family doctor with his big heart and little black bag − part healer, part priest and part family counsellor' has been replaced by the highly trained and impersonal specialist. The Somers quote *Time* magazine as complaining that a 'balkanisation' in specialisms has developed − each a separate kingdom staking a separate territorial claim to a part of the human body − asking 'Who's to start working up the "God only knows" diagnosis?'[30]

More recently in Britain, there have been complaints of 'lack of fit' between the organisation of the professions and the needs of clients. One of the key areas for this argument has been that of hospitals for the mentally handicapped − staffed primarily with doctors and nurses, though the needs of the patients are widely acknowledged to be primarily educational and social. Pauline Morris proposed that the situation should be remedied by the introduction of a 'training arm' as powerful and prestigious as the medical and nursing arm.[31] This would be composed of social workers, physiotherapists and other non-medical specialists. She saw that such a development would mean a good deal of intra-professional conflict, but took the orthodox conflict theory view that this could be a preliminary to growth. Jones, Brown *et al.* thought this proposal unrealistic, since the existing staff could not be dismissed, hospitals could not afford to double their treatment costs, and all the 'training' staff were in short supply.[32] They followed the Briggs Committee's recommendation that nursing for the mentally handicapped should evolve into a separate 'caring profession'[33] but foresaw many practical difficulties in developing this from the established procedures of the General Nursing Council on one side and CCETSW on the other. The most hopeful sign in the whole situation, paradoxically, was the fact that large numbers of staff caring for the mentally handicapped both in hospitals and in the community had no training at all, so that at least some schemes could be developed without transgressing professional boundaries.

A key example of the restrictiveness of professionals in hospitals is provided by Eda Topliss, [34] who, writing of a ward experiment in a geriatric hospital, describes how an occupational therapist and a physiotherapist successfully taught simple elements of their own skills to nurses and nursing auxiliaries; but they were aware that they were infringing the professional codes of their own organisations in doing so, and were only able to defy professional norms of conduct — even in the interest of the patients — because they happened to be married women with no particular career aspirations.

The social services tried to get away from 'balkanisation' through the development of generic social work, but there are uneasy signs that there are still 'clients who don't fit' because their needs do not match the organisation of the service, and the service will not or cannot change to meet their needs. The more refined and esoteric the techniques of social work become, the more the contention that there ought to be a residual service for people who are dirty, feckless and unappreciative of these techniques builds up. Some authorities tend to use Family Service Units on contract for just these cases, on the argument that what they really require is 'long-term case-work'.

Phoebe Hall, concluding her study of the development of the personal social services through the late 1960s and early 1970s, comments:[35]

The remarkable degree of solidarity achieved by social workers when lobbying for the Local Authority Social Services Act has been eroded to some degree. Many younger workers seem reluctant to join a professional body which they feel places the interest of the profession far higher than those of the clients they are supposed to be helping.

Autonomy and responsibility

Many people seek professional status because it provides a degree of autonomy and personal discretion in work, the freedom to do a job well for its own sake, and without detailed direction. Elliott suggests that professionalism[36]

> provides a measure of insulation from other role-groups — employer, client, society at large — which can be bought by emphasising knowledge and occupation.

However, there are times when autonomy carries risks, and when another element in the professional situation — professional organisation — is invoked to protect the practitioner and spread the risks. Medical men have a long experience in defending their right to make a clinical judgment in good faith — even though the decision may prove to be wrong. Social workers are only just beginning to realise that they may need similar protection. This has been particularly evident in cases of non-accidental injury to children, where a particular social-worker's handling of a case may be held in question by press and television long before a committee of enquiry finds the answers in poor co-ordination, over-heavy case-loads, and too little training. Some local authority social work teams have closed ranks to protect individuals against this kind of scapegoating, declaring that all decisions on cases are the responsibility of the team; but the instinct of press and television is always to personalise — to find the answer in one person's alleged incompetence. It is notable that when such cases occur (and they will continue to occur as long as social services departments are understaffed and undertrained) social work students who have enthusiastically advocated autonomy and personal discretion at the field level suddenly perceive the advantages of supervision and organisational protection.

Nevertheless, there is considerable concern among social workers, not about professional supervision, but about bureaucratic management. It is remarkable in retrospect how little the discussions about the new social services departments in the Seebohm Report and after took into account the fact that they would be departments within the local authority structure, and therefore subject to all the regulations, the norms and the devices for public accountability which the wider organisation had already developed. Discussion about 'free-standing departments' may have obscured this. Many commentators wrote about them as though they would exist in a vacuum, oblivious of the fact that, during the same period, local authority structure was being streamlined and controls tightening. In the classic Weberian sense, authority in a local or central government department is basically structural, while professional authority is charismatic. A member of a bureaucracy holds his postion because he is placed there to carry out certain defined responsibilities, and is expected to carry them out *sine ira et studio*. A professional holds power by social definition, and his expertise is a blend of innate capacity, acquired knowledge and skills, and willingness to use his own personality as a tool. Many sociologists have followed Etzioni[37] in seeing a potential conflict between the 'enforced and sanctioned values' of the former, and the internalised values of the latter. Loeb and Smith[38] thought that in a hospital setting, there was

> always something of an unstable balance between administrative and professional contingencies, and many conflictful areas are usually present. . . . each may tend to see the other's position as possible only for a fool or a rascal.

However, Kogan and Terry take, at least initially, an optimistic view of the situation:[39]

> The department would expect its professionals to work professionally, according to their professional norms: and indeed it would not go to the trouble and expense to employ professionals if it wanted work done any other way.

In further discussion, they qualify this position considerably: the department will not expect professionals to work outside the law; or outside publicly sanctioned limitations of expenditure; or so as to conflict — at least knowingly or irresponsibly — with the professional norms of other professionals employed by the same department. The tone of the original statement and the qualifications are so much at odds with each other that one is left wondering whether Kogan (a university professor) wrote the first, and Terry (a Director of Social Services) wrote the second. But their conclusion is a sensible one: professionals are not the only people to have norms of working behaviour. The lay administrator may find the norms of the social worker 'too case-oriented, charismatic and lady bountiful, or too revolutionary', and his views may also be legitimately held. The ingenious 'polyarchic' system of Jimmy Algie[40] is an attempt to give organisational expression to the inherent dilemmas of this situation in such a way as to make room for team development, room for growth, and room for the lateral communication on which both depend; but, despite extensive and continuing discussion, we may have to come to terms with the fact that this is one of the questions which is not capable of clear resolution: the tension between different value systems is in-built. It will always be capable of resolution where individuals are prepared to be flexible and to agree on common goals, and will always cause friction where they are not.

Meta-professions?

Paul Halmos, in a well-known study[41] took the view that teachers, social workers, psychiatrists and other workers in the helping professions, despite their differences of academic discipline and professional organisation, in fact belonged to a single profession — that of 'counsellors'. These were people who administered 'help to others through the medium of intimate personal relationship', and he suggested that this delineation was a greater social reality than delineation by professional organisation or original training.

A somewhat similar line of argument was followed by Dr Arie Querido, Medical Officer of Health for Amsterdam, in a speech to the International Federation for Mental Health in 1964, when he argued that all the participants, whether their basic training was in medicine, psychology, social work or education, had in fact become members of a more specialised profession: they were 'mental hygenists' (a phrase which may sound more attractive in Dutch than in English). The thought is an interesting one: now that we have come to recognise that education and training are not only appropriate to the young, that professional boundaries need to change in response to changing social conditions, is the whole concept of a professional grouping as involving a life commitment, possibly from the early twenties, outdated? The concept of *education permanente*, or continuing education, suggests at least the possibility of refining skills and changing direction in mid-career.

Possibly the most common 'meta-profession' is management. The assumption of the 'Grey Book' on Management within the Reorganised National Health Service[42] is that senior doctors, nurses and health service administrators are all 'managers'. This is at once a reconciling mechanism for groups in potential conflict and a recognition that professional status and skill are not fully matured at the time of initial qualification.

Some professionals would contend, with Smith and Levinson,[43] that each profession is built on 'some hard core of inviolate skill and knowledge', but there are at least two difficulties attached to this view. One is that the 'hard core' may be very difficult to define. Social workers find it extremely difficult to answer the question 'What is social work?', and a Ministry of Health committee once sat for two years trying to define the essential core of nursing – only to break up without conclusions or recommendations. If Halmos is right, the core activities of a number of professions may in fact be very similar. The other difficulty is that if the core is defined in terms of the existing professions – medicine, nursing, teaching, social work and the rest – these tend to get left behind as the individual progresses in his career, and it is the 'peripheral' activities – signing forms, reading memoranda, going to committees, addressing public meetings and being responsible for other people's work – which assume a greater importance. The work of a medical houseman, a ward nurse, a classroom teacher and a basic grade social worker has fairly obvious differences. They are not so apparent in the work of a Regional Medical Officer, a Regional Nursing Officer, the head of a large comprehensive school, and a Director of Social Services.

Most senior professionals retain an attachment to their original training. Some – notably doctors and teachers –are often able to keep in practice, so that a consultant still sees patients, and a head teacher or a university professor still teaches students. Social workers and nurses do not have this opportunity, and both professions have been concerned to find some organisational means by which nursing adminstrators may still nurse, and social work administrators may still see clients. One Director of Social Services took advantage of his secretary's absence to answer his own telephone and take his share of intake calls – and was given much food for thought by the variety of human problems which landed on his normally protected desk. The attachment to the original professional training is not merely a matter of sentiment – if a Director of Social Services is to administer the work of social workers, he needs to know what social workers do, not what they did fifteen or twenty years ago. The system by which nurses cease to do bedside nursing almost as soon as they are qualified, becoming 'first-line managers' as ward charge nurses, has frequently been criticised, but so far there is no solution to the problem.

Talking to other professionals

To join a profession is to join a group with its own private vocabulary. The patient who goes to the doctor with a sore throat will be told that he has laryngitis. Lawyers talk about 'speeding a case', which merely means seeing it through the courts without any implications of undue haste, and 'inquisitorial procedures', which are concerned with finding out the truth, not with the use of rack or thumbscrew. The clergy have their own curious vocabulary, mostly of Greek origin (*koinonia, diakonia, agape)* and administrators develop odd bits of jargon ('visiting fireman', 'wearing two hats'). Social workers have tended to use ordinary words with extraordinary emphasis — 'family', 'relationship' — but are now building up their own vocabulary with terms like 'non-directive relationship', 'presenting problems' and 'client self-determination'. Words can also be used to exclude — e.g. it is very probable that anyone claiming to be a social worker and using the words 'welfare' or 'counselling' will not be recognised as such by members of BASW.

Much of this special language is functional in that it provides a more exact description of a phenomenon or process than is possible in ordinary language, or it provides a quick shorthand reference to something rather complicated which would take a long time to explain. Often special terms carry undertones which assume a universe of shared values and assumptions. However, they become dysfunctional when they are used to blind the general public with science (a practice which often provokes adverse reactions); when they are used inaccurately by people whose knowledge of the skill and experience represented by the profession is only partial (witness the mishandling of a sociological vocabulary by some clergy, or the misuse of psychiatric classification by some former mental welfare officers); or when they are used to exclude members of another profession.

'In a certain sense', wrote Smith and Levinson, 'each profession faces members of another profession as laymen.'[44] Doctors, clergy and lawyers all talk of 'laymen' — and include each other in their own particular definitions. One of the less desirable aspects of professionalisation is the tendency for this kind of occupational arrogance to grow and to find linguistic definition.

The health and social services have now reached the stage of development where communication across professional boundaries is of prime importance if the professions are to meet the changing needs of the public. In order to keep public credibility, they must learn again to talk to each other, and perhaps to build up new meta-professions with vocabularies of their own.

Professionals and the public

In the last resort, professional status — with all its opportunities, pitfalls and dangers — is a matter of public recognition, expressed through accepted training procedures and statutory regulation. Dr Ronald Bodley Scott, in a classic paper,[45] suggested that the general public was highly ambivalent about the power and status accorded to professionals. Their superior knowledge and skill was respected; but their claims to professional competence were sometimes treated with scepticism, and their assumedly superior way of life envied. This emotional conflict was dealt with by splitting them into 'good' and 'bad' groups. Thus in the medical profession, the adjectives applied to general practitioners tended to be accepting adjectives — 'competent', 'stolid', 'cheerful' — while the adjectives applied to consultants were rejecting adjectives — 'elegant', 'polished', and even 'sinister'. Dr Bodley Scott suggested that

> It is possible . . . to discern a certain hostility to the specialist. His appearance is too distinguished, his manners are too perfect, and he is too well-groomed. This glittering figure fills his patients with feelings of their own inferiority.

It is not difficult to find similar accepting and rejecting stereotypes for the other health and social services professions; and the story of the universities since the time of the Robbins Report might be seen as one of ambivalence in time — a period of high acceptance and prestige being followed by one of near-rejection. The point is not whether public stereotypes about doctors and nurses, teachers and social workers are soundly based; it is simply that they do exist, and the professionals ought to be aware of the ambivalence which often underlies them. Brian Abel-Smith writes:[46]

> The policies of professional groups are matters which concern the community as a whole. At its very least a profession represents a quasi-monopoly of labour services, and as such the terms of admission to it raise questions of the public interest. When a profession is given powers by statute, Parliament must watch to see that these powers are not used to the harm of other people. Where the major employer of the profession is the state itself, government is inevitably involved in wider questions of policy.

Ultimately, the position, the work opportunities and the identity of the professions are matters of credibility. If they lose that credibility through irresponsibility, inflexibility or lack of response to public need, they are unlikely to survive.

References

1   Under the Social Work (Scotland) Act 1968. The Seebohm Committee's terms of reference excluded probation: see *Report of the Committee on Local Authority and Allied Personal Social Services,* Cmnd 3703, HMSO, 1968, para. 704.

2   Calouste Gulbenkian Foundation, *Community Work and Social Change: a Report on Training,* Longmans, 1968. *Social Work Curriculum Study: the Teaching of Community Work,* CCETSW, 1975 (the Pinker Report).

3   CCETSW, Report of Working Party on Education for Residential Work, Novemeber 1973.

4   CCETSW, *Day Services: an Action Plan for Training,* November 1975.

5   CCETSW, *People with Handicaps Need Better Trained Workers:* report of a Working Party on social work with handicapped people, November 1975.

6   R. G. S. Brown, 'Lessons from the National Health Service Reorganisation: A Reorganisation in Retrospect', in K. Jones and S. Baldwin (eds), *The Year Book of Social Policy in Britain 1975,* Routledge & Kegan Paul, 1976.

7   Harvey L. Smith and Daniel J. Levinson, 'Major Aims and Organisational Characteristics of Mental Hospitals', in M. Greenblatt, D. J. Levinson and R. H. Williams (eds), *The Patient and Mental Hospital,* Free Press, Chicago, 1957.

8   M. L. Cogan, quoted in P. Elliott, *The Sociology of the Professions,* Macmillan, 1972, p. 8.

9   G. Millerson, *The Qualifying Associations,* Routledge & Kegan Paul, 1964.

10 E. Sutherland, 'Professionalisation in Illegitimate Occupations: Professional Theft', in H. M. Vollmer and D. L. Mills (eds), *Professionalisation,* Prentice-Hall, Englewood Cliffs, 1966, p. 33.

11 H. Wilensky, 'The professionalisation of everyone', *American Journal of Sociology,* 70, 1964, pp. 142-6.

12 A. Chaplin, *Medicine in the Reign of George III,* Fitzpatrick Lectures, Royal College of Physicians, 1919.

13 Report of the Royal Commission on Medical Education, Cmnd 3569, HMSO, 1968, paras 8 and 12.

14 R. Stevens, *Medical Practice in Modern England,* Yale University Press, 1966, p. 22.

15 B. Abel-Smith, *A History of the Nursing Profession,* Heinemann, 1960, p. 242.

16 Stevens, op. cit., pp. 17-18.

17 Abel-Smith, op. cit., p. 84.

18 Sir Alfred Mond, 22 March 1922, quoted by Abel-Smith, op. cit., p. 104 and note 3.

19 Abel-Smith, op. cit., p. 156.

20 The first was a degree of community nursing started in the University of Manchester in 1958.

21   Report of the Working Party on Social Workers in the Local
     Authority Health and Welfare Services, HMSO, 1959, para. 49.
22   Elliott, op. cit., p. 96.
23   Ibid.
24   H. Eckstein, *The English Health Service*, Harvard University Press,
     1958, pp. 141ff.
25   R. G. Walton, *Women in Social Work*, Routledge & Kegan Paul,
     1974.
26   J. G. Rosen and K. Jones, 'Profile of the Male Nurse', in *Problems
     and Progress in Medical Care No. 7*, Nuffield Provincial Hospitals
     Trust/Oxford University Press, 1972.
27   Evidence to the Royal Commission on Doctors' and Dentists'
     Remuneration, quoted in Elliott, op. cit., p. 67.
28   C. Wright Mills, *White Collar: the American Middle Classes*, Oxford
     University Press, 1951, p. 112.
29   Ivan Illich, *Medical Nemesis: the Expropriation of Health*, Calder
     & Boyars, 1975.
30   H. and A. Somers, *Doctors, Patients and Health Insurance*, Brook-
     ings Institution, Washington, DC, 1961, p. 33.
31   P. Morris, *Put Away: a Sociological Study of Institutions for the
     Mentally Retarded*, Routledge & Kegan Paul, 1969, p. 307.
32   K. Jones, J. Brown *et al.*, *Opening the Door: a Study of New
     Policies for the Mentally Handicapped*, Routledge & Kegan Paul,
     1975, pp. 195–202.
33   Report of the Committee on Nursing, Chairman, Professor Asa
     Briggs, Cmnd 5115, HMSO, 1972, paras 557–65 and recommenda-
     tion 74.
34   E. M. Topliss, *Staff Communications, Relationships and Deploy-
     ment in a Geriatric Hospital*, paper presented to the Medical
     Sociology Section of the British Sociological Association, York,
     November 1972.
35   Phoebe Hall, *Reforming the Welfare: the Politics of Change in
     the Personal Social Services*, Heinemann, 1976, p. 130.
36   Elliott, op. cit., p. 142.
37   A. Etzioni, *Modern Organisations*, Prentice-Hall, Englewood
     Cliffs, 1964, chapter 8.
38   Martin Loeb and Harvey L. Smith, 'Relationships among Occupa-
     tional Groupings within the Mental Hospital', in Greenblatt,
     Levinson and Williams, op. cit., p. 10.
39   Maurice Kogan and James Terry, *The Organisation of a Social
     Services Department: a Blue-print*, Bookstall Publications, 1971,
     p. 17.
40   J. Algie, 'Management and organisation in the social services, and
     structuring a social services department', *British Hospital Journal
     and Social Services Review*, 26 June and 10 July 1970.
41   P. Halmos, *The Faith of the Counsellors*, Constable, 1965.
42   *Management Arrangements for the Reorganised National Health
     Service*, HMSO, 1972.

43 H. L. Smith and D. J. Levinson in Greenblatt, Levinson and
    Williams, op. cit., p. 4.
44 Ibid.
45 R. Bodley Scott, 'Occupational Images and Norms: Medicine', in
    Vollmer and Mills, op. cit., pp. 114-19.
46 Abel-Smith, op. cit., p. 240.

Chapter five

The Voluntary Sector

As a topic for discussion within the framework of social policy, 'the voluntary social services' is still likely to raise protective hackles. There is a tendency to consider social policy primarily in terms of statutory services, and tack the voluntary sector on as an afterthought — one lecture at the end of a course, one paragraph in a government report, beginning 'the voluntary services also have a role to play'.

The reasons for this are largely historical. Memories of Victorian philanthropy, of the patronage of the poor, of complacency about the facts of poverty and human misery, die hard. Much of the development of welfare provision over the past hundred years, the growth of services 'as of right' and of the concept of the welfare state, has been associated with the replacement of patchy, fragmented voluntary effort with responsibilities laid squarely on a public authority. The conflict between those who believed in the voluntary principle and those who believed in statutory services and public responsibilities had had a political tinge: voluntary services have often been strongly encouraged by Conservative governments (as encouraging individual initiative and saving on public expenditure) while Labour governments have been less than enthusiastic.

Often, voluntary organisations have pioneered some kind of provision, establishing a service which has then been taken over by the state. Perhaps inevitably, stereotypes have grown — the voluntary services seeing statutory intervention as 'bureaucratic', 'official', 'run by the Town Hall', while the new professional workers have seen their voluntary predecessors as 'inefficient', 'amateurish' and 'woolly'. Mike Thomas comments:[1]

> Too often the fight resulted in a kind of apartheid between what have come to be known as the statutory and voluntary 'sectors' — a term in itself reminiscent of military and diplomatic practice . . . . The most encouraging development in the past ten or fifteen years has been the gradual breakdown of this model.

Thomas is not alone in the view. In 1965, T. H. Marshall wrote that the antithesis between public and private services was gradually disappearing.[2] In 1973, R. H. S. Crossman, a former Labour Secretary of

State for the Social Services went further in prophesying 'a volunteer takeover':[3]

> I am convinced that community services — professionally trained, but manned largely by part-time volunteers — will within a decade be running a large part of our welfare state. In a chaotic, haphazard, English way, the volunteer takeover has started already.

Clearly the old stereotypes about voluntary social service are no longer applicable, and the political element in the debate has disappeared. Both Labour and Conservative governments are now keen to encourage voluntary service as a way of increasing public participation in the social services, breaking up the rigid structures which statutory agencies can develop, and providing a better quality of service for those in need.

Voluntary social service takes many forms, and is constantly changing. Some writers, like Lord Beveridge,[4] have seen this chameleon-like quality as a source of strength, providing a flexibility and adaptability, which the statutory services, because they are subject to public accountability, find it hard to match. But chameleon-like qualities do not aid definition. We have some difficulty in finding modes of analysis which cover such diverse activities as those of Oxfam or the International Red Cross, Alcoholics Anonymous, membership of a government working party or Royal Commission, the Campaign against Racial Discrimination, the neighbourliness of small Church groups or Rotary, students working on a Community Development Project, school groups who work in hospitals or tidy up old people's gardens, a sponsored walk for Mencap, groups which organise conferences at Oxford, groups which address thousands in Trafalgar Square, the housewife who bakes a rice pudding for a sick neighbour, the accountant who spends a couple of hours a week sorting out the funds of the Community Council, and the old lady of eighty who knits woollen socks for lifeboatmen. These are not vague activities; but it is not easy to generalise about them.

To start with, we need to make a distinction between voluntary *workers,* who are not paid for the work they do, though they may receive expenses; and voluntary *organisations,* which are independent of government control and free to make their own policy. Voluntary workers may work for a voluntary organisation or a statutory one — many local authorities now have a Community Work Organiser, and many hospitals have an Organiser or Co-ordinator of Voluntary Services. Voluntary organisations may recruit volunteers, but it they are of any size, they probably have a paid professional staff.

Voluntary work and voluntary workers

We can distinguish six main types of voluntary work:

  (i) Direct service-giving of a philanthropic kind, such as visiting old people, helping on a hospital ward, taking mentally handicapped children on an outing, cleaning up the physical environment.

 (ii) Helping to run a voluntary organisation — committee membership, keeping records, doing the accounts, manning the telephone, organising meetings.

(iii) Participation in self-help groups for people with common problems, e.g. Alcoholics Anonymous, the Parents of Thalidomide Children, Chiswick Family Rescue.

(iv) Financial assistance — fund-raising and the giving of money.

 (v) Public service: e.g. membership of a local authority,[5] a Regional Health Authority or a Government Working Party or Commission. Work as a non-stipendiary magistrate or a member of a Consumer Council.

(vi) Pressure-group activity — leafletting, holding meetings, writing policy statements, making representations to central or local government.

Any one organisation may be involved in several of these activities, and any one individual may offer assistance to different organisations at different levels.

This list suggests the inappropriateness of two other stereotypes about voluntary work: all voluntary workers (or even the majority) are not middle-aged, middle-class and female; and all voluntary workers are not unskilled in contrast to the skilled professional.

Middle-aged, middle-class housewives have a good deal to offer in some kinds of voluntary work. Anyone who has brought up a family and perhaps looked after an elderly relative has a head start in the personal care of handicapped children or old people; but the pool of such women is drying up. Today, most married women have jobs, and little time to spare from the double role of worker and housekeeper. Volunteers are increasingly likely to be found among other groups in the community — particularly the young (sixth formers or students) who have periods of comparative freedom in their educational careers, and the early retired, who, freed from the pressures of work and raising their families, often have administrative, financial or craft skills to offer.

We are moving away from a concept of skill as something which belongs only to the paid professional, and recognising that many personal gifts and bits of experience can be utilised in voluntary service, if there is someone to organise the matching between needs and resources.

Voluntary organisations

Voluntary organisations may be international, like the International Red Cross or the World Federation for Mental Health or UNICEF; or national, like Age Concern or the Spastics Society; or purely local, like the Yorkshire Association for the Disabled. International organisations may relate directly to agencies of the United Nations, and act as a super-structure for national bodies in various countries. National organisations may relate directly to central government, and have their own local and regional branches. The National Council of Social Service, set up in 1918, acts as a co-ordinating body for many organisations (though not all), and large towns usually have their own Council of Social Service, affiliated to NCSS, or an independent Community Council. Rural areas may have a Rural Community Council.

Smaller, local organisations may be affiliated to a larger body, or be independent. Some exist purely for social service; others may represent the social service interest of an organisation with another purpose — Rotary, the Women's Institute, a Church or political group — which provides its own co-ordination. No administrative chart would do justice to the complexities of relationship, the degrees of dependence and the constant shifts of responsibility involved. One of the important aspects of voluntary social service is that it represents a spontaneous movement which has a habit of defying bureaucracy. One of the problems is that this makes it very difficult to bring it into relationship with the bureau-cracies of central and local government. While there is now a fair degree of co-ordination at the top (described later) there is no structure for voluntary societies which corresponds to the new county authorities which were set up in 1974.[6] Any Director of Social Services must deal with a tangle of national, regional and local bodies, some representing particular client groups, some attempting a partial co-ordination for a part of his area, and many in competition with each other.

In the past few years, many of the larger national voluntary organisa-tions have become highly professionalised. Their methods of fund-rais-ing have changed as high taxation has reduced the possibility of the large legacies on which many of them formerly depended. In approach-ing the small giver, they have turned to new methods of fund-raising, such as Christmas cards, second-hand shops, sponsored walks, covenants, and occasionally football pools or raffles. They have acquired new, trendy titles — Shelter, Mind (formerly the National Association for Mental Health), Age Concern (formerly the National Old People's Welfare Association). Their General Secretaries (now usually called Directors) have learned to use the media. The Child Poverty Action Group did this admirably by taking their petition on the plight of low-income families to 10, Downing Street on Christmas Eve 1965 — utilising the popular sentiment about Christmas and children. A cold snap in February will produce the Director of Age Concern on radio and television, explaining the dangers of hypothermia to old people living alone. A hospital scandal will lead to interviews with the Director of Mind, a debate about Child Benefits will almost inevitably involve a spokesman from CPAG. Such publicity has become an important part of the work of large organisations in reaching and educating the public, and their executive officers have become regarded as experts in their own particular field.

National voluntary organisations may act as pressure-groups for particular groups of clients, collect and disseminate information, offer assistance and advice to their branches, promote new projects, run conferences and courses for both volunteers and professionals, and perhaps run their own specialised casework service. They may receive grants from central government, and many local organisation or branches receive grants from local government. Technically, such financial aid is free of strings, but local government in particular is likely to attach some conditions: for instance, it may offer premises or the payment of a salary for a trained worker rather than a money grant. Kathleen Slack, writing in the 1950s of the relationship of statutory and voluntary agencies for old people's welfare, noted cases where the Town Clerk or the Treasurer became chairman of the local branch in a supposedly private capacity, and was thus able to ensure that Town Hall money was spent on purposes which the Town Hall would approve.[7]

The development of Educational Priority Areas, Community Development Projects and Urban Aid Programmes has led to new possibilities of voluntary-statutory partnership at the local level, as a web of services in which the two are barely distinguishable has been developed. Voluntary bodies have acquired a highly professional, full-time leadership, paid for out of public funds; statutory agencies have acquired new dimensions with volunteer help. The development of community work in the 1960s has led to the appointment of community workers in both voluntary and statutory agencies with common social goals and barely distinguishable roles. Philip Bryers, writing about community work in

1972, comments:[8]

> Voluntary agencies have been used by statutory agencies as one way
> of reducing the monolithic nature of the welfare state, and achieving
> unofficial results with official funds.

Why voluntary social service?

There are three standard justifications for the existence of voluntary
social services:[9]

(i) *They have an initiating role.* Most of our social services — schools,
hospital, community agencies — were in fact started by voluntary effort.
Some owe their origin to medieval piety, others to eighteenth-century
rationalism (which produced a remarkable crop of hospitals and dispen-
saries, for example) and some to nineteenth-century benevolence. It
was not until the twentieth century that the state possessed either the
knowledge or the support of the public will necessary to develop statutory services. Even today, much pioneering work in the social services
is done by voluntary agencies because they have the freedom to move
quickly. Services for immigrants, for battered wives and battered babies,
for homeless single men, for rootless young people, have all been started
in the last few years by voluntary groups which saw a need and went
out to meet it with a simplicity and an immediacy which statutory
organisations cannot match in the initial stages.

(ii) *There is a need for continuing partnership.* One example of this
is in the care of old people in their own homes. The statutory services
can provide medical care, visits from the social worker and the health
visitor, financial support, and increasingly fringe services such as laundry
and chiropody (formerly pioneered by Old People's Welfare); but it
cannot provide somebody to pop down to the post office and draw the
pension, somebody to drop in with a cake or a rice pudding, somebody
to make sure that there is coal in the coal-bucket, somebody to be a
companion and a listener and a friend. Statutory services are typically
skilled and episodic. The continuous work of support and friendship is
best done by voluntary visitors — and thousands undertake it every week
of the year. Meals on Wheels provide a good example of statutory/volun-
tary co-operation: the local authority provides the food and usually the
transport: the volunteers undertake delivery — and report back if
someone is in special need or difficulty, and needs a visit from a social
worker.

Another kind of partnership is that which exists in the field of youth service, where statutory and voluntary clubs and other activities run side by side and pace one another. One reason for this in the danger of political domination in a service wholly run by the state — there are nasty examples like the Hitler Jugend to act as a warning. Another is that state provision is not always acceptable — young people like to form their own groups and to attach themselves to a variety of causes and activities. So there is room for the Young Liberals and the Young Farmers and the church groups and the Boy Scouts and a variety of voluntary efforts aimed at reaching the unattached.

(iii) *There are jobs which the statutory services cannot do.* Perhaps this is more debatable than it used to be. In the days before the Second World War, when most trained case-workers worked for voluntary agencies, it was frequently contended that it was impossible to do 'real' social work in a statutory agency. Now the balance has shifted, and the local authorities are the main employers of qualified social workers; but there are still groups — meths drinkers, heroin addicts, closed cultural groups like the Chinese or Pakistani women — who do not expect or want contact with the statutory authorities, and who can best be reached by volunteers, at least in the first instance.

To these arguments, we can perhaps add the following:

(iv) *There is virtue in diversity.* Nobody really wants a 'monolithic welfare state'. The essence of social service is essentially personal, derived from face-to-face contact, and it is this personal element which voluntary social service — with all its untidiness and its contradictions — essentially preserves. It ensures that the services do not become top-heavy, remote from the needs. It has a spontaneity which is valuable, and ensures a wider spread of provision.

(v) *It preserves 'the gift relationship'.*[10] In his last book, Richard Titmuss argued with passion the case for social exchange rather than commercial exchange as the basis of human society. Crossman comments:[11]

Mr. Titmuss was convinced that one of the diseases from which
modern society is suffering is the frustration of the altruistic motive.
True enough, we all want to live well, to have sex, to dominate, but
we want just as deeply to feel we are needed by other people, and
to spend some of our time doing good. And the community needs to
get our voluntary contribution just as much as we need to give it.

(vi) *All the needs cannot be met by the state.* There are limits to the amount which any government can raise through direct and indirect taxation. Both are unpopular, because nobody likes paying rates and taxes. A government which goes beyond those limits is going to lose power. Voluntary social services can tap the public pocket and organise the public in a way which is acceptable, and which supplements the work of the statutory services. They can draw on local goodwill, personalise a cause, give the assurance that *this* service or *this* sum of money is going to *this* need. In a period of rising costs paralleled by rising expectations, any government, of the Left or the Right, needs the voluntary social services.

(vii) *It offers a critical dimension.* Shortly after taking up appointment as Secretary of State for Health and Social Services David Ennals stated:[12]

> It is your [the voluntary organisations'] job to criticise the performance of government, to speak out loud and clear. I am not talking about incessant, petulant, carping criticis, implying that we are deliberatly setting out to grind down the underprivileged, but constructive criticism based on experiences and a shared concern. Voluntary bodies should be the Minister's conscience, constantly reminding him of his responsibility in the field in which they are operating.

(viii) *There is a strong information-giving role in relation to the public.* Voluntary organisations can provide constructive criticism for statutory bodies; they can also have a valuable contribution to make in informing the public over issues and in developing a more considerate attitude to many groups in society who, perhaps through fear or ignorance, have been stigmatised.

Difficulties of voluntary social service

So far we have looked at the advantages: now let us look at some of the problems which voluntary societies have to face.

Many have difficulties in selecting workers. Unlike statutory agencies, which can appoint people of specified skills from a short-list of candidates, they have to take who comes, and it is extremely hurtful for a volunteer to be told that he/she is unsuitable for a particular task. Volunteers offer what they have, and often expect it to be acceptable. A few organisations like the Marriage Guidance Council do screen applicants carefully, and the growing development of Volunteer Bureaux (described later) means a more sophisticated matching of people to jobs.

Volunteers come into service with motivation as mixed as that of any other group, and sometimes with very unsuitable attitudes.[13] If we are to make use of the houseproud suburban lady who wants 'to clean up some of the old dears', the budding young novelist who sees meths drinkers as copy, the schoolboy who finds a couple of hours on a ward for the mentally handicapped the only alternative to Corps or organised games, they need to be screened, and they need to be trained. Again, the Marriage Guidance Council is a notable exception; but few voluntary organisations offer training, and where it exists, much of it is still of the 'six lectures by experts' variety. The volunteers sit on hard chairs, getting increasingly bored, while six local notables talk about their own work and indicate patronisingly that there may be a small (unqualified and amateur) place in it for the volunteer too, provided he does exactly as he is told. We are beginning at last to see another pattern of training, sponsored by Volunteer Bureaux, in which volunteers are encouraged to do the talking — to identify their own skills and weaknesses, to analyse their own contribution — while the experts listen. Ideally, one would like to see the development of extended case-discussions in which volunteers could learn by getting expert consultation week by week as they analysed their on-going work — a sort of social work supervision process. But that is time-consuming, and few professionals have yet either the time or the will to attempt it.

Most volunteers want the human rewards of face-to-face contact with clients. That is what they volunteer for and if they are set to clear out the old filing-cabinets they will soon drift away. Many organisers of voluntary service have found difficulty in getting volunteers for administration or office work, where they are often badly needed. To some extent this situation is now being eased by the early retired, who sometimes actually like office work and administration, and may have skills developed in their working life to offer.

Often there is confusion and inconsistency at the local level as to how statutory bodies should use and involve volunteers. In *Bargain or Barricade?* Giles Darvill presents five different attitudes to volunteers held by social services departments. Interestingly the attitude that is seen as facilitating interdependence and interaction is termed by Darvill the 'intimate-enemy' attitude'.[14] While volunteers and voluntary organisations can offer useful criticism, local councillors who themselves are 'volunteers' may be highly ambivalent about receiving it. Possibly this is one reason to account for a recent Volunteer Centre finding that only 30 per cent of social services committees that it surveyed were co-opting representatives from voluntary organisations.[15]

Voluntary organisations do not always provide services at the point of need. (The obvious retort to this is that statutory organisations do not do this, either.) But only the largest and most sophisticated voluntary agencies have any system of evaluation, and the spirit of public service can go badly astray in social diagnosis. Kathleen Slack mentions an Old People's Welfare Committee in a London Borough which spent 95 per cent of its annual income on Christmas parcels — though the peak period of need for old people in their own homes is in January and February. Others spent much of their income on seaside outings for the fit elderly, and ignored the needs of the housebound. Rotary and Woman's Institutes often give parties for the over-60s (many of them quite able to organise thier own entertainment, and still working full-time) while making no provision for the frail and lonely over-80s.

Some voluntary organisations are legally tied in the use of their resources. If a worthy citizen left the sum of 8s. per annum to provide indigent old ladies with red flannel petticoats every Michaelmas in 1623, it is not easy to break the trust, even though old ladies no longer wear red flannel petticoats, and Marks and Spencer's does not provide anything suitable for the sum of 40p. There are tens of thousands of small trusts of this kind, and many thousands of pounds still locked up in their execution. At one time, it needed a private Act of Parliament to break such a trust. Today, the Charities Act of 1960 applies, and it is possible to get a fairly wide application of the doctrine of *Cy près*, which literally means 'the nearest appropriate thing'. For example, several funds for red flannel petticoats might be combined to provide a clothing fund, or money designed for the purchase of tallow candles might be used for fuel debts. But the process is slow and cumbersome, and riddled with legal complications as to the intentions of the testator.[16]

On a much larger scale, needs change faster than organisations. St Dunstan's Association for the War-blinded (a popular cause with a vivid appeal — it is much easier to imagine being blind than being deaf or epileptic) has considerable reserves, while the number of the war-blinded in Britain diminishes yearly. The public is often generous, but makes curious moralistic judgments. It is nearly always easy to raise money for children, who are generally appealing; much more difficult to do so for the mentally ill or prisoners' wives. It is notable that a number of organisations which in fact deal with clients of all ages stress the 'child' appeal — the Child Poverty Action Group in its title, and bodies like the Spastics Society and some of the societies for the mentally handicapped in their advertisements.

Voluntary societies can outlast their usefulness. A classic example is

the home for unmarried mothers which began its annual report with
'It is regrettable that the need for this kind of accommodation seems
to be declining.' There are many small societies, kept going by devoted
adherents who do not realise that the social services have changed, and
that the very real purpose which attended their foundation no longer
exists. The Annual Meeting is still held, the Duchess continues to preside,
but the tide of social change has long since swept past them. It would
be cruel to give examples.

At the other end of the spectrum, there are voluntary groups — perhaps not very highly organised — which have a valuable job to do, but
simply run out of funds. Among the younger groups, concerned with
newer needs like those of immigrants or meths drinkers, a great deal of
time and energy has to be spent on shaky finances and the problem of
how to keep in operation for the next few months. Some take on jobs
for which they do not have suitable resources — for instance, it is not
advisable for school or student groups to undertake the task of befriend-
ing lonely individuals. When the examinations or the vacation come
along, the friendless ones are going to be left unvisited. Groups of this
kind, which can only offer help for limited and disparate periods, are
much better occupied on specific tasks like decorating or gardening,
because they cannot provide the continuity necessary for a more generalized social support.

The Seebohm Report

A good deal of modern thinking about voluntary social service — and
some of its contradictions — stems from the thinking of the Seebohm
Committee.[17] Chapter XIV of the Report published in 1968 develops
the idea of reciprocal giving: every member of the community gives
what he has to offer, and accepts what he needs in time of need.

> Such a conception spells, we hope, the death-knell of the Poor Law
> legacy and the socially divisive attitudes and practices which
> stemmed from it.

The community is 'both the provider and the recipient' in 'a network
of reciprocal social relationships'. The social services department, with
its professional staff, is a focal point in that network, and the community worker 'a source of information and expertise, a stimulator, a cata-
lyst and an encourager'.

It is a pity that this concept is not highlighted at the beginning of the Report, because it is the Seebohm Committee's main theoretical contribution – though marred by some rather sentimental thinking about the nature of 'community'. 'Citizen participation' is their motif – 'the maximum participation of individuals and groups in the community in the planning organisation and provision of the social services' (para. 500) – and they see it as cutting through the traditional distinctions between 'voluntary' and 'statutory'. The whole community provides the resources for social service – partly through rates and taxes, partly through direct service – and the whole community consumes them.

From these noble heights, the Committee descends, unfortunately, into some rather confused thinking. Voluntary social services are an essential part of this network, and though the old philanthropic forms may be withering, the new participatory ones are flourishing. Volunteers may work directly for the social services department (para. 500 states that ' the responsibility for using voluntary help wisely must rest with the Principal Officer of the Social Services Department') and they may be supported by the social services department if they are 'vigorous and outward-looking' and offer 'good standards or service' (para. 496). They may 'reveal new needs' (the initiatory role mentioned earlier) and 'expose shortcomings'. The local authority 'will need to tolerate and use the criticisms made by voluntary organisations, and not expect the partnership to be without conflict.'

At first sight, it looks as though there are two quite different philosophies at work here – one in which individual volunteers are firmly harnessed to the purposes of the social services department, and one in which voluntary organisations are seen primarily as pressure groups or protest groups. Drafts which are subject to alteration in committee are seldom as coherent in philosophy as the writing of individuals. Another explanation would be that members of the Seebohm Committee were thinking of different types of voluntary organisation – for while the concept of working under the guiding hand of the statutory authority fits quite well with the aims and purposes of organisations like the Samaritans and Family Service Units, it is scarcely appropriate to more vociferous groups like the Claimants' Union, or to anti-establishment groups like Release or PROP.

Subsequent enquiries of members of the Seebohm Committee suggest that they were unaware of any possible contradictions. They thought in terms of local authorities with the farsightedness and lack of undue sensitivity which would make it possible for them to support organisations which were sometimes highly critical of local authority services, and to learn from the criticism. In an ideal world of 'citizen participation', perhaps this is the way it would be. At present, it is probably only the largest and most affluent local authorities who possess these admirable qualities — and even they must be concerned with the limits of public accountability.

The Aves Report

While the Seebohm Committee was sitting, the National Council of Social Service and the National Institute for Social Work Training set up a joint committee under the chairmanship of Miss (later Dame) Geraldine Aves, a retired senior civil servant from the Ministry of Health, to consider the role of the voluntary worker.[18] The Aves Committee was concerned that the aims of voluntary work in the personal social services should be clarified: volunteers should not be used in public services to do manual or domestic tasks for which paid workers were normally employed. They should complement the role of paid workers, and not be regarded as unpaid substitutes. In a worsening employment situation, this was a necessary gesture to the trade unions, who were begining to regard volunteers as a threat to jobs. It was recommended that volunteers should have a better status: they should normally receive expenses if they worked for a public service, be covered by insurance and carry some form of authorisation. There should be training (set down in para. 223 under the triple heads of Information, Skill and Understanding), and respect for the volunteer's own personal qualities and attitudes. The difficult question of motivation is seen as capable of modification in training:

> Motives deriving from experience of disability or loneliness, seeking a means to a career and other personal circumstances, can have positive value. With training and continuing guidance it is often possible to make constructive use of other motives which are sometimes frowned upon, such as underlying feelings of guilt or conflicts regarding authority, provided that the volunteer is helped to some awareness and acceptance of these feelings . . . it should not be forgotten that professional workers have similar motives, though their longer training provides more opportunity to deal with them (para. 225).

There is recognition of the widening field of recruitment for voluntary work, with special mention of the recruitment of the recently retired (perhaps through pre-retirement courses) and that of school children (provided that it is genuinely voluntary work, and not a substitute for a school subject). They expect the 20 to 40 age-group to provide few volunteers, and the service of younger people to be of relatively short duration.

There is a rather gingerly handling of the question of working-class volunteers: the vexed question of why voluntary social service has remained a predominantly middle-class activity. For some work 'a certain educational standard is necessary', but 'the expansion of educational opportunities and the widespread influence of mass media' have greatly increased the field of possible recruitment. Nevertheless, the argument that people who are in difficulties can more easily be helped by those who share their background of experience is an 'assumption that cannot be accepted wholesale . . . it seems to us that it is attitude rather than social background which is important, and the main object of extending the field of recruitment is to obtain more volunteers with understanding, sensitivity and the will to help' (paras 165 and 167). One is left with the impression that the Aves Committee does not expect a massive exodus from the Bingo halls and the Working Men's Clubs.

Perhaps the most important recommendations are those relating to the administrative structure of voluntary service. The Aves Committee recommended the setting up of Volunteer Bureaux — whether as part of the work of a Council of Social Service or some other organisation — to act as centres of recruitment, advice and information, and to match individuals and groups to the developing and changing needs of the community. At the national level, they recommended a Volunteer Foundation of independent status. The Committee considered the possibility of grafting this work on to some existing organisation, such as the National Council of Social Service, the National Institute of Social Work Training, or the Social Work Advisory Service, but concluded that for differing reasons, the aims of these bodies were incompatible with what they had in mind: an organisation which, given 'a generous grant from public funds' and a small staff, could assemble information, promote studies and pilot projects, advise on training schemes and methods and provide 'impetus and guidance'.

The Volunteer Centre

The 'national volunteer foundation' recommended by the Aves Committee was set up in London with the support of the VSU in 1973. It had, according to Mike Thomas, its first Director, 'a simple message: that increased and more effective community involvement in all the social services — health, social work, probation and after-care — would benefit those who use the services, those who work in them, and the community as a whole.[19]

The work of the Centre started with four main strands: the collection and dissemination of information, advice and technical assistance to projects and organisations, direct development work, and 'the role of acting as a focal point for people and issues'. Publications of the Volunteer Centre, like their *Directory of Current Research* and Giles Darvill's lively and controversial *Bargain or Barricade?* on the relationship between social services departments and voluntary agencies in their areas, are by now well known.

Volunteer bureaux

The relationship between the Voluntary Services Unit (statutory) and the Volunteer Centre (voluntary, but supported from public funds) is a prototype of the kind of two-way relationship which can be developed at local level.

As a result of the recommendations of the Aves Report, volunteer bureaux have now been set up in many towns, often attached to a Council of Social Service or a similar body. There were over 200 by 1973. As 'employment bureaux' for volunteers, they deal with many enquiries from both voluntary and statutory agencies, and are able both to direct volunteers where they can be most useful and to mount campaigns for volunteers for particular purposes.

The Voluntary Services Unit

The VSU, a small unit of civil servants in the Home Office, was set up in 1972 as 'Lord Windlesham's Unit'. It was experience of the early work of this unit which prompted R. H. S. Crossman's now well-known article in *The Times,* quoted earlier. One of its early members, Andrew Rowe, has described its formation as part of Conservative government policy[20] following Mr Heath's announcement that an additional £3.5 million would be provided over four years for support to voluntary organisation (this announcement led to considerable misunderstanding, because some of the voluntary organisations thought that they would be able to draw on the money direct; in fact, it was distributed through government departments, and one of the VSU's early tasks was to confirm that Mr Heath had spoken in good faith, and that at least this amount of money had been made available through different channels).

Another early task was to implement the major recommendation of the Aves Report by setting up the Volunteer Centre, described above.

The Voluntary Services Unit also defined four main on-going tasks — co-ordination with Whitehall, general support and assistance to the voluntary sector, financial support to particular bodies, and extending the opportunities for voluntary service. Co-ordination at the central government level is necessary because the shape of responsibility within the statutory structure does not match the shape of the voluntary services. Departments of State — the Department of Health and Social Security, the Home Office, the Department of Education and Science — have generalised responsibilities for areas of administration, and the position is complicated by the separate existence of the Welsh, Scottish and Northern Ireland Offices. Voluntary organisations exist to serve interest-groups or client groups which may need to contact any or all of these statutory organisations. Hence it was decided that the departments of state and the regional offices named above should have a liaison officer at assistant secretary level to work with each other and with the VSU.

The VSU exhibits the belief, common to both the Aves and the Seebohm Reports, that there is a large pool of potential volunteers for social service, and that the opportunities of extension are almost unlimited. Andrew Rowe treats this idea with caution, pointing to the difficulties in the employment of volunteers:[21]

> As any volunteer organiser knows, finding, employing and keeping volunteers is not a simple task. If a recruiting campaign brings in large numbers of would-be volunteers, jobs may not be available for them. Supporting a volunteer, defining his job and helping him to learn how to do it takes a good deal of time, especially at the beginning, and many professional workers, however enthusiastic in principle, shy away from the added burden, unable to sustain the idea of the extra load in the short term, despite the likelihood of an improved service and possibly diminished load in the longer term. Many volunteers grow quickly bored or respond to inadequate supervision with damaging unreliability. Some will find particular jobs distasteful or gravely disturbing. Others will try to work out their own problems on those they are meant to help. For all these reasons, great care has to be taken before setting out on a programme of expansion.

The work of the VSU as 'a friend to voluntaryism' takes the forms of both personal contact and financial assistance. We read of Lord Windlesham, during his brief period as co-ordinating Minister for Voluntary Social Service, inviting 'the heads of voluntary organisations to lunch in his room in the Old Admiralty building', or wide contacts by VSU staff with voluntary workers in the field to build up a store of first-hand knowledge; of regional meetings, conferences and seminars. Considerable financial support has been given to the National Council of Social Service (which now derives 60 per cent of its income from government sources), the Young Volunteer Force Foundation, and a large number of smaller organisations threatened with closure as the economic crisis developed, and whose work was thought to be of 'high social priority'.

Developments in hospitals

The organisation of voluntary service in hospitals, one of the traditional fields, started somewhat earlier than the developments traced above, and requires special mention. The new movement started in 1963, when the Nuffield Provincial Hospitals Trust financed a three-year project at Fulbourn Hospital, Cambridge, which is a psychiatric hospital. In the same year, St Thomas's Hospital in London appointed its first Organiser of Voluntary Services. By 1966, there were enough similar appointments for the King's Fund to organise a conference; and in the following year, the King's Fund set up an investigation which was reported in Jan Rocha's *Organisers of Voluntary Services in Hospital.*[22] Jan Rocha described how a number of hospitals, mainly in the London area, were appointing these staff on the model of hospitals in the USA. There was no one pattern of organisation, and no one training, but with the confidence of the hospital staff (particularly the ward staff) an organiser could increase the number of volunteers and ensure their active use for the benefit of patients. She ends her pamphlet with a detailed list of suggestions on how to handle the work. In 1971, Finzi, King and Boorer published *Volunteers in Hospitals*[23] which goes over some of the same ground, but has an extended discussion on the goals and methods of the new service.

The movement was given additional impetus in 1974 by the decision of the Secretary of State for the Social Services to transfer the employment of hospital social workers to local authority Social Services Departments. Though existing staff are secure in post, there is in some areas a very great imbalance between the proportion of social work staff with medical social work or psychiatric social work experience or training in hospitals, and those in the community. Hospital administrators perhaps fearing a reduction in their social work teams, have turned to volunteer organisers as a new way of keeping contact with the community.

Training is at present of a very rudimentary kind — no more than two or three days' orientation — and, in the absence of qualified social workers, hospital authorities have appointed volunteer organisers with a variety of backgrounds. This is not generally seen as a suitable post for community workers, though the advantages of a community work training seem considerable, and it will be a pity if voluntary work in hospitals develops in a narrower framework than that in local authorities and community agencies. At the end of 1975, there were 295 posts full-time or part-time, then designated 'Voluntary Service Co-ordinators'.[24]

Voluntary services or community involvement?

The Report of the Wolfenden Committee on the Future of Voluntary Organisations has underlined both the variety of causes which these organisations serve, and the importance of their work in a situation where public expenditure on the social services is unlikely for many years to keep pace with rising public expectations.[25] The Committee stresses the responsibility which the organisations owe to the public which supports them:[26]

> We urge them to be eternally vigilant in this matter if they are not only to deserve, but to be seen to deserve, their freedom. There is more to be done than is done at present in self-criticism, keeping up to date, monitoring performance, studying how far users and consumers are satisfied with what they receive.

The Wolfenden Committee makes no clear recommendations for the future. Perhaps we have reached the stage where we should stop talking about 'voluntary social service', with its dated philanthropic connotations, and talk instead in terms of 'community involvement'. The new movement has many dimensions, political as well as social, moral as well as administrative. It offers a means of escape from the rigidities of statutory systems which come to be self-maintaining, a defence against bureaucracy, a mode of participation in community living, a passionate assertion that there is more to life than getting and spending.

When T. H. Marshall forecast in 1965 that the antithesis between voluntary and statutory services would disappear, the movement was at its beginning: the Seebohm Committee in the early stages of its deliberations, the Aves Committee not yet set up, the first few organisers of voluntary services in hospitals struggling with a new remit, community work training no more than a good idea, all the development of EPAs and CDPs ahead of us.

The new ideas came out of Seebohm and Aves fed by rapid developments in the field. The Voluntary Services Unit, the Volunteer Centre and the volunteer bureaux have given them administrative expression. Now we have to see whether they can maintain their impetus and stand the test of time. Does that large untapped pool of volunteers really exist? Are we mature enough for 'citizen participation'?

References

1   M. Thomas, 'The Volunteer Centre', in K. Jones (ed.), *The Year Book of Social Policy in Britain 1973*, Routledge & Kegan Paul, 1974, chapter 14, p. 235.
2   T. H. Marshall, *Social Policy*, Hutchinson, 1965, 3rd edn, 1970, p. 97.
3   R. H. S. Crossman, 'None so fair as can compare with the British volunteer', *The Times*, 8 August 1973.
4   W. Beveridge, *Voluntary Action*, Allen & Unwin, 1948, part IV, *passim*, especially p. 301.
5   Since the implementation of the Local Government Reorganisation Act, 1973, local authority councillors are paid a small sum for attendance at council and committee meetings, but this is compensation for loss of earnings, not a salary.
6   J. Lansley, *Voluntary Organisations Facing Change*, Gulbenkian Foundation, 1976.
7   K. Slack, *Councils, Committees and Concern for the Old*, Occasional Papers in Social Administration no. 2, Bell, 1960, pp. 66-7.
8   P. Bryers, 'Community Work in 1972', in K. Jones (ed.), *The Year Book of Social Policy 1972*, Routledge & Kegan Paul, 1973, chapter 15, p. 219.
9   These are not explicitly listed, but are implicit in the papers which make up the Nuffield Symposium – A. F. C. Bourdillon (ed.), *Voluntary Social Services: Their Place in the Modern State*, Methuen, 1945.
10 R. M. Titmuss, *The Gift Relationship*, Allen & Unwin, 1970.
11 Crossman, op. cit.
12 Quoted by D. Wilson in 'Slaves of the status quo or a force for change?', *Social Work Today*, vol.7, 22 July 1976.
13 Recent developments in relation to Community Service Orders illustrate a situation where 'voluntary' work is undertaken by people who are not volunteers.
14 G. Darvill, *Bargain or Barricade?*, Volunteer Centre, 1975.
15 *Encouraging the Community*, Volunteer Centre, 1976.

16 B. Nightingale, *Charities,* Allen Lane, 1973, pp. 13ff.
17 *Report of the Committee on Allied and Personal Social Services,*
    Cmnd 3703, HMSO, 1968.
18 *The Voluntary Worker in the Social Services,* Allen & Unwin, 1969.
19 Thomas, op. cit., p. 234.
20 A. Rowe, 'The Voluntary Services Unit', in K. Jones (ed.), *The
    Year Book of Social Policy in Britain 1974,* Routledge & Kegan
    Paul, 1975, chapter 12, passim.
21 Rowe, op. cit., p. 193.
22 J. Rocha, *Organisers of Voluntary Services in Hospitals,* King
    Edward VII Hospital Fund, 1968.
23 J. Finzi *et al., Volunteers in Hospitals,* King Edward VII Hospital
    Fund, 1971.
24 *Voluntary Service Co-ordinators in the Health Services, 1975,* The
    Volunteer Centre, July 1976.
25 *The Future of Voluntary Organisations,* Report of the Wolfenden
    Committee, Croom Helm, 1977, p. 74.
26 Op. cit., p. 191.

Chapter six

Citizen Participation

As Sherry Arnstein was prompted to observe, 'the idea of citizen participation is a little like eating spinach: no one is against it in principle
because it is good for you.'[1] It also gives you a lot to chew over. We
need to analyse the apparently universal acceptance of participation, to
study underlying assumptions and values and to ask fundamental
questions. Who is being encouraged to participate? The answer is not
immediately self-evident.

The idea of citizen participation in the social services has gathered
momentum over the last ten years.[2] This growth of interest has not
evolved in a social or political vacuum. The rise of organisations such as
claimants' unions, tenants' associations and neighbourhood councils has
been informed by general concerns about the distribution of power and
decision-making ability in our society. They reflect growing anxiety
about the encroaching bureaucracy of the welfare state and its apparent
inability to respond effectively to complex and varied needs. Earlier,
we discussed the role and function of the voluntary social services.[3]
This analysis will concentrate on participation initiatives developed by
statutory authorities.

Citizen participation has been taken to signify the right of consumers
to ensure adequate delivery of services, to have a say in deciding what
these services should be, or how they affect the quality of the environment. The Seebohm Committee,[4] for example, distinguished between
three forms of participation in the personal social services:

(a) where people are engaged in providing services or help;
(b) participation in the decision making process;
(c) participation in the form of pressure groups publicising needs or
shortcomings in provision.

These three areas obviously overlap. A pressure group may also provide a service and be consulted by decision makers. We will focus on
participation in the decision-making process, which underpins all three
areas. In particular, values and interests of government and 'the public'
need to be identified. The structure and process of decision making
need to be explored.

Some recent government initiatives which have invoked the concept of participation provide a starting point for analysis. The trend towards increasing public involvement is evident along the whole spectrum of social policy: from housing to health, from education to community relations. To avoid sacrificing depth of analysis for breadth of coverage, it is appropriate to select a few of these developments, with the intention of tracing issues of wider relevance. Therefore the role and function of participation programmes will be analysed in the spheres of town and country planning, the health services and the personal social services. From this empirical base we can consider more generally the various attitudes and premises which frame the ideal and its operationalisation in policy making.

People and planning

The publication of the Skeffington Report in 1969 was a landmark in the development of citizen participation as a central issue in the planning process. It represented explicit statutory recognition that opportunities for people to be involved in decision making were too limited. The Committee's brief was 'to consider and report on the best methods including publicity, of securing the participation of the public at the formative stages in the making of development plans for their area'.[5]
The Committee's recommendations made concrete proposals on the use of the media to disseminate information and established the post of Community Development Officer to initiate participation in designated areas. The Report also advocated that 'community forums' should be established, as a kind of workshop for those 'already active' in community life.

Given the fanfare of 'participation in planning', it is hardly surprising that reaction to Skeffington was generally tepid. The recommendations were considered vague and insubstantial.[6] The lack of clarity over the CDO's role, the anomalies of his position in the employing organisation, were given scant regard — was he to be a 'trouble-maker' or 'trouble-shooter'? As for community forums, the Report actually lists reasons why planning authorities would not follow its recommendations:
 (a) 'community forums' might emasculate the identity of independent groups;
 (b) they might become talking shops;
 (c) they might become a focal point of opposition to the local authority;
 (d) they might become a centre of political opposition.

Such factors obviously play a part when assessing the enthusiasm of the local authority to expose its plans to public discussion.

The tenor of the above criticisms is that Skeffington had good, if unclear, intentions but was all bark and no bite. Others took a less sanguine view. For example, Damer and Hague contend that the recommendations reflected only the interests of planners and administrators. 'The purpose of public participation in planning is to make life easier for the planners.'[7] They point out that, during the 1960s, bottlenecks had developed in the administrative processing of plans due to constant appeals and ministerial approvals. Thus Skeffington attempts to relieve the congestion by leaving minor planning issues to be settled locally and, by means of a token participation programme, to remove public antagonism to major plans. 'Participation was an administrative necessity if the whole British planning system was not to disintegrate.'[8]

The Skeffington proposals have yet to be widely adopted.[9] To be fair, this is as much a consequence of the Committee's restricted terms of reference as the actual content of the recommendations. The Committee could only advise on participation practice and programmes. It could not set out legal requirements which local authorities would have to fulfil. Nevertheless, Skeffington did seem to confuse participation with public relations.[10] Recently there have been well-publicised instances of public enquiries into planning issues which have been marked by frustration and dissent. Objections have not been limited to the content of the planning proposals. The whole nature and structure of DoE enquiries has been challenged. One imagines that the stormy scenes, ejections and bitter arguments were far from what Skeffington envisaged as the outcome of his proposals. The image of participation as a miracle ingredient — which cleanses the system of inefficiency, promotes rational planning and resolves conflict — was never far from the surface.

Participation in the health and social services

The reorganisation of health and social services provided further opportunity for the idea and potential of participation to be given official sanction. The Seebohm Report mentioned measures to promote consumer involvement in running services, such as involving mothers in caring for their own children in hospital, or encouraging pensioners to take part in the management of their clubs. The Committee also gave qualified encouragement to consumer representation on social service committees and sub-committees.[11] The theme of citizen participation was integral to the Seebohm ideal of a community-based, family-oriented service. Beyond that, there were few guidlines for practical implementation and procedure. 'We would hesitate to prescribe detailed patterns of organisation to secure participation but suggest, nevertheless, that it may be fruitful to experiment with new forms of bodies advisory to the area offices of the department.'[12] Consequently, a formalised participatory structure (or set of procedures) was not incorporated in the 1970 Social Services Act. Social service authorities have followed different paths to give expression and form to the participation ideal.

Some authorities (such as the London Borough of Lambeth) have initiated Social Service Liaison Officer schemes, whereby local voluntary organisations are contacted by an area officer. The function of these co-ordinators varies considerably, and the relationship between the officer and local groups may range from 'close support' to a 'reasonably efficient system of bureaucratic links'.[13] Some aspects of the Liaison Officers' role resemble Skeffington's Community Development Officers; and perhaps it is open to similar ambiguities. Other developments of participation in the social services bear affinity with the idea of 'community forums'. Seebohm referred to advisory bodies which 'would function as a forum for the discussion of local community needs and services and would include in their membership local councillors and other people from the areas, including direct consumers of the services and other volunteers.'[14] North Yorkshire County Council, for example, have established a Social Services Advisory Panel, composed of District and County councillors and representatives of voluntary organisations. However, in general developments of this kind have been sluggish, diffuse and fragmented. Any overall assessment is also hampered by the scarcity of co-ordinated information and research into their impact or effectiveness. The Seebohm recommendations left room for flexibility of interpretation and style, according to local needs and resources. They have also meant that any initiatives are wholly dependent on the complexion, and whim, of the local social services authority. In contrast, the role of participatory structures in the National Health Service was conceived rather differently.

The 1973 National Health Service Reorganisation Act[15] laid down guidelines to establish a specific structure where the views and complaints of consumers could be made known. Community Health Councils were set up as consumer consultative councils for each region in the country. Coming three years after social services reorganisation, CHCs implicitly acknowledged that the notion of citizen participation had entered the mainstream of political debate. It could be faced less tentatively, and written into legislation.

After a period of considerable doubt and confusion, a government circular in 1974 clarified some aspects of the role and composition of CHCs.[16] Membership ranges between eighteen and thirty people. Half the members are nominated by the local authority, a third by voluntary organisations and the remainder by the Regional Health Authority. Each CHC has access to information from health authorities, and the right to visit health service premises. The circular also suggested areas in which CHCs had the right to be consulted by the Area Health Authority: the effectiveness of service provision; service planning; and changes in services, such as hospital closures. CHCs were to act as a 'patient's friend' in complaints made about the service, and to involve the public in their activities and assessments of local standards.

In outline, criticisms of Community Health Councils have often followed similar lines to those lodged against Skeffington. The hierarchy of RHAs, AHAs and District Management Teams makes organisational sense without the inclusion of CHCs.[17] The role of CHCs is purely advisory — they have no responsibility for management. They are in the health service, but not of it. It is difficult to escape the feeling that, in reorganisation plans, CHCs were little more than a charitable afterthought. The ethos of managerialism, which characterised Sir Keith Joseph's period of office as Social Services Secretary, is clearly evident. Set in the context of a service where the tradition of clinical freedom (or professional jealousy, depending on your point of view) bites deep, it is perhaps not surprising that CHCs were conceived as in no way limiting the executive functions of the professional administrator.

The problem of incorporating consumers' opinions and demands was viewed in terms of 'on the one hand, the taking of right decisions and then carrying them through and, on the other hand, the need for a system by which the community's reactions to decisions and the carrying them through may be effectively ventilated.'[18] In other words, the power of management is not compromised. Consumers, as represented through CHCs, can only *react* to decisions that they do not have responsibility for. They only have the right to be *consulted* by health service management.[19] Participation is construed narrowly and equated with consultation or 'ventilation'. As Denise Wynn pointed out in a review of CHCs they 'don't automatically have the right to participate in health care planning teams . . . and, when it comes down to it, they are at the mercy of their own health authorities' views on CHC participation. Some authorities refuse to let CHCs near the planning teams because they maintain that they are just exploratory discussions.'[20]

Indeed, the role of CHCs is shot through with ambiguity. Their independence from the administrative structure could sharpen their critical edge, but on the other hand, CHCs depend on good relations with the authorities for getting information quickly and in comprehensible form. We referred earlier to the dilemma of Community Development Officers, as 'trouble-shooters' or 'trouble-makers'. The choice facing CHCs is often of similar dimensions. Does 'being the patient's friend' mean acting as aggressive advocate or docile consoler? In effect, most CHCs probably attempt to walk the tightrope; between being 'for' the public or 'for' the health service. The perils of falling off are, on the one hand, assiduously fighting shy of any controversy and, on the other, risking complete breakdown of communications with the authority.

It is too harsh to dismiss the CHCs as nothing more than managerial tokenism. They *can* present prospects for influence, effecting change and reordering priorities. The full benefits of public participation in health service management might not become clear for some time. Ruth Levitt, for example, takes an optimistic view: 'In one or two years an awful lot of laymen have become well informed about the NHS and are already being an influence on NHS thinking. My impression is that they are affecting the way that the NHS goes about its work. It now always has to take into account that it must consult the CHCs.'[21]

The effect of these initiatives in the health and social services does not lend itself to sweeping judgment. Social service authorities have evolved a variety of procedures. Different CHCs have interpreted their function in different ways. Critics have suggested that the challenge of developing participatory services has either been evaded or not gone beyond safe concessions. Others might argue that it was unrealistic to expect decision makers to grasp the participation nettle with both hands. Have the kind of measures discussed above done any more than shine a chink of light through the bureaucratic monoliths? The answer remains open to debate.

The role of values and interests in participation

From this brief outline of some government initiatives which have embraced the idea of citizen participation,[22] we can move to a broader canvas. Participation cannot be plucked off for analysis — or application — in isolation from wider social processes and structures. One fundamental theme common to many discussions and programmes is that they are forwarded in terms of an assumed *consensus of interest*; consensus both *between* decision makers and ' the public' and *within* 'the public' itself. Accordingly, the main problem is identified as achieving *communication* between the parties involved; of ensuring that sufficient consulting and informing lead to harmony and satisfaction. The Skeffington Report expressed it well: 'we see the process of giving information and opportunities for participation as one which leads to a greater understanding and co-operation rather than a crescendo of dispute.'[23]

Of course, better communication *is* an important aspect of exercises in participation, interests *may* coalesce, a happy compromise *may* be reached which dissolves differences of opinion. Indeed, the pressures to compromise are often difficult to resist.[24] But one should not assume a consensus of values *a priori*. Bland assertions that participation promotes harmony — or dispute — need to be replaced by a critical examination of the interests of the parties concerned: both those initiating the process, and those being exhorted to participate. The rest of the paper is devoted to exploring more fully these values and assumptions; of the planners and the planned; the representatives and the represented.

Participation and the public

The question was posed earlier — do people want to participate? Sometimes, it seems, not many do. Disappointed authorities often blame poor response to intensive, and expensive, exercises in participation on 'public apathy'. The term 'apathy' deserves analysis, for if participation is forwarded as an important tenet of democracy, apathy is its corollary. It implies that the opportunity to participate was offered and not taken up. Apathy suggests that people have to some extent forfeited their democratic rights. It is the corollary of participation because if participation justifies involvement, apathy justifies exclusion.

Empirical information can be adduced which appears to support this image of a largely apathetic populace, uninterested in promptings to 'get involved'. The Maud Report found that about a third of adults in England and Wales are not members of any voluntary organisation. A further quarter belong to only one.[25] Polling rates in local government elections usually range between 30 per cent and 40 per cent (and, as a rule of thumb, the more local the area, the smaller the turn-out). In a survey undertaken by Northallerton Community Health Council, the results showed that 97 out of 110 people had never even heard of

CHCs.[26] Furthermore, the results cannot be explained by reference to the fact that the British are 'naturally reserved' — or any other peculiar 'national disease'. The American community activist Saul Alinsky once reckoned that not more than a 2 per cent involvement could be expected from the most active community.

S. E. Finer comments:[27]

In the Kingdom of the Blind the one-eyed man is King. In the democracy of the common man, the professional is Prince. If you have nothing better to do with your own time than organise and conspire, it is you who will end up making the laws for your neighbour, who may be no worse than you and . . . is usually a far sight better. But in the fashionable quest for participation, this workaday little fact has been overlooked.

We are left with a small group of 'joiners' running the show for the mass of 'non-joiners'. The idea has come to take on dimensions of an unalterable natural law. Political scientists such as Schumpeter and Dahl have enshrined the idea in their theory of pluralist democracy.[28] The non-participation of the many most of the time is necessary to ensure the stability and continuity of the democratic system. It is a pluralist system for competing élites, contending for support of the masses. Participation is reduced to a choice between different decision makers. These perspectives perhaps prompt caution over accepting visions of a participatory Utopia: a pretty claustrophobic place where everyone scurries around busily participating with other people. But how do they *explain* differences in involvement? Is the label 'apathetic' an adequate representation to account for this apparent unwillingness to participate?

Reasons for apathy are often sought in the characteristics of the individual. Wider social processes and structures pass unexamined. Alternative explanations identify failures of achieving citizen involvement as indicative of the alienation and anomie of modern industrial society.[29] In this context, the benefits of participating are seen as lying in the *process itself,* as much as the end-product of rewards and costs. Involvement becomes a way of achieving 'personal fulfilment', to use a phrase from the first Gulbenkian Report.[30] It provides a sense of purpose and control over the environment. It counteracts the alienating tendencies to industrialisation. These arguments direct the focus to wider themes and issues: but they are still open to criticism. They may foster the romanticised mythology of an organic, pre-industrial community. Second, in delineating *universal* trends, they can gloss over the harsh fact that rates of participation *vary*; and vary according to social class.

Closer examination of empirical data bears out the premise that rates of participation in decision making are not evenly distributed throughout the community. Membership of formal voluntary organisations, for example, is directly related to class. Middle-class people tend to be more active; joining a voluntary organisation is pre-eminently a middle-class activity.[31] Furthermore, the middle class is even more heavily over-represented as office-holders in voluntary organisations.[32]

In this light, the apathy of some sections of the community may indicate not an abrogation of democratic rights, so much as the feeling that 'participating' is a futile exercise where nothing can be gained. Past experience may reinforce this response. People will only start getting involved if they see that possibilities for effecting change are open to them.[33] For example, Norman Dennis[34] shows that rehousing in Sunderland was seen as inevitable, and this fatalism was buttressed by the cursory treatment enquirers received at the Town Hall. The same process was vividly portrayed by George Orwell, some thirty years earlier:[35]

> this business of petty inconvenience and indignity, of being kept waiting about, of having to do everything at other people's convenience is inherent in working-class life. A thousand influences constantly press a working man down into a passive role. He does not act, he is acted upon. He feels himself the slave of mysterious authority and has a firm conviction that 'they' will never allow him to do this, or that or the other.

Orwell's remark shifts the focus of the argument towards 'them', towards structures of decision making which can inhibit involvement. The irony and paradox of the situation is that the same politicians and officials who complain about 'apathy' may, through the content and structure of the values and assumptions written into participation exercises, in fact be feeding that apathy.

Participation and government

Three aspects of statutory initiatives in citizen participation can be outlined which may deter a broadly based public response. The first concerns the nature of the *procedure*. Institutionalised measures of participation may ensure continuity and regularity which encourage more than sporadic public involvement. On the other hand, formal procedures can inhibit or compress the terms of debate. Rigidly controlled discussion and communications may come more easily to officials and councillors enmeshed in rounds of committee and sub-committee meetings. It can stifle and frustrate people who find that their views are swallowed up in a mire of procedural nit-picking.

Second, the *content* of information and discussion at public meetings and forums may consist of a plethora of technical or obscure terms; even where the issue under discussion is relatively straightforward. Couching fundamental, but uncomfortable, questions in esoteric jargon can mislead, confuse and ensure professional exclusiveness. Jon Gower Davies' 'evangelistic bureaucrat' is a caricature of government officials who take part in these processes of mystification and exclusion.[36]

> The exercise of power precludes discussion. It restricts the partners to the debate to fellow-officials and colleagues; and in doing so immunises the official or councillor to the clarity of thought and logic or argument that characterises policy that have to be justified in the face of scepticism, in the heat of controversy, and under the permanent threat of an effective consumer veto.

From this basis, decision makers can present the interests of the local authority as 'scientific' and far-sighted, in contrast to the narrow or parochial attitudes of 'the community', which can then be ignored.

In local government, the development of a battery of techniques in corporate management, such as PPBS and cost-benefit analysis, has also defused the *political* components of policy making.[37] Critics have argued that these techniques, originally forwarded in response to the growing complexity of local government tasks and legislation, represent 'a shift of social power and prestige towards managerial and professional experts and away from local politicians save those who subscribe to managerial values'.[38] Too often, the thrust of these developments emphasises the long-term and abstract, rather than the immediate and concrete aspects which affect people's day-to-day experiences. The true impact of the decisions thus only becomes apparent when it is too late, and the chance of participating has passed.

Some local authorities (Islington Borough is probably the most celebrated example[39]) have taken steps to avoid some of the pitfalls mentioned above. As one Islington councillor said, 'First we just held meetings and said, "Well, this is what the council proposes to do",' whereas now 'the best public consultation I've seen is when it's in the terms of the people being consulted. They organise the meeting.'[40] The form and content of public meeting and forums can be altered and improved.

The third aspect, decision makers' *interests* and their *attitudes* to groups of individuals involved, are less amenable to change.

Community Health Councils, Social Services Advisory Panels and community forums all encourage involvement of voluntary organisations – but *which* organisations will be consulted? John Dearlove found that local organisations in Kensington were classified by councillors as 'helpful' or 'unhelpful'.[41] 'Unhelpful' groups tended to make 'unacceptable' demands on the local authority, by challenging it to take on new commitments, or reverse present policy. 'Helpful' groups did not rock the boat by threatening to upset the inertia of local government policy-maintenance. Newton has made a similar distinction between 'well-established' and 'non-established' pressure groups in Birmingham. 'Well-established organisations probably have easy access to decision makers and, in many cases, have been incorporated in the decision making machinery.'[42] 'Non-established' groups have to resort to channels other than those structured for them by government; 'they have to take a more roundabout route into the political system, using such tactics as petitions, protest marches and public meetings to make their voice heard.'[43] These tactics are likely to reinforce the original conception of decision makers that such groups are 'irresponsible'; and 'irresponsible' groups are generally ignored.

Consequently 'participation by local organisations in decision making' can receive a highly selective interpretation. Groups may be excluded if their interests and demands do not conform to pre-ordained criteria of what constitutes an opinion 'worth consulting'. The binary distinction – between 'inclusion' and 'exclusion from' formal participatory forms and structures – is ideal-typical. In practice, there are gradations in the level and degree of consumer involvement.

Arnstein's ladder of citizen participation takes up these issues.[44] Each rung in the ladder represents a level of involvement. Arnstein develops her analysis from a definition of participation as 'the redistribution of power that enables the have-not citizens presently excluded from the political and economic processes, to be deliberately included in the future'.[45] The bottom rungs of the ladder are *manipulation* and *therapy* – these describe levels of 'non-participation' which have sometimes been construed to substitute for genuine participation. The objective of these exercises is to 'educate' or 'cure' the participants. Rungs 3 and 4 involve *informing* and *consulting*. The 'have-nots' are given a voice, but it is not necessarily heeded. The next level, *placation,* allows participants the right to advise, although power holders retain the right to make decisions. These three levels represent varying degrees of tokenism. 'Participation' is expressed in terms of the top three rungs. Rung 6, *partnership*, is characterised by negotiation and bargaining. Next, we come to the dizzy heights of *delegated power* and, finally, *citizen control*, where the 'have-nots' have gained full managerial power.

Arnstein's formulation has its faults: the 'have-nots' are compressed into a homogeneous mass, the designation and ranking of the various levels is open to question, Yet it does contain the germs of a sensitive scheme to assess statutory forays into the realm of participation. (Thus we might suggest that the Skeffington proposals fall somewhat between therapy and informing, or that CHCs and social service forums range from rungs 3 to 5.) More fundamentally, the analysis places questions about the role and degree of participation firmly in the context of the distribution of political power.

Developing this analysis, it is suggested that participation often delivers less than it promises for two further reasons. The area of decision which invites involvement can be limited to relatively safe issues, reinforcing existing social and political attitudes, and curtailing the field of discussion.[46] Second, to get their name down on the unwritten political agenda, groups may downscale their demands: representatives risk 'co-option', organisations risk 'encapsulation'[47] in the formal structure. They may be 'forced to change the pattern of their activities in such a way that they cease to pose any substantial challenge to government'.[48] The alternative is often a political wilderness. In this way, 'non-established' organisations sometimes lose if they participate and lose if they do not participate.[49]

Citizen participation, in effect, may connote only those citizens broadly conforming to the values and interests of decision makers. The preceding analysis sheds a different light on the questions posed earlier. It challenges assumptions of 'the community' as an organic, homogeneous entity, and steers away from Burkeian, blanket terms like 'the public interest'. Indeed, the terms 'citizen' and 'consumer' which often prefix participation carry undertones of the consensual approach. Reasons for widespread 'public apathy' are also challenged. Some of the processes which serve to inhibit, stifle or redirect involvement are outlined above. This is not meant to signify that nothing can be gained from participation in decision making. Some of the initiatives mentioned earlier do not, for example, foreclose access by 'non-established' groups or their representatives. (The stormy passage of some CHCs bears witness to this.) What the analysis does suggest, however, is that, in a society marked by inequalities of power and conflicts of interest, policy attempts to promote participation face an uphill struggle; and that half-hearted measures are not enough.

The parameters of the foregoing discussion have been largely confined to statutory initiatives in the social services. Hilary Rose, for example, has drawn the useful distinction between 'participation in' and 'participation against'.[50] This paper has analysed 'participation in' decision making in social policy. 'Participation against' bypasses or challenges the traditional courses, the formal procedures of government. Richard Bryant has written of community action:[51]

> if it is a genuine expression of popular feeling, [it does not] necessarily conform to the models of participation embodied in statutory programmes. Fundamental conflicts, which often reflect contrasting sets of cultural and class values, can occur between official conceptions of 'participation' and actual expressions of 'participation in action'.

In this sense, manifestations of 'public participation' may be fairly widespread, but fall outside, or conflict with, the official definition of the term. The notion of unchanging 'public apathy' begins to look even more brittle. Gunnar Myrdal once noted that 'Political participation . . . is pretty much restricted to intermittently recurring elections. Politics is not organised to be a daily concern and responsibility of the common citizen.'[52] Thirty years later, the role of 'participation in' the social services is all too often open to a similar charge.

Recently, arguments about the function and potential of citizen participation in social policy have been thrown into sharp relief against the background of cutbacks in public expenditure. Hilary Rose has asked, 'in a situation of resource constraint in a material sense, is participation being offered to us as the one infinite resource?'[53] Or, on the other hand, does participation become the most easily expendable resource? The arguments and counterarguments that arise from consumer involvement in decision making can cause revisions, redrafts and delay in implementation. Perhaps government can stomach this, if it is dealing with priorities for extra resource allocation. Sometimes participation is no doubt politically and practically expedient for this very reason. But in the context of cutbacks and 'crisis talk',[54] where firm decisions need to be made quickly, consultation can easily fly out of the window; and some of the cutbacks have been made in the most autocratic and peremptory fashion. In this context, the need for an effective (that is, loud) consumer voice becomes even more vital. John Bennington and Paul Skelton write, 'there is certainly strong evidence to suggest that people want to govern and control their own affairs and show no lack of initiative in doing so when real opportunities are opened up.'[55] As pressure mounts on the resources — and ideals — of the welfare state, the political challenge intensifies: to 'open up real opportunities', and to fulfil the promise of citizen participation.

References

1   S. Arnstein, 'A ladder of citizen participation', *Journal of the American Institute of Planners,* July 1969, p. 216.
2   See R. D. Scott, 'Political science, planning and participation', *Planning Outlook,* vol. 12, 1972, pp. 17-21.
3   See the chapter, 'The Voluntary Sector'.
4   *Report of the Committee on Local Authority and Allied Personal Social Services* (Seebohm Report), Cmnd 3703, HMSO, 1968, paras 491-4.
5   *People and Planning,* Report of the Skeffington Committee on Public Participation in Planning, Cmnd 2274, HMSO, 1969, para. 1.
6   For a general, wide-ranging critique see A. Kay, 'Planning, Participation and Planners' in D. Jones and M. Mayo (eds), *Community Work One,* Routledge & Kegan Paul, 1974
7   S. Damer and C. Hague, 'Public participation in planning: a review', *Town Planning Review,* vol. 42, no. 3, July 1971, p. 224.
8   Damer and Hague, op. cit., p. 221.
9   E. Butterworth and R. Holman (eds), *Social Welfare in Modern Britain,* Fontana, 1975, p. 124.
10 R. Batley, 'An exploration of non-participation in planning', *Policy and Politics,* vol. 1, no. 1, 1972.
11 Seebohm Report, para. 628.
12 Seebohm Report, para. 506.
13 R. Deakin, 'Study of Consumer Participation', Interim Report to the Working Group on Consumer Participation, Personal Social Services Council, Institute of Community Studies, November 1976 (unpublished).
14 Seebohm Report, para. 506.
15 National Health Service Reorganisation Act 1973.
16 DHSS, National Health Service Reorganisation Circular, HRC(74)4, 1974 (Guidance).
17 See P. Bryers, 'Community Work in 1972', in K. Jones (ed.), *The Year Book of Social Policy in Britain 1972,* Routledge & Kegan Paul, 1973, p. 224.
18 Sir Keith Joseph, quoted in D. Phillips, 'Community Health Councils' in *The Year Book of Social Policy in Britain 1974,* p. 106.
19 Ibid.
20 D. Wynn, 'Consumer watchdogs — all bark and no bite?', *Mind Out,* no. 18, September/October 1976, pp. 8-10.

112   Citizen Participation

21 Quoted in Wynn, op. cit., p. 10.
22 And other examples, such as Community Development Projects, can easily be added to the list.
23 Skeffington Report, para. 20.
24 See P. Marris and M. Rein, *Dilemmas of Social Reform*, Routledge & Kegan Paul, 1967. They provide an eloquent testimony of such pressures in the US Anti-Poverty Programme.
25 *Management of Local Government*, no. 3, *Community Attitudes Survey* Ministry of Housing and Local Government, HMSO, 1967, p. 114.
26 Quoted in Wynn, op. cit., p. 8.
27 S. E. Finer, 'A hive of busy bees', *New Society*, vol. 39, no. 745, 13 January 1977, p. 73.
28 See C. Pateman, *Participation and Democratic Theory*, Cambridge University Press, 1970, chs 1 and 2.
29 For a discussion of these terms see R. Horton, 'The dehumanisation of alienation and anomie', *British Journal of Sociology*, 15, 1964, pp. 283-300.
30 Calouste Gulbenkian Foundation, *Community Work and Social Change*, Longmans, 1968, p. 4.
31 K. Newton, *Second City Politics*, Oxford University Press, 1976, p. 84.
32 Ibid. See also T. B. Bottomore, 'Social Stratification in Voluntary Organisations', in D. V. Glass (ed.), *Social Mobility in Britain*, Routledge & Kegan Paul, 1954, p. 374.
33 S. Alinsky, *Rules for Radicals*, Random House, New York, 1971, p. 105.
34 N. Dennis, *People and Planning*, Faber & Faber, 1970, p. 347.
35 G. Orwell, *The Road to Wigan Pier*, Gollancz, 1937, p. 43.
36 J. G. Davies, *The Evangelistic Bureaucrat*, Tavistock, 1972, p. 227.
37 See, for example, Bains Committee, *Report of Working Party on Local Authority Management Structures*, HMSO, 1972.
38 Peter Self, quoted in J. Bennington and P. Skelton, 'Public Participation in Decisionmaking by Governments', Institute of Municipal Treasurers and Accountants Seminar Programme Budgeting in 1984, August 1972 (unpublished), p. 6.
39 R. le B. Williams, *Islington Borough Plan and Public Consultation: A Review of the Issues Stage*, Open University, 1976.
40 Quoted in P. Chamberlayne, 'The political context of community action', *Social Work Today*, vol. 7, no. 13, 16 September 1976, p. 360.
41 J. Dearlove, *The Politics of Policy in Local Government*, Cambridge University Press, 1973.
42 Newton, op. cit., p. 46.
43 Newton, op. cit., p. 47.
44 Arnstein, op. cit., p. 216.
45 Ibid.
46 P. Bachrach and M. Baratz, 'Two faces of power', *American Political Science Review*, 56, 1962, pp. 947-52.

47 See H. Rose and J. Hanmer, 'Community Participation and Social
    Change', in D. Jones and M. Mayo (eds), *Community Work Two*,
    Routledge & Kegan Paul, 1975.
48 J. Dearlove, 'The Control of Change and the Regulation of Com-
    munity Action', in *Community Work One*, p. 32.
49 E. A. Krause, 'Functions of a bureaucratic ideology: "Citizen
    participation"', *Social Problems*, 16, 1968–9, pp. 129–43 (p. 140).
50 H. Rose, 'Participation: The Icing on the Welfare Cake?', in
    K. Jones and S. Baldwin (eds), *The Year Book of Social Policy in
    Britain 1975*, Routledge & Kegan Paul, 1976, p. 63.
51 R. Bryant, 'Community action', *British Journal of Social Work*,
    vol. 2, no. 2, Summer 1972, p. 212.
52 G. Myrdal, *An American Dilemma*, Harper, New York, 1944, p.717.
53 Rose, op. cit., p. 63.
54 J. Hearn and I. Roberts, 'Planning under Difficulties: The Move to
    Decrementalism', in *The Year Book of Social Policy in Britain
    1975*.
55 Bennington and Skelton, op. cit., p. 6.

Chapter seven

Community Care

To the politician, 'community care' is a useful piece of rhetoric; to the sociologist, it is a stick to beat institutional care with; to the civil servant, it is a cheap alternative to institutional care which can be passed to the local authorities for action — or inaction; to the visionary, it is a dream of the new society in which people really do care; to social services departments, it is a nightmare of heightened public expectations and inadequate resources to meet them. We are only just beginning to find out what it means to the old, the chronic sick and the handicapped.

In order to separate out this tangle of meanings and the patterns of thought which they represent, it is necessary to look at the emergence of community care as a policy objective, and to place alongside it the accumulation of evidence on the undesirable features of institutional care. Curiously, the policy development came first. Only after the decisions were taken and the policy objective settled did the sociological evidence begin to claim attention. The term 'institutional care' is nearly always used in a pejorative sense, as implying that it is undesirable and avoidable. 'Residential care' usually carries the opposite connotation.

Community care and mental health

The origins of the modern community care movement can be traced back to the Royal Commission on Mental Illness and Mental Deficiency of 1954-7,[1] which considered at some length the problem of our out-dated mental hospitals, and the stigma still attached to in-patient treatment. There were already some developments in care outside the hospital: for instance, the Mental Deficiency Act of 1913 contained provisions for voluntary and statutory supervision of the mentally handicapped in the community, and these were widely used. The 1930 Mental Treatment Act recognised a growing movement for out-patient clinics; the National Health Service Act of 1946 contained a curious enabling clause (section 28) which stated that

local authorities may, and to such extent as the Minister may direct shall, make arrangements for the care and after-care of illness and mental defectiveness.

Under this clause, local authority health departments had set up their mental health sub-departments, with a staff of mental welfare officers and occasionally a psychiatric social worker, under medical direction.

In this period, nobody used the term 'community care'. The statutory reference to 'after-care' was soon balanced by the concept of 'pre-care', but it was generally assumed that hospitalisation was the central part of the process of treatment, even if it was no longer the whole. Only slowly did the idea of 'alternative care' — in which the patient did not need to go into hospital at all — gain ground.

The earliest reference to 'community care' seems to have come in the Royal Commission's Report of 1957. Chapter 10, 'The Development of Community Care', was concerned only with the spelling-out of local authorities' rights and duties in relation to section 28 of the National Health Service Act, and with recommending the expansion of services. This was given legislative effect in Part II (sections 6-13) of the Mental Health Act 1959. The Act did not mention community care — only 'local authority services'. It contained no innovations in respect of these services, since section 28 already gave local authorities very wide enabling powers. An attempt to have these powers made mandatory at the Committee stage of the Bill was unsuccessful.

The real shift of emphasis came in 1961, when Enoch Powell, as Minister of Health, announced in a somewhat intemperate speech 'the run-down of the mental hospital'. With references to 'the defences we have to storm' and 'setting the torch to the funeral pyre', he announced that the country's 150,000 mental hospital beds (about 42 per cent of all hospital beds) would be reduced to about half that number by 1975, and that it was envisaged that most of these would be in units in general hospitals.[2]

Professor Richard Titmuss, speaking to the same conference on the following day, was frankly doubtful about the government's intentions. He thought that the primary motive was economic, and that while mental hospitals would be run down, there was no real intention of developing adequate community care facilities. Patients would be 'transferred from the care of the trained to the care of the untrained'. He challenged the government to show evidence that it 'really meant business' by providing a specific earmarked grant for the development of mental health services in the following year.[3] There was no official reply.

The new policy was based on some rather limited statistics of doubt-ful interpretation, and relied chiefly on the effect of the new range of psychotropic drugs introduced in the mid-1950s. These were often successful in suppressing the more distressing symptoms of mental ill-ness, but again there was comparatively little research, and psychiatrists were divided as to whether they contributed to recovery or merely alle-viated symptoms.[4]

The Community Care Blue Book 1963

In 1962, the Ministry of Health published *A Hospital Plan*.[5] This was complemented a year later by *Health and Welfare: the Development of Community Care*,[6] commonly known as the Community Care Blue Book. Between them, these two documents marked a radical departure in policy affecting the whole of the health and welfare services. District general hospitals, probably of about 600-800 beds, and serving all the hospital needs of a population of 100,000-150,000, would replace the country's scattered and often antiquated hospital stock. The total number of beds would not increase commensurately with the growth expected in population. In future, the emphasis in hospital provision would be on acute care, non-acute phases being dealt with in the com-munity:[7]

> In drawing up the hospital plan, it has been assumed that the first
> concern of the health and welfare services will continue to be to
> forestall illness and disability by preventive measures; and that where
> illness or disability nevertheless occurs, the aim will be to provide
> care at home and in the community for all who do not require
> the special types of diagnosis and treatment which only a hospital
> can provide.

Those mainly affected by the shift in policy were geriatric patients, the mentally ill, the physically and mentally handicapped, and women in childbirth, and it was to the question of provision for these four groups that the Community Care Blue Book was addressed. The difficulty was that the issues could not be approached in the unitary manner possible in *A Hospital Plan,* since the services involved in community care were local authority services. Each local authority jealously guarded its own autonomy from central government, and had a wide freedom in spending its rate support grant — special earmarked grants had been abolished at the end of the 1950s. The Blue Book therefore consisted of some 46 pages of generalised guidance in the four areas of service, eight pages of expensive but rather unnecessary pictures showing patients making toys, learning braille, sitting in a hostel lounge and so on, and over 300 pages of local authority plans which showed a remarkable diversity in both existing provision and proposals for provision in ten years' time. There was no consensus about what provision was required, or what it would be possible to provide.

At this stage, the community care policy had widened to include a number of different conditions; but it was still purely a matter of central government policy and local authority provision — there was no sense that relatives, neighbours or voluntary social services might have any part to play. Michael Bayley was later to make a very useful distinction between care *in* the community and care *by* the community.[8] This was care *in* the community with no sense of using the community's own resources or even getting the community's approval. (Many local communities were in fact particularly resistant to the idea of having hostels for the mentally ill sited in their vicinity. No attempts at all were made to create a favourable climate of opinion for these.)

Further, motivation behind the policy was still primarily economic. Many of our hospitals had been built in the mid-Victorian period when an expanding Empire meant expanding exports. The same degree of capital outlay could not be envisaged in the 1960s — particularly by a government dedicated to cutting public expenditure.

The sociological evidence

Up till this time, a community care policy had generally been welcomed by the political Right and questioned by the political Left, which suspected that it was a polite name for a second-class service. But evidence was beginning to come in from the sociological field which suggested that large institutions were inherently depersonalising and should be run down on humanitarian grounds. This appealed to the revolutionary element on the Left, which had not lost the spirit of 1789, and saw fresh Bastilles to be destroyed. The seminal work was Goffman's *Asylums,* published in 1961, which analysed the nature of the 'total institution', relatively cut off from the world outside, and creating pathological conditions for the inmates. Goffman's concepts of 'binary management' (the split between staff and patients), 'batch living' and 'the institutional perspective' — whereby the institution itself becomes of apparently greater importance than the individuals it is designed to serve, resulting in 'the assault on the self' — were developed in the American context, but found a ready response in British sociological circles. One of its notable features was that it provided for the first time a theoretical basis for cross-service comparison — its findings were as applicable to the prison or the old people's home as the mental hospital, and could be extended to apply to the school, the barracks or the concentration camp. (Perhaps Goffman's main weakness was that he noted the way in which all these institutions were alike, and neglected to explore the many ways in which they were unlike.)

A few English writers had been working independently towards the same sort of conclusions though not with Goffman's breadth of theoretical grasp. A distinguished voluntary worker, Lady Allen of Hurtwood, had written a pamphlet *Whose Children?* in 1945 which exposed the unimaginative and depersonalising treatment of children in children's homes. A psychiatrist, Dr Russell Barton, had written a small training manual for nurses called *Institutional Neurosis* (1959), claiming that many long-stay mental hospital patients had two illnesses — the one which caused their admission, and the one which hospital life gave them. A university lecturer, John Vaizey (now Lord Vaizey) had written, at the suggestion of Richard Titmuss, a painful account of his own experiences as a boy of fourteen in a series of war-time orthopaedic hospitals, entitled *Scenes from Institutional Life* (1959).

Vaizey's conclusions express his personal political philosophy:

> Army officers, hospital sisters, prison warders — many of these people are inadequate and unfulfilled, and they lust for power and control . . . they mask their insecurity and insufficiency with rigid rules and authoritative discipline.
> . . . Somewhere I feel that there must be a body of people who genuinely feel that to exercise power is wrong, and should only be done reluctantly and with a sense of guilt, and strangely, my adolescent belief that it is the Labour Party still persists.

The publication of Goffman's *Asylums,* which raised the issues to a more theoretical level, found an immediate response in British sociology, and the policy of community care, which had originated in a rightwing desire to cut public expenditure, received support from the other half of the political spectrum.

The Institute of Community Studies at Bethnal Green had already developed a strong interest in the needs of the under-privileged. Peter Townsend followed *The Family Life of Old People* (1957) with *The Last Refuge* (1962), a study of residential care for the elderly, in which he drew on Goffman's findings, and included in what was primarily an empirical study a theoretical chapter on 'The Effects of Institutions on Individuals'. Terence and Pauline Morris followed with *Pentonville* (1963), in which they describe the effects of the exercise of total power over prisoners in a closed environment, giving a detailed account of social and personal deterioration. Pauline Morris followed this with a major study of hospitals for the mentally handicapped, entitled *Put Away* in 1969. King, Raynes and Tizard in *Patterns of Residential Care* (1971) again drew on Goffman's analysis to study the administration of homes for mentally handicapped children, and from their work came the theory of 'normalisation'. They were able to show that mentally handicapped children who were given the same sort of living and learning opportunities as normal children in children's homes improved in individual and social capacity as against those who were kept in an institutional, hospital-type environment. Miller and Gwynne, in *A Life Apart* (1971) a study of provision for the physically disabled, distinguished between the 'warehouse model', where the residents are simply put away into storage, and the 'horticultural model', where they are encouraged to grow.

The hospital inquiries

A new phase in the protest against institutional conditions started in 1967 with an immediacy which brought the subject off the library shelves and into the headlines. AEGIS — the Association for the Elderly in Government Insitutions — was set up by a group of London Fabians to investigate the plight of old people in hospital. A letter to *The Times* asking for information released a 'pent-up rage and misery' as relatives, patients, nurses and social workers wrote to tell of callousness, squalor, neglect and violence, psychological and physical. The resultant book, *Sans Everything* (1967) is a powerful indictment of institutional conditions. The case was somewhat damaged by the refusal of the editor, Mrs Barbara Robb, to give evidence before one of a series of official inquiries set up by the Department of Health and Regional Hospital Boards to examine the evidence. The inquiries were painstaking and thorough. Unfortunately the trail was cold by the time they took place — staff had moved, or refused to give evidence — so that only a few of the allegations were proved, and only a comparatively small number were disproved. Many senior hospital staff took the view that, even if such practices had occurred in the past, they were unthinkable by the time the investigations took place.

Whether incidents of institutional cruelty and ill-treatment were unthinkable or not, allegations continued to be made after 1968. In the following four years, dozens of cases occurred in which neglect or cruelty was alleged in different hospitals, mostly for the mentally ill or mentally handicapped. All were investigated and three of the inquiries — those at Ely, Farleigh and Whittingham — were published and widely publicised.[9] The Ely Inquiry started as a result of an article in the *News of the World*. Many of the charges were proved, and in some instances criminal proceedings against nursing staff followed.

Originally, the protest movement was a theoretical attack on the institution as such by sociologists. By 1968, it had become a very practical attack on actual instances of ill-treatment and maladministration. *Sans Everything* provided the bridge between two movements which were very different in character.

For a time, the movement against the institution captured the attention of press and television, and many voices were raised in indignation. Unfortunately, the publicity did not last. Other subjects captured the headlines and the allegations and the inquiries have continued long after the indignation has died away. A report which was briefly mentioned by the press but which would repay careful study is that of the Committee of Inquiry at St Augustine's Hospital, Chartham, Canterbury.[10] This was published in 1976, the chief complainant being a chemist who had worked at the hospital while completing his PhD at the University of Kent. The Committee's analysis of the situation and the problem is honest and perceptive.

But the movement as a whole has been basically destructive — it has shaken the morale of staff in long-stay hospitals badly, but has never reached the constructive stage of demanding better community care as an alternative. It is easy to say 'Get the patients out', but the question is 'To what?'

Care in the community

Local authorities continued in the main to be both bewildered and somewhat resentful at the magnitude of the task which was being thrust upon them. Often they were genuinely in the dark as to the type of provision which ought to be made, and the sort of resident who would be involved. In particular, they were worried about increased costs, and the proportion which would have to be borne from the rates. A good example of the problems involved occurs in the building of hostels: many local authorities were prepared to build hostels for patient reha- bilitation, but they expected the provision to be small and the turnover to be rapid. When it became apparent that hostels were in fact providing a permanent environment for patients who had nowhere else to go, and who were incapable of living alone, the ominous phase 'silting up' began to be used. Local authorities had not expected to have to house a long- stay population.[11]

Research by R. Z. Apte in 1968 suggested that the hostel could pro- duce an environment just as depersonalising as that of the hospital — and with less opportunities for social stimulus. Hostels could easily be- come dumps within the community.[12] In some cases, patients were being discharged to 'community care' which consisted of a hostel at night and a training centre during the day: the effect was simply that of a two-part institution.

It was in this situation that Michael Bayley's distinction between care *in* the community (which might be institutional in type), and care *by* the community (which is essentially non-institutuional, and involves the recipient in the life of the community itself) was made. His study of *Mental Handicap and Community Care* (1973) led to the new concept of 'a structure for coping' for the mentally handicapped individual to be not simply a statutory service provided by the local authority, but a pattern of services using whatever resources are available in com- bination: family, friends, neighbours, voluntary and statutory resources. This broadens the concept of community care. It also makes new de- mands on the social worker, whose task may consist more in construct- ing a support system than in offering personal insights in the case-work tradition.

Dr Gerald Erickson, in a recent thesis, has proposed the use of net- work theory as a treatment tool in the care of the mentally ill in the community. Many mentally ill persons do not have a normal network of supportive friends and relatives — and whether this is a cause or a consequence of their illness is less important than the task of activating passive relationships and creating new ones.[13]

Gradually, our idea of what community care might be is becoming more sophisticated. We are moving from a mere desire to save money or to smash the institutional system to a more positive appreciation of the opportunities and difficulties of providing good care in the community without routinisation and regimentation. For all its limitations, the

Community Care Blue Book of 1963 had foreseen this:[14]

> services . . . should be so organised and administered as to meet precisely the varying needs of special groups and even of different individuals. In the past, the emphasis was on the provision of a range of services; now it is on ascertaining and meeting particular needs. In the future, the services will be increasingly sensitive to the specific needs and individual characteristics of the people they are designed to serve.

The arguments summarised

It may be useful at this stage to set out the major points which have been made for and against both the institution and community care.

Against the institution, it can be argued that:

total institutions create pathological situations: the system takes precedence over the individual;

staff attitudes are authoritarian, and patients are made to feel inferior;

institutional living collapses different spheres of life experience (work, play, domestic existence) into a single experience under an 'overall rational plan' (Goffman's argument);

many institutions are old and unsuitable for modern treatment; and

many instances of cruelty and ill-treatment have been brought to light.

The arguments in favour of residential care (the acceptable term) are that:

in fact, very few hospitals or residental homes are 'total institutions'. A careful re-reading of the first five pages of *Asylums* will show that Goffman recognised this, and did not attack all residential establishments;

residential living can be organised on democratic lines — therapeutic community experiments in mental hospitals have indicated this;

only modern suburban man expects to have different spheres for work, play and domestic existence, and town planners find commuter living socially undesirable;

one cannot condemn the principle of institutional (or residential) care on the basis of bad examples. The Scandinavian countries have excellent new hospitals. If we had the will to build, we could find the money;

finally, every allegation of cruelty and ill-treatment was thoroughly and fairly investigated. The reports of the enquiries make it plain that such instances were specific to particular wards or even particular shifts, and that the general level of care even in the hospitals investigated was good.

In the same way, we can make out a case against community care, and make rejoinders to that. It can be argued that:

community care is an ideal, but in fact it is not happening. Fifteen years after the Powell policy, community provision for the mentally ill, the group with the longest history in this respect, is still 'minimal';[15]

the impetus for community care has to come from local authorities. Many local authorities give this low priority, and will not act;

there are considerable theoretical and practical difficulties in estimating the need for community care and in according priorities among the various possibilities in provision. These tend to produce inter-professional conflict which hinders development;

hospitals and other residential institutions can be inspected. There is a greater chance of cruelty or neglect passing unobserved in the community;

good community care would be more expensive than good institutional care because it involves the dispersal of scarce skills and resources rather than their centralisation;

the move to community care has fragmented the compaign for good standards of care. It is now necessary to conduct many local campaigns instead of one national one.

On the other hand community care can be defended:

in fact, if one looks back over fifteen years, a great deal has happened. Local authorities are experimenting with sheltered housing, group flats, and many other schemes;

as the movement for public participation grows, local Councils of Social Service and other voluntary agencies are taking the initiative, and prodding local authorities into action;

many campaigns are better than one, because there is a greater chance of success;

the community will provide its own watchdogs — friends, relatives and neighbours; and

good community care need not be more expensive because it has new resources to draw on: all care need not be paid, professional care.

Community attitudes

Much depends on whether the community (whatever that means) is prepared to provide care. The community care philosophy involves a fairly rosy view of human nature, and the acid test is whether it can be translated into positive action on a national scale. Are human beings, as the economists believe, motivated only by considerations of personal greed and private profit? In that case, we had better build more institutions quickly, because there is no hope of reasonable standards of care in the community. Or are they, as Richard Titmuss believed, capable of making social exchange — the reciprocity of gifts and services freely offered and freely received — the basis of social interaction?[16] In that case, community care stands a chance — though there is still the problem of stigma. Some people are going to need to receive a great deal, and to contribute very little. Their appearance or behaviour may be unattractive or even frightening, and offend ideas of the 'normal'.[17] Is it realistic to expect that they will be accepted as part of the brave new community world? Or are there limits to public tolerance — limits which ought to be recognised and respected for fear of a back-lash?

Public education, much of which is carried out by the voluntary societies for the aged, the mentally ill and the handicapped, can do a certain amount to lower the threshhold to tolerance and enable more of their clients to live fulfilled lives in the wider society; but even so, there are limits. Consider the following case:

> Peter is 25. He is an only child, his parents are dead, and there are no near relatives. He was in hospital for some years, being spastic and confined to a wheelchair. He has also had a colostomy, and is sensitive about the smell. He cannot work, does not get on with his landlady, and has no friends. He is quite intelligent and desperately lonely. The social services department is looking for a family who will befriend him and take him out occasionally.

Peter may be lucky, or he may not. He may be brought into contact with a family who will 'adopt' him for life: or one which will be enthusiastic for six weeks, and forget all about him when the novelty wears off; or one which returns him promptly to the social services department saying that they are sorry, but they are very sensitive people, and they simply cannot stand it; or there may be no offers at all. It is a question whether Peter, and people like him, would not be happier in the small artificial community of a hostel or even a hospital ward than in the outside world. To talk of the outside world as 'the community' is to assume a level of social support which may not in fact exist.

Slowly, we have come to recognise that the issues are not a matter of 'institutional care versus community care'. The dichotomy is false. No responsible observer would condone the cruelty and neglect which were found in institutions at the end of the 1960s. The setting up of the office of Health Service Commissioner (one of the recommendations of *Sans Everything*) is one guarantee that such conditions can be checked. Another is the growing practice of inviting voluntary helpers to work on the wards, where they can help to supplement the work of hard-pressed staff and be around to see that petty cruelties are not practised in private.

But equally, few now contend that we run services entirely without residential centres. The hospital, no less than the local authority home or hostel, is part of the community care spectrum rather than being set over against it. The choice is not either residential care *or* community care, but some elements of both. The residential setting may be used more flexibly than in the past to provide care for short periods — perhaps for active treatment, perhaps to give friends and relatives a rest or a holiday. Efforts can be made to provide community contacts and outings for those who need to stay long-term. In these and many other ways, the walls of the former 'total institutions' may be breached.

There is another possibility which stands between residential care and home care: that of day care. Day hospitals and centres for the mentally ill started in the 1950s, and while they have not fulfilled all the hopes of their early protagonists, they have provided a valuable intermediate means of treatment and care. Day care for the elderly and the physically handicapped is newer, but has a considerable potential. Clients can live in their own homes, but are picked up by ambulance or sitting-case car perhaps one or two days a week and taken to a 'club' where they receive all their meals, join in handicrafts or games or other activities, receive minor services like hairdressing or chiropody, and perhaps are taken shopping or out for a drive. The client keeps his independence and self-respect; the social services are in touch with him and can provide for his needs; and the cost to the statutory services is considerably lower than that of the most minimal kind of institutional care.

The question is now not 'institutional care versus community care' but what kind of care for what kind of patient in what kind of circumstances. The important thing is that we should build up structures appropriate to the needs of individual men and women, and foster a sense of community involvement in different kinds of provision. This needs skill and dedication, and better techniques for social intervention than we have so far evolved. The period of rhetorical debate is over.

References

1   *Report of the Royal Commission on Mental Illness and Mental Deficiency*, Cmnd 169, HMSO, 1957.
2   *Report of the Annual Conference of the National Association for Mental Health*, 1961.
3   Titmuss, op. cit.
4   See K. Jones and R. Sidebotham, *Mental Hospitals at Work*, Routledge & Kegan Paul 1962, chapter 2, for a contemporary assessment.
5   *A Hospital Plan for England and Wales*, Cmnd 1604, HMSO, January 1962.
6   *Health and Welfare: the Development of Community Care*, Cmnd 1973, HMSO, April 1963.
7   *A Hospital Plan*, para. 31.
8   M. J. Bayley, *Mental Handicap and Community Care*, Routledge & Kegan Paul, 1973.
9   *Report of the Committee of Inquiry into Allegations of Ill Treatment . . . at the Ely Hospital, Cardiff*. Cmnd 3795, HMSO, 1969; *Report of the Farleigh Committee of Inquiry*, Cmnd 4557, HMSO, 1971; *Report of the Committee of Inquiry into Whittingham Hospital*, Cmnd 4861, HMSO, 1972.
10   Published by the South East Thames Regional Health Authority, March 1976.
11   E. Durkin, *Hostels for the Mentally Disordered*, Fabian Pamphlet no. 24, 1971, for an account of problems of definition in hostel care.
12   R. Z. Apte, *Half-way Houses*, Occasional Papers in Social Administration, Bell, 1968.
13   G. Erickson, 'Personal Networks and Mental Illness', DPhil thesis, University of York 1976, as yet unpublished.
14   *Health and Welfare: the Development of Community Care*, para. 9.
15   *Better Services for the Mentally Ill*, Cmnd 6233, HMSO, 1975: foreword by the Secretary of State for the Social Services, Mrs Barbara Castle.
16   See R. M. Titmuss, *The Gift Relationship*, Allen & Unwin, 1970.
17   For a full treatment of this theme, see E. Goffman, *Stigma: the Management of Spoiled Identity*, Prentice-Hall, Englewood Cliffs, 1963.

Perspectives on Deviancy

The movement which is variously known as 'deviancy theory' or ' the alternative perspective', with its derivatives of radical criminology, anti-psychiatry and radical social work, came from American sociology, and began to have a major effect on the social sciences in the mid-1960s. It was quickly taken up by some British schools of sociology, and in the main treated with polite disinterest by those concerned with the development of social policy and social work, who thought that it contained little that was new. When told that it was wrong to label people as 'lunatics', 'criminals' or 'inadequates', they pointed out that they had long been trying to get rid of such stigmatising terms, speaking more gently of 'mental ill-health' or 'delinquent acts' or 'under-achievement'. When informed that there was much wrong with the organisation of society, and that it cramped and distorted the lives of those who were sick or poor or uneducated, they replied that they were aware of this, and that was why they were in business. When told that 'misfits' were defined by society, or that 'deviance is a property conferred upon rather than inherent in behaviour'[1] they made it clear that they had read Ruth Benedict's classic *Patterns of Culture*,[2] and that there was nothing very new in the view that behaviour which was stigmatised in one society might be accepted as normal in another. Further, they pointed out that the rejection of judgmental attitudes was basic to social work teaching, and that social administration had long been known (at least to public administrators) as 'the worm's-eye view' because it looked at the public services from the consumer end rather than from top administration down. So they concluded that the new perspective had little to teach them, and was based on a misconception of the work which they did and the value-positions which they held; and in this they were wrong.

The new movement was not a rational development from accepted positions. It was an academic whirlwind, a new way of looking at people and events which involved something like a conversion experience. It was difficult to define, because its proponents distrusted labels, categories, frames of reference and mental constructs of all sorts. It defied rational analysis, and introduced into academic life a kind of higher unreason which bewildered many and alienated some. It added up to a fundamental attack on established assumptions and established traditions, and neither the assumptions nor the traditions will ever be quite the same again.

Labelling theory is the study of how and why people are defined by the wider society, and the effect of labelling on their subsequent lives — often in the form of a self-fulfilling prophecy. It involved attacking the dominant explanation of deviant behaviour in the 1950s and early 1960s, structural-functionalism, in two ways: first, structural-functionalism assumed that there was a consensus about the nature of society, and its goals, and accepted the existing structure: labelling theory challenged that assumption with the contention that values and goals were diverse, and that one should ask 'deviant to whom?' and 'deviant from what?'[3] What is regarded as vandalism in working-class boys may be dismissed as high spirits in undergraduates; what is regarded as gross psychosis in the poor may be seen as lovable eccentricity in the rich. Second, structural-functionalism concentrated on the static concepts of criminality or mental illness or poverty, whereas the new approach concentrated on process. Erving Goffman's essay on 'The Moral Career of the Mental Patient' is a classic study of how a person is first defined as mentally ill, then led through 'the betrayal funnel' into hospitalisation, and finally committed to a pattern of living in which all his acts are construed in the light of the definition. Any unusual or bizarre behaviour is methodically recorded. His many commonplace and normal acts are not. Further, the fact that he is in a mental hospital will be taken as prima facie evidence that he is the sort of person mental hospitals exist for.[4]

This process leads to what is known as *deviancy amplification*: the labelling process actually creates deviant behaviour because it alters the self-concept of the deviant, and he sees himself as belonging to a stigmatised class.

Deviancy theory is the wider study of individuals and social groups whose lives are in some respects at variance with the norms of the society in which they live. It rejects the official perspective — the perspective of police and courts and psychiatrists and social workers — insisting that the perspective of those who are subjected to their ministrations is at least as valid as that of the professionals, and that the professionals actually create deviancy in their own interests. They are basically 'agents of social control'. Behind this view lies a political critique which challenges the basis of power and authority structures in society.

Both labelling theory and deviancy theory owe much to *ethnomethodology,* which is concerned with the perceptions of individuals and the

meanings assigned to everyday events.[5] Basically, ethnomethodologists have tried to look afresh at the ordinary actions of ordinary people, and to decipher the codes of conduct and meaning which rule their actions and responses. Garfinkel[6] implicitly distinguishes between 'normative paradigms' in which the meanings are taken for granted, and 'interpretative paradigms' in which meanings are assumed to be problematic, or to be other than they appear. Beneath the formal verbal exchange of people in everyday situations may lie currents of meaning and emotion which are never openly articulated.

Ethnomethodologists have employed shock methods to throw light on accepted behaviour. In one of Garfinkel's experiments, students were told to behave like lodgers in their parents' homes, responding to all assumptions of a shared life of common meanings with a studied and impersonal politeness. A few students refused to undertake the experiment. Those who did were able to report that in most cases the effect was one of confusion, irritation and bad feeling, which was precisely the hypothesis employed.[7] This was very much in the mood of intergenerational warfare which characterised the mid-1960s — novels like *The Catcher in the Rye* and *The Graduate* provide more extreme examples of the same sort of process. Some commentators have seen this kind of experimentation as at best trivial and at worst deliberately disruptive and even cruel. Gouldner writes:[8]

> The message seems to be that anomic normlessness is no longer something that the sociologist studies in the social world, it is now something that he *inflicts upon it,* and this is the basis of his investigation.

But the analysis of what was assumed to be simple and ordinary began to yield patterns of great complexity. Ethnomethodology and the related study of *symbolic interactionism* (which concentrates on what occurs between individuals without prior reference to what is assumed to be the character and history of those individuals) have their roots in the philosophical studies of phenomenology and existentialism, which ask such fundamental questions as 'How do I know that I exist?', 'How do I know that what I perceive is reality?', 'How can I perceive anything but the present?' (questions at least as old as Socrates). One result is the use of a method of analysis which ignores the rules of space and time, jumbling together apparently disparate phenomena in order to study new facets of human experience without prior constructs relating to culture or historical context. Lévi-Strauss in anthropology calls this the 'synchronic method' in contradistinction to the 'diachronic method' which regards cultures and periods of history as separate and distinct.[9]

Radical criminology

The rigidities of much legal thinking about crime, which focuses not upon the actor but upon the act itself, have long been apparent to many criminologists and probation officers. Theirs was the task of constructing explanations for criminal behaviour — explanations which might incur the wrath of the police and the courts. Policemen, magistrates and judges have often taken a highly moralistic and static view of human behaviour — a division of society into good citizens and 'villains'. Such attitudes may be deeply embedded in concepts of personal identity, and difficult to modify.

Even liberal criminologists have exhibited their own rigidities of thought. In the second edition of *Social Theory and Social Structure,* R. K. Merton criticises contemporary criminology for 'assigning a term such as crime or delinquency to a class of behaviour' on the grounds that such blanket-theories lead to the expectation of simplistic theories of causation.[10] The idea of a delinquent sub-culture is basic to such standard works as Thrasher's *The Gang* or Whyte's *Street Corner Society.*

Howard Becker's symposium *The Other Side,* based on contributions to the Fall 1962 issue of *Social Problems,* was the first of a number of imaginative attempts to avoid such formulations. The contribution of the 'new criminology' has been to stress the 'naturalness' of much law-breaking, the arbitrariness of selecting certain people as law-breakers, since almost everyone breaks the law in some way sooner or later, the class bias often inherent in this selection, and the effects of the labelling process through the procedures of arrest, trial and sentence in creating 'deviancy amplification'. There is much emphasis on the importance of listening to the law-breaker, and on appreciating the significance of what he has done within his definition of the situation. There is a belief that much crime is simply a diversity of behaviour which society can and ought to tolerate, and that the results of doing so would be less damaging than the charade of public condemnation. A British contribution, Taylor, Walton and Young's *The New Criminology,* traces the development of these ideas.[11]

Much of the emphasis of the new movement is on juvenile delinquency — Edwin Schur's slogan of 'leave the kids alone' typifies this emphasis.[12] It is particularly applied to victimless crimes, such as marijuana smoking and other forms of drug abuse, but is extended to crimes against property, which are seen largely as formulations by the property-owning classes to protect an inequitable distribution of wealth. It is more rarely invoked in relation to crimes against the person, such as assault and battery or murder. However, Taylor and Cohen's *Psychological Survival,* based on a study of prisoners with life sentences in E wing of Durham Prison, develops the approach in an extreme form. The authors, in the guise of adult education lecturers, were able to get to know a group of men who had been convicted of serious crimes, and who were thought by the prison authorities to require special security arrangements. They found them as heterogeneous a collection of men as any other, with a variety of personal qualities and talents, and apparently better company than most. They have a fundamental point to make: when society sends a man or woman to prison, it imprisons the whole person, though the act which leads to imprisonment may result from only one facet of personality and relate to only point in time. This reduction of all roles (parent, child, spouse, worker, neighbour, citizen) to the single role of prisoner is profoundly damaging to the personality, and benefits nobody, since it further alienates the prisoner from the society which inflicts the role upon him.

Taylor and Cohen's identification with the prisoners leads them to take a patronising attitude to prison staff (invariably referred to as 'screws') and to a certain satisfaction in prison élitism:[13]

> The prisoners . . . felt in some danger of being contaminated by what they regard as the dull, prejudiced, lumpen-proletarian nature of their guards. Their jokes were often at the officers' expense.

It seems reasonable to conclude that the 'new criminology' has filled a gap in criminological knowledge by emphasising that the offender has a point of view and an experience which must be taken into account if the aim is rehabilitation rather than deterrence. The extreme views in which the existence or relevance of anti-social acts is totally denied or ignored are referred to by Becker as 'unconventional sentimentality'.[14]

Anti-psychiatry

In the psychiatric field, the deviancy perspective has been adopted by a few psychoanalysts, notably R. D. Laing, David Cooper and Thomas Szasz, who have developed the argument of Freud's *The Psychopathology of Everyday Life* that the behaviour regarded as pathological in mental hospital patients is merely an exaggeration of traits to be found in the rest of the population. They deny the reality of diagnostic labelling and the efficacy of medical treatment for what they see basically as 'problems in living'. The attack is concentrated on what Szasz calls 'institutional psychiatry' — the organic school which sees psychiatric treatment essentially as a branch of medicine and treatment primarily in terms of medication and shock treatment to 'cure' or 'relieve' an 'illness'. The movement has very little following in psychiatry, but has been given wide publicity. The film *One Flew Over the Cuckoo's Nest,* based on Ken Kesey's novel of the same name, drew packed audiences, and led to protests from members of the Royal College of Psychiatrists on the grounds that it was recreating the traditional fear of psychiatric treatment which the mental health movement had long laboured to overcome. The story of R. P. McMurphy, the all-American gambling, wenching, fighting (=normal?) male who takes on the staff of a mental hospital single-handed and is drugged, forced to attend 'group therapy' sessions which only call forth and deepen human anguish, subjected to shock treatment and finally lobotomised into a human vegetable, to be the subject of a mercy killing by another patient is special pleading of a compelling kind.

R. D. Laing's *The Divided Self* is a perceptive study of some classic double-binds in human living[15] — almost a verbal version of Feiffer's cartoons. We are all 'disturbed personalities' — sick, sick, sick.[16] Life consists of learning to cope with one's own problems, and those of other people. *Knots* extends this argument.[17] The approach is strongly pheno-menological — an attempt to look at human situations without prior constructs, and to see what lies between people as well as in them. The concept of the dichotomy between 'I' and 'Me' owes much to the existentialists.

Sanity, Madness and the Family[18] consists in the main of a series of case-histories indicating that families scape-goat teenagers when the 'real' problem is one of parental disturbance or an insupportable family situa-tion. While the analysis was limited, the proposition that families may 'elect' one of their members to be labelled as mentally ill, and thus to bear the weight of all the family problems, has been widely accepted in family therapy. Though it provides a sufficient explanation in some cases, it should be remembered that Laing and Esterson refer specifi-cally to 'schizophrenic' patients, and the weakness of the case in sup-porting a general proposition lies in the fact that individuals are not only members of families: they have other roles in peer groups and work groups, and disturbed behaviour originating in relation to these other groups needs to be taken into account.

Laing's later work, notably *The Politics of Experience and The Bird of Paradise,*[19] bears the marks of rhetorical excess and exhibits some confusion of thought, possibly associated with the 'research into varieties of experience including mind-expanding drugs' mentioned in his brief biography:[20]

> We who are still half alive, living in the often fibrillating heartland of a senescent capitalism — can we do more than reflect the decay around and within us? . . . We are all murderers and prostitutes, no matter to what culture, class or society one belongs, no matter how normal or moral one takes oneself to be.

But behind such language is an authentic social ethos and a human concern for the indignities which professionals can inflict on patients, particularly in the name of medical progress.

David Cooper, working, like Laing, from the Tavistock Institute of Human Relations, focuses on the pathological aspects of family life: perhaps a necessary corrective in a period when social workers and family therapists saw the family as inevitably supporting and enabling. There was a need for a reminder that family life can also be crippling, warping and destructive.[21] The family is the one 'total institution' of which we all have experience in childhood. Many of our earliest memories are of the world seen from behind bars, those of the cot or play-pen, and perhaps this explains some of the force of the anti-institutional movement.

Geoffrey Pearson makes a valuable point when he says that, though Laing and Cooper belong to the 'soft Left', Thomas Szasz is of the 'hard Right.'[22] Szasz writes of the 'myth of mental illness' — a myth invented by 'institutional psychiatrists' for their own porfessional ends[23] — and argues, like Laing and Cooper, that there is no such entity: society needs the 'madman' in order to define the boundaries of human conduct, and mental treatment, like the Spanish Inquisition, is basically a means of social control, organic methods of treatment taking the place of the *auto-da-fé*.[24] But Szasz, also a psychoanalyst by profession, believes firmly in the cash nexus between therapist and patient on the grounds that it preserves the patient's freedom of choice.[25] He does not indicate that freedom of choice might be somewhat limited if the patient is poor, and he has no patience with mental illness as a defence against charges of criminality. If people break the law, he believes that they should be tried by the law, irrespective of their mental condition.[26] We can ask in all seriousness whether the effects of the new perspective are not sometimes harsher than those of the older liberal philosophy which saw all or most crimes as 'sickness'.

Radical social work

In social work, the movement took several different forms. There was the protest movement against the conditions of residential care referred to in the previous chapter. There was a wave of 'grass roots' involvement which came from the American Poverty Programme of the 1960s, concentrated around the political iconoclasm of Marcuse[27] and the flinty opportunism of Saul Alinsky:[28]

> I have learned not to confuse power patterns with the personalities of the individuals involved, in other words to hate conditions, not individuals . . . understanding these forces enables one to develop the strategy which my opponents describe as Alinsky-style mass ju-jitsu. The opposition is always stronger than you are, and so his own strength must be used against him. I have repeatedly said that the status quo is your best ally if properly goaded and guided.

There was the experience of the British Community Development Projects, started in 1970, where twelve teams of action and research workers in selected areas began to insist, one after the other, that the problems of their area were not to be solved by local and ameliorative measures, but required a radical reorganisation of a society in which some people were condemned to lives of bleak deprivation.[29] There was much dissatisfaction with the case-work approach in social work, which, though overtly 'value-free' assumed that problems originated in individuals and families, and could be dealt with without reference to a crippling social framework.[30] There was an unease resulting from the sudden expansion of social services departments in local authorities, which meant higher salaries and better promotion prospects for social workers, but seemed to offer little to their clients but the possibility of confrontation with yet another bureaucratic machine. An innate distrust of 'the glossy approach to social welfare'[31] and of the increasing professionalisation of social workers often led to problems of commitment for those whose first loyalty was to their clients. The situation was typified by an annual dinner of the newly-formed British Association of Social Workers when members were lobbied outside the entrance to their four-star hotel by junior colleagues collecting on behalf of the Child Poverty Action Group.

Much of the feeling behind the movement is summed up in Herbert Gans' trenchant paper on 'The uses of poverty'.[32] In a static and inegalitarian society, the poor have a purpose. They do the dirty jobs. They provide employment for professional groups such as police and social workers who protect society from them and ensure that they do not threaten the rest of society. They use up inferior goods (second-hand clothing, stale bread) which the rest of society does not want, and cannot bear to throw away. They can be stigmatised as lazy, spendthrift, dishonest and promiscuous, thus reinforcing the norms of the respectable. Because they are powerless, they can be made to absorb the greater part of the cost of change, being the first to be laid off from work in time of recession, or to have their homes and communities destroyed in urban renewal projects.

As in the 'new criminology' there is an emphasis on making the imaginative effort to see what the process looks like to the client, and not only to the worker. The slogan of 'power to the people' is overtly political. In some cases, it has led to the creation of forms of citizen participation – or at least to the attempt to set them up; though the difficulties of creating genuine welfare programmes which are popularly based were well described by Marris and Rein in their analysis of the American Poverty Programmes,[33] and British experience seems to have added little in the way of further enlightenment.

For a time, it appeared that community work might develop as a separate profession alongside case-work-based social work. That now appears unlikely, for several reasons: the activities of some community workers, particularly on the experimental Community Development Projects, were so politicised that they raised a good deal of opposition in Town Halls and government offices: less because they were radical, than because they ignored or actually destroyed local initiatives which were meant to help the people of the poorer areas, and achieved nothing in their own right. The Association of Community Workers decided that the potential dangers of professionalisation were too great for them, and adopted a non-professional stance.[34] Their motives were worthy of respect, but they lost the tactical battle in a period when only professional strength ensured the survival of a body of knowledge and the power to put it into practice. Social work teaching itself expanded, and community work began to be taught as a social work method – one kind of intervention alongside others, such as case-work and groupwork. What is left is a new awareness of the client's own perspectives, and a broader kind of social work practice.

The deviancy critique reconsidered

The new deviancy theorists drew the same criticism which Gouldner made of Garfinkel: that they were inflicting anomic normlessness on society by championing crime, aberrant behaviour, drug-abuse and rebellion against all forms of authority in the name of objectivity. Many social scientists were prepared to accept the contention of Robert Dentler and Kai Erikson as early as 1959[35] that deviant acts were both defined by society and induced by it as a means of maintaining group equilibrium; they could accept Erving Goffman's serene conclusion that stigma resided in societal attitudes rather than in individuals, and that almost any kind of behaviour or physical attribute was capable of being stigmatised in some society;[36] but they found unacceptable the suspension of all judgment about the consequences of human behaviour, and the total reversal of all accepted standards. Geoffrey Pearson acknowledges the subjectivity and excess in statements that 'gay is good, black is beautiful . . . deviance is the norm, madness is hypersanity' which can lead to 'the counter-stigmatisation of the good, the clean and the healthy'.[37] He also points to a basic contradiction in the movement: the deviant is seen as a hero — a sort of Robin Hood figure challenging the values and standards of the smug citizenry — and as society's victim. Thus at one and the same time, the deviant can boast of his superior insight and sensitivity, while crying, 'You made me the way I am — what are you going to do about it?'[38] Deviancy theory is often profoundly ahistorical — Jack Douglas is able to write a short history of the American black population without paying any attention to the fact of slavery.[39] Vieda Skultans and Roger Bastide write of 'madness' as though the days of Bedlam and the private madhouse were still with us, ignoring the long and patient process of reform in mental health.[40] Dr Szasz jumbles together examples of the ill-treatment of the mentally ill from such diverse cases as those of King Ludwig of Bavaria and Sylvia Plath, without any indication of the different cultures against which they were reacting.[41]

The movements which have been briefly described here are already taking on an historical colouring. They arose in the 1960s in the context of a much wider movement of disenchantment with the acceptance world, and in particular in the context of a troubled America which faced simultaneously the assassination of some of its leading political figures; the disintegrative effects of the Vietnam war — which, by presenting two polar views of reality, typified the moral conflict of a generation; the rapid expansion of the universities and student unrest, culminating in the deaths at Kent State University; the growth of the drug culture; the explosive early days of the movements for civil rights and women's rights. It was inevitable in such a situation that there should be some search for the radical promise.

Patterns of cause and effect in the movements which swept the USA, and indeed much of the non-Communist world, are complex, and will have to wait a balanced evaluation; but the deviancy critique, for all its anti-historicism, was itself part of an historical situation, and part of the experience of an age. Behind it was the promise of a Marxist or neo-Marxist critique of capitalist society. Works like Marcuse's *One-Dimensional Man,* Debray's *Revolution of the Revolution* and Fanon's *The Wretched of the Earth* fed it with political fire. Illich's outright rejection of the medical system and the school system,[42] a turning away from all the devices and constructs of technological sophistication to a simpler and supposedly purer peasant economy, gave it a social rationale.

The attack was shrill, and sometimes unbalanced. This was its immediate strength, because it combined old and new knowledge in a passionate and forceful attack on established ways and established views, articulating disillusion, rebellion and a genuine idealism. It produced its cult figures — Goffman, Laing, Szasz, Illich and Paolo Freire, and perhaps some of the lack of balance can be explained by the fact that they all, perhaps paradoxically, made use of the technological developments of the twentieth century to make their views known: they used the mass media. In an age when press, television and radio drench us daily in trivialities, when this week's best-seller is next week's forgotten text, perhaps one has to be shrill to be heard at all.

The concept of 'the deviant imagination' — the ability to look at social problems from the perspective of those involved rather than from a reified professional view — is valuable. The helping professions do often serve their own professional interests rather than the interests of the clients or patients they were trained to serve — a fact that troubles many thoughtful medical and social work students. They cannot help people effectively unless they try to understand the rationale behind their actions. And far too much social research is geared to agency needs and perceptions.

But the immediate strength of the movement — its sharpness of attack — was in the long run its main weakness, because it offered no bridge from theory to practice, and no means of integrating the new insights with existing knowledge. One of the difficulties about deviancy theorists is that they *are* theorists, and they are not interested in possible alternatives. They are content to condemn the welfare professions without giving them any guidance as to how to find their way through the morass which they have substituted for the old moralistic certainties. Indeed, any attempt to find solutions invites the charge of being a liberal reformer, a group for whom a special scorn is reserved. Yet it is questionable how many deviancy theorists really believe that there would be no crime without criminal law, no disturbed behaviour without psychiatrists, no social problems without social workers; or that political revolution would automatically solve all human ills, restoring society to a kind of primal innocence.

Deviancy theory started as a message, and became an industry. A fuller estimate of its importance to social policy will have to wait on what practitioners in the welfare professions are able to make of it. At its worst, it has been self-indulgent, subjective and irrational. At its best, it has offered valuable criticism of our social institutions which rightly troubles us and ought to lead to greater insight and better practice.

References

1 L. J. Taylor, 'Labelling and Social Interaction', paper presented to the Fourth National Conference on Research and Teaching in Criminology, University of Cambridge, 1970.
2 R. Benedict, *Patterns of Culture*, Routledge, 1935.
3 This theme is developed by several writers in Howard Becker (ed.), *The Other Side: Perspectives on Deviance*, Free Press, New York, 1964. See especially papers by Kai Erikson and J. I. Kitsuse.
4 In E. Goffman, *Asylums*, Anchor, New York, 1961.
5 A useful introduction to the concepts is R. Turner (ed.), *Ethnomethodology*, Penguin, 1974.
6 H. Garfinkel, *Studies in Ethnomethodology*, Prentice-Hall, Englewood Cliffs, 1967.
7 Garfinkel, op. cit., pp. 47-9.
8 A. Gouldner, *The Coming Crisis of Western Sociology*, Heinemann, 1971, pp. 393-4.
9 C. Lévi-Strauss, *Structural Anthropology*, Penguin, 1972 (first edn in French, Librairie Plon, 1958).
10 R. K. Merton, *Social Theory and Social Structure*, 2nd edn, Free Press, Chicago, 1957, p. 177.
11 I. Taylor, R. Walton and J. Young, *The New Criminology: for a Social Theory of Deviance*, Routledge & Kegan Paul, 1973.
12 E. M. Schur, *Crimes Without Victims*, Prentice-Hall, Englewood Cliffs, 1965.
13 L. J. Taylor and S. Cohen, *Psychological Survival: the Experience of Long-term Imprisonment*, Penguin, 1972, p. 66.
14 Becker, op. cit., Introduction.
15 R. D. Laing, *The Divided Self*, Tavistock, 1960.
16 Jules Feiffer's cartoons, published as *Sick, Sick, Sick* by Collins in 1959, originally appeared in *The Village Voice*, a radical weekly published in Greenwich Village, between 1956 and 1959.

17 R. D. Laing, *Knots*, Tavistock, 1970.
18 R. D. Laing and A. Esterson, *Sanity, Madness and the Family*, Tavistock, 1964.
19 R. D. Laing, *The Politics of Experience and The Bird of Paradise* (published as one volume), Penguin, 1967.
20 Laing, op. cit., p.11.
21 D. Cooper, *Psychiatry and Anti-Psychiatry*, Paladin, 1970; *The Death of the Family*, Allen Lane, 1971.
22 G. Pearson, *The Deviant Imagination*, Macmillan, 1975, pp. 31 and 38-45.
23 T. Szasz, *The Myth of Mental Illness*, Harper & Row, New York, 1962.
24 T. Szasz, *The Manufacture of Madness*, first published in New York, 1970; Paladin edn, 1973, pp. 89-90.
25 Szasz, op. cit., pp. 22-7.
26 Szasz, op. cit., pp. 261-4.
27 H. Marcuse, *One-Dimensional Man*, Routledge & Kegan Paul, 1964.
28 S. Alinsky, introduction to the Vintage Books edn of *Reveille for Radicals*, Random House, New York, 1969, p. x.
29 See R. Lees and G. Smith (eds), *Action-Research in Community Development*, Routledge & Kegan Paul, 1975; D. Jones and M. Mayo (eds), *Community Work One*, 1974, and *Community Work Two*, 1975, both published by Routledge & Kegan Paul.
30 See, for example, H. Throssell (ed.), *Social Work: Radical Essays*, University of Queensland Press, 1975.
31 Throssell, op. cit., p. 13.
32 H. Gans, 'The uses of poverty', *Social Policy* (USA) July/August 1971, pp. 20-4.
33 P. Marris and M. Rein, *Dilemmas of Social Reform*, Routledge & Kegan Paul, 1967. See especially chapter VII, 'The Voice of the People'.
34 See D. J. Cox and N. J. Derricourt, 'The De-professionalisation of Community Work', in Jones and Mayo (eds), *Community Work Two*.
35 R. Dentler and K. Erikson, 'The functions of deviance in groups', *Social Problems*, vol.7, 1959/60, pp. 98-107.
36 E. Goffman, *Stigma: Notes on the Management of Spoiled Identity*, Prentice-Hall, Englewood Cliffs, 1963.
37 Pearson, *The Deviant Imagination*, p. 112.
38 Pearson, op. cit., p. 24.
39 J. Douglas, *American Social Order*, Free Press, New York, 1971, quoted in Pearson, op. cit., p. 13.
40 V. Skultans, *Madness and Morals*, Routledge & Kegan Paul, 1975; R. Bastide, *The Sociology of Mental Disorder*, trans. J. McNeil, Routledge & Kegan Paul, 1972, first edn in French, 1964.
41 T. Szasz, *The Age of Madness*, 1970, Paladin edn, 1975.
42 See I. Illich, *Medical Nemesis: the Expropriation of Health*, Calder & Boyars, 1975, and *Deschooling Society*, Calder & Boyars, 1971.

Chapter nine

Legalism and Discretion

While there is probably fairly general agreement that the system of individual welfare rights that has been built up over the years should not be dismantled, there is still dispute at the margin about whether the right balance has been achieved between legalism and discretion, and thus 'between precedence and innovation, precision and flexibility and between equity and adequacy'.[1] By legalism is meant the allocation of welfare benefits or services on the basis of legal rules and precedent. By discretion is meant the allocation of welfare benefits or services on the basis of individual judgments.

Tawney has said that:[2]

> The services establishing social rights can boast no lofty pedigree.
> They crept piecemeal into apologetic existence, as low grade
> palliatives designed at once to relieve and to conceal the realities
> of poverty.

Nevertheless the development of social policy can be characterised as a movement from discretion to legalism. Even up until the Second World War 'welfare' — whether alms, charity, poor relief or unemployment assistance — was allocated for the most part on the basis of discretionary judgments about the deserving nature of each individual case. There was no sense of legal entitlement — the applicant was a supplicant and the poor law guardians, the charities and the officials of the Unemployment Assistance Board would not have conceived that their beneficiaries should have rights.

The turning point in the movement from discretion to rights came with the great spate of social legislation in the late 1940s — the Family Allowance Act 1945, the National Insurance Act 1946, the National Health Service Act 1946, the Education Act 1944 and the National Assistance Act 1948. The broad aspiration of this legislation was to ensure a minimum standard of living for all as of right: everyone would be entitled to free medical treatment, everyone would have equal access to education, contributors would receive social insurance benefits as of right, and there was even an entitlement to national assistance once need had been proved. The consumer of welfare was no longer a supplicant beholden to the giver but a citizen claiming his legal entitlement. These at least were the aspirations.

T. H. Marshall has distinguished between three components of citizenship in Britain:[3] civil, political and social rights. During the eighteenth century we had achieved (at least on paper) civil rights — those necessary for individual freedom such as liberty of person, freedom of speech, thought and faith, the right to own property and make valid contracts, and the right to justice. During the nineteenth century we achieved political rights through adult suffrage. During the twentieth century we have begun to introduce social rights — the right to live the life of a civilised person according to the standards of society. While civil and political rights are for the most part recognised and enforced, social rights such as the right to a decent standard of living, to a reasonable house, to an adequate education, are frequently neither recognised nor enforced.

Neither are these basic social rights declared in any general way in Britain because we have no written constitution or Bill or Rights. However we are signatories of the Universal Declaration of Human Rights which states *inter alia*:[4]

Every human being has a right to a standard of living adequate for the health and well being of his family.

The United Nations' Covenant on Economic, Social and Cultural Rights 1966 declares more specific rights to insurance, family benefits, adequate food, clothing and housing and physical and mental health, and education. But the European Convention on Human Rights (1966) (which has specific articles dealing with social rights) is the only covenant for which citizens have access for the redress of grievances (through the European Court of Human Rights). Britain is a signatory to both of these international agreements.

The movement from discretion to rights in social policy has been associated with the increasing intervention of the state in human affairs. It has been part of the movement away from the *laissez-faire* individualism of the nineteenth century. Citizens' welfare is no longer only (or mainly) left to the private market or charity. The state's role is no longer residual but institutional. It is the state that has responsibility now for maintaining basic social rights. This shift in the relationship between the individual and state has brought about the fundamental change in the principles of English law which are at the root of much of the discussion about legalism and discretion. It is to this, the relationship between justice and administration, that we now turn.

Justice and administration

Writing at the turn of the century Dicey claimed:[5]

> It would be a grave mistake if the recognition of the growth of
> official law in England . . . led any Englishman to suppose there
> exists in England as yet any true administrative law.

Dicey believed that the only true justice was legal justice characterised by the application of a body of law within an institutional framework by a judicial mind. However, with the extension of government
from one field to another there arose a need for a technique of adjudication better fitted to respond to the social requirements of the time.
It was impossible for the State to extend the functions of government
as long as its activities were limited by the individualistic ideas which
prevailed in the courts of law. One result of this has been that administration has made inroads on what was previously the preserve of the
legislature and the courts.

In fact as Robson[6] points out there has been a long tradition in the
English constitution of a mingling of administrative and judicial func-
tions from the time of the King's Council and the Star Chamber, in the
Court of Requests and Courts of Chancery and later in the work of
Justices of the Peace who, according to the Webbs, mixed judicial deci-
sions, administrative orders, and legislative resolutions.[7]

> Though many of the orders were plainly discretional and determined
> only by the justice's view of social expediency, they were all assumed
> to be based on evidence of fact and done in strict accordance with
> the law.

The gradual separation of judicial and administrative functions never
reached completion. Coroners and Returning Officers still have both
judicial and administrative functions and judges still have extensive administrative duties. Most of the administrative functions of JPs were
transferred to local government but they still retain some administrative
functions in prisons, the probation service and the police authority.

However with the vast extension of the work of government there
developed a new body of administrative law that gave discretionary
judicial powers to the administration outside the traditional structure
of legal institutions.[8]

> The revival of administrative law in England is very largely due to
> the creation of new types of offences against the community, the
> growth of a new conception of social rights, an enhanced solicitude

for the common good and a lessening of a belief in divinity of extreme individualistic rights which was evinced in the early nineteenth century.

Dicey would have viewed this growth of discretionary powers by government officials, even if they were subject to control by administrative tribunals, with disdain. He would have held that administrative justice would sap the foundations of precedence and judicial case law and be subject to political influence. However Robson defended the development of administrative law.[9]

Again and again in the history of civilisation what appeared at first as an arbitrary discretion wielded by an irresponsible official gradually crystallized into a body of known, ascertainable and consistently applied law.

He thought that as long as administrative discretion retains the character of justice and the spirit of justice there is no reason why the administration should not be as capable as the judiciary in administering justice. Justice demands that the decisions made by authority are comparatively regular and stable, are more or less consistent, and that self-interest and emotion are as far as possible eliminated. Judges are trained to administer law with consistency; impartiality and judicial discretion must be exercised, as Halsbury said, in accordance with[10]

the rules of reason and justice, not according to private opinion, according to law and not humour. It is to be not arbitrary, vague and fanciful but legal and regular.

Modern Diceyists attack administrative discretion on two fronts. These are that:

(1) Administrative discretion undermines substantive rights. The bureaucracy intervenes to thwart the aspirations of legislators so that rights enacted in law do not get implemented; and

(2) Administrative discretion does not meet the requirements of consistency and impartiality and in practice is either amateurish, inquisitorial and moralizing; or in an attempt to match judicial discretion, a mass of rules are created which result in wooden uniformity. The procedures of administrative discretion do not meet the criteria of justice.

Those who continue to defend the exercise of discretion by the administration are inclined to make the distinction between proportional (equitable) justice and creative (individualised) justice. Any system of welfare requires the capacity to respond to the special needs and circumstances of each individual. It needs this element of flexible individualised justice as Titmuss says:[11]

> In order to allow a universal rights scheme, based on principles of equity, to be as precise and inflexible as possible. These characteristics of precision, inflexibility and universality depend for their sustenance and strength on the existence of some element of flexible individualised justice. But they do not need stigma. The essential problem is to find the right balance.

and Olive Stevenson says:[12]

> It is somewhat ironic that in a shift from eligibility to entitlement and in the reaction against the degrading procedures by which eligibility was sometimes established, there may be a new kind of injustice in which the individual finds there is no rule to fit his own case.

Discretion as a threat to substantive rights

The actual nature of social or welfare rights is difficult to discern. It is doubtful if some of them exist in law (there is for example no law providing the right of the homeless to a house). Even where there is a right in law, the mode of delivery may turn a right into a discretion (and *vice versa*). A category of the population may have a right to a benefit or service but the test of category may involve a discretionary judgment and the actual service provided may be limited by discretion. Most welfare rights are fenced in by qualifying conditions and those qualifying conditions inevitably involve discretionary judgments. In some cases that discretion is more or less governed by rules and not left to human caprice. Thus a decision on national insurance about whether an unemployment benefit claimant is eligible for benefit is made on the basis of his contributory record, whether he is available for work and for what reasons he is unemployed. All this is governed by the legislation itself and by precedents determined by the National Insurance Commissioners and the High Court. If he is not satisfied with the decision made on his claim he can appeal to a local tribunal and upward through the Insurance Commissioners to the High Court. On the other hand what does the right to health care on the basis of medical need mean? It is certainly not enforceable through the courts and it is subject to administrative discretion: a clinical judgment is made about diagnosis and treatment

and the care which is received is not only dependent on the judgment of doctors but the availability of facilities.

One example of how the stated intentions of legislators can be mediated by the executive is the Chronically Sick and Disabled Persons Act. Alfred Morris MP obtained all-party support for a comprehensive Private Member's Bill giving local authorities mandatory duties to trace the handicapped in their area and ensure they are informed of the help available under the Act. Local authorities were also required to make services available to those disabled in need in their area. However, when it came to enforcing this legislation, things began to go wrong. First, its implementation was delayed because Sir Keith Joseph felt that social services departments were too busy. When he did issue the order, it recommended not full identification of the disabled, but sample surveys. In the absence of a clear lead from the government, the County Councils' Association and Association of Municipal Corporations issued a circular to local authorities which Alfred Morris described as 'a disturbing and shocking manoeuvre' — 'a hard-faced and cynical blueprint for diluting and evading the purpose of the law'. The associations recommended that before local authorities gave a disabled person a telephone, he must be unable to leave home *and* at risk when left alone *and* have no family or friend within reach of the house *and* be physically and mentally capable of using the telephone *and* unable to afford the cost himself *and* it would be unreasonable to ask relatives *and* he must know someone he can telephone!

The Chronically Sick and Disabled Persons Act was implemented unevenly between different authorities; though the Act gives authorities a mandatory duty to provide services where need exists it leaves it to them to decide what constitutes need. If an authority admits a need and refuses to provide assistance, then a case may lie for the Secretary of State to seek an order of mandamus to enforce the local authority. In practice a local authority is unlikely to be silly enough to accept that a need exists and risk court action, and no case has been taken.[13] The legislation may have been unrealistic and ill conceived but nevertheless the discretion left to the administration had the effect of overturning the intention of reformers.

During the late 1950s and early 1960s in almost every area of social policy it became clear that the hopes that had been invested in the reforms of the previous decade were not being achieved. The evidence of widespread and continuing poverty, poor housing, educational deprivation, difficulties of access to health and welfare, even the failure of the legal system to reach out to all, brought disillusion. These problems arose partly as a result of the shortage of resources and partly as a failure of legislation to cover certain groups adequately. However part of the fault lay at the delivery stage — at the interface between the client, claimant or patient and the service. The authorities were less than energetic in selling their service and benefits, and many are unaware of their rights. (A recent example of this is the finding by Rosemary Newnham that half of the council tenants evicted by Edinburgh Corporation for rent arrears were eligible and not claiming rent rebates.[14]) Others were deterred by the organisational form of the service.[15] For example the condition of supplementary benefit offices and those forbidding hatches common in council offices which have to be leaned through at waist level to obtain attention, seem designed as a symbolic deterrent. These are trivial examples, but what they reflect is the ambivalence with which many social policies are implemented, financed and administered. As Titmuss said:[16]

> Many need-eligibility programmes are basically designed to keep
> people out; not let them in. Moreover, they are often so administered
> as to induce among customers a sense of shame, guilt or failure in
> using a public service.

One suggested reason for the fact that entitlements for the poor are not being effectively enforced is that the poor have been and still are seen as in some way blameworthy.[17] The attempts by the 'welfare rights movement' to affirm or reaffirm the existence of these rights is a reflection of their belief that poverty is primarily the consequence of impersonal forces. We shall return to this conflict in values at the end of the chapter.

Discretion as a threat to procedural rights

> Every measure which produces the possibility of beneficent state
> action necessarily produces at the same time the possibility of the
> abuse of power.[18]

The discretionary power that has been invested in administration has raised a host of issues concerning the rights of welfare recipients. Much of the criticisms of discretion in relation to procedural rights have been directed at the supplementary benefit scheme, but in local government and particularly in social work, discretionary judgments are made with less regard to principles of justice and with less adequate procedures for the redress of grievance.[19]

The law of social welfare grew up on the theory that welfare is a 'gratuity' furnished by the state and thus may be subject to whatever conditions the state sees fit to impose.

Recipients are therefore subject to forms and procedures and control not imposed on other citizens. They are subject to the tendency of moralists to prescribe what is best. The administration may seek to impose moral standards on welfare recipients: Louisiana cut off aid in cases where mothers gave birth to an illegitimate child, and discrimination between categories of single parents in the provision of exceptional need payments may be influenced by the moral valuation of officers.[20] Investigation of eligibility necessarily and inevitably results in some invasion of privacy, but procedures for investigation for cohabitation and the policy of a housing department that keeps press cuttings of criminal charges on its tenants may be invasions of privacy. Two common invasions of rights derive from the Elizabethan poor law: the attempt to impose duties for financial responsibility beyond those normally expected[21] and the practice of insisting on residence qualifications for benefits — still a common requirement on housing waiting lists. Welfare authorities may also seek to control other aspects of a recipient's life beyond what is acceptable to non-recipients — they can decide what work the recipient can be compelled to do, they can impose standards of behaviour on their tenants and even in some States in America require loyalty oaths in order to receive benefits. Perhaps the most common characteristic of the welfare process is that of secrecy. In justice the law must be known or at least ascertainable, but much decision making in social policy is based on secret criteria or no criteria at all. The Cullingworth Committee[22] was critical of local authorities' reluctance to divulge the basis of their schemes for allocating council houses and every day the staff of social service departments make 'professional' decisions about whether to provide aid to the handicapped or help under section 1 of the Children and Young Persons Act,[23] or a home help to an old person, without ascertainable criteria and without redress. Redress is perhaps the key to these procedural issues. As de Smith has said:[24]

> Public authorities are set up to govern and administer and if their every act or decisions were to be reviewable on unrestricted grounds by an independent judicial body, the business of administration would be brought to a standstill.

Nevertheless rights lawyers argue: that because administrative discretion in welfare involves important decisions over the people's lives they should be subject to basic safeguards; that there are fewer opportunities for a fair hearing in welfare decisions; and that of all areas of administrative discretion, the opportunities for the redress of grievance are least developed.[25] Where in the exception there is access to tribunals such as in supplementary benefits, these tribunals do not meet the criteria of openness, fairness and impartiality that natural justice demands.[26] (See also the chapter on 'The Redress of Grievance'.)

Welfare rights movement

It is against this background that a new assertion of legalism in welfare has developed in Britain. Many diverse influences have gone into this 'welfare rights movement'. It has been developed in Britain by social workers influenced by the writings of Wootton[27] and Sinfield[28] and disturbed by the material problems of their clients, by lawyers concerned that a large section of the public does not get access to the legal advice and assistance that they need, and principally by the Child Poverty Action Group. The antecedents of the movement are in the USA where through action in the courts, lawyers and social workers managed to get laid down what low income families should get, item by item. It is an attempt to define poverty in terms of a denial of rights and to alter the status of the client from a supplicant appealing for handouts to a claimant demanding his entitlements. It is based on the principle that society has through legislation accepted a commitment to provide certain benefits and services, and if people are not getting those rights then the agencies of the law are failing in their repsonsibility. Thus the welfare rights movement is concerned with the manipulation of the law in clients' favour and the pushing of the law to its furthest limits to extend the generosity of the service. As Tony Lynes has said, it is a classically Fabian strategy.[29]

The hotchpotch of pressure groups, claimants and community groups and advice services that make up the welfare rights movement have been active in three main areas.[30] First, they have been concerned to *enforce* welfare rights through the provision of information and advice. They have sought to improve the availability of benefits directly through advice and information and indirectly by revealing to local and national agencies their failure to publicise the benefits and services. Second, welfare rights workers have begun to advocate on behalf of claimants. The American welfare rights movement thought that:[31]

> campaigns to double and triple the relief rolls would produce significant pressure for national reforms in the relief system, perhaps along the lines of a national guaranteed common income.

The British welfare rights aspirations have been less ambitious. Their activities have varied from writing letters asking for written explanations of how benefits are assessed, or for exceptional needs payments, to representing claimants at tribunals. Tribunals, through their advocacy have been persuaded to take a different view from the Supplementary Benefits Commission on such things as monthly visits of prisoners' wives, school sports kits, and fees for heavy goods vehicle driving lessons. Third, the welfare rights movement has sought to extend poor people's rights by using the law. This strategy developed in the USA where a written constitution which guarantees safeguards to their citizens and a Supreme Court is able to interpret that constitution and to bind by its decisions both Congress and the State legislatures.[32]

> The lawyers expected that as a result of their successful cases the world would change in favour of the poor. Unfortunately the high hopes have not been fulfilled. Crucial decisions by the Supreme Court have been open to varying interpretations and there has been a backlash. In welfare rights, particularly, state legislatures, in order to abide by the letter of the decisions, have reduced benefit entitlement to save the public purse.

In Britain with no written constitution and no supreme court, it has been necessary to take social legislation in a piecemeal fashion. In some precedent-making cases, rights lawyers have revived forgotten laws to extend rights. In Nottingham Corporation v Newton (1974 2 AER 760) the court affirmed the right of tenants to use section 99 of the Public Health Act 1936 to summon local authorities before the magistrates' courts in order to obtain orders for repairs to be carried out on their houses. Another type of precedent-making case has been the attempt by lawyers to challenge official interpretations of the law. The Child Poverty Action Group has sought leave to take a series of test cases to the High Court challenging the decisions of supplementary benefit appeal tribunals and in effect the SBC's interpretation of social security legislation. In R v Greater Birmingham Appeal Tribunal (ex p. Simper) (1973 2 WLR 709) the court held that the commission's use of discretion in relation to allowances for heating was wrong and as a result extra heating allowances were paid to thousands of new claimants.

Another case successfully challenged the commission's interpretation of the Family Income Supplement Act.[33] A series of cases have also been taken to the National Insurance Commissioner which have extended the Attendance Allowance Board's interpretation of the eligibility criteria.[34]

The use of test cases to maintain or extend rights is only in its infancy and its achievements have been limited. As well as the successes there have been harmful results.in McPhail v Persons Unknown (1973 3 WLR 71) a case which originated as an attempt to extend the rights of squatters, their rights were in fact greatly restricted. Legislation used in the courts to advance rights can be repealed or amended by policy makers — this occurred in the Simper case. The legal procedures for getting prerogative orders of certiorari, prohibition or mandamus from the High Court are complex and expensive[35] and it is not at all clear that judges are really prepared to become involved in vetting administrative discretion: in one recent case[36] the judges indicated their unwillingness to interfere with a tribunal's decision *even if it was erroneous in law*.

The defence of discretion

Much of the debate about legalism and discretion in the last decade has centred on the supplementary benefits scheme. One in thirteen of the population of the UK are dependent in whole or part for their income on supplementary benefits and far from becoming a residual service for those who failed to qualify for insurance benefits as Beveridge intended, the supplementary benefit scheme has become the prop for the whole social security edifice. As with most assistance schemes supplementary benefit has an area of flexibility at the margin and this flexibility is embodied in the discretionary powers of the officials to meet needs not covered by the scale rates of benefit. Claimants desperate to supplement the scale rates have turned to these discretionary additions for extra help. At first little was known about what could be obtained in the way of these additions and in what circumstances because the SBC administrative rule used by officers (the A code) was governed by the Official Secrets Act. As a result of pressure from the welfare rights movement more and more information has been published in hand books and guides and over a third of claimants now obtain Exceptional Needs Payments and Exceptional Circumstances Additions each year. The expansion of discretionary payments has been a source of continual dispute and presented the Commission with an enormous extra administrative burden. David Donnison, the Chairman of the Supplementary Benefits

Commission, has argued[37] that the Commission cannot go on providing these additions on an individual basis. The current government review of supplementary benefits is likely to standardise policy and procedures. This may reduce the area of discretion and increase the area of right but it may also reduce the capacity in the system to relate benefit to need. Titmuss, when vice chairman of the SBC, in a biting attack on the 'pathology of legalism' stoutly defended this area of flexible individualised justice.[38]

Just where the line should be drawn between legalised basic rights and discretionary additions is a problem which a fully legalised system based on case law and precedent cannot even begin to consider. It is however a constant challenge to any system like the supplementary benefits scheme which continues to recognise the need for individualised justice.

The other area of dispute on supplementary benefits concerns the conflict inherent in the scheme between providing a humane service to those cast aside by the economic and social system and the need to maintain the values which maintain that system. In practice the supplementary benefit scheme maintains social values through a set of controls. Two of these controls are concerned with the work ethic and the family ethic. Procedures for unemployment review, rules about benefit for strikers, and the level of benefit itself all operate as incentives to return to work. The activity of the rights movement was successful in getting two other procedures concerned with the work ethic — the four week rule and the wage stop — abolished. The supplementary benefits system also bolsters the family with powers to pursue erring husbands and putative fathers (liable relatives) and more controversially through the cohabitation rule. The Commission have been at pains to argue that the rule is intended to ensure that no unmarried couple living together as man and wife are better off than married couples.[39] Although they have refined and reviewed the procedures governing the rule more than once, in practice the rule still results in many single mothers having their benefit withdrawn without a hearing and as a result of a judgment about the nature of their relationship with a man.[40]

The discretionary basis of these controls has satisfied no one. Claimants and their representatives identify them as the principle source of injustice in the system and yet there is still a bitter chorus of vilification against scroungers and the workshy, and demands for stiffer controls. Officials administering their discretion find it the most difficult and odious part of their work. So far attempts to get the courts to intervene, to provide for instance a legal definition of cohabitation, have so far been unsuccessful. The supplementary benefits tribunals do not provide a satisfactory mechanism for the protection of rights and the scrutiny of official discretion. The Ombudsman cannot give a ruling on the justice of a discretionary decision, only on maladminstration. The success of the Commission's own attempts to clarify the basis for their decisions and get some consistency in decision making has been reduced by high staff turnover, overwork and, because of the size of the operation, the inevitable difficulty of getting uniform decisions by hundreds of officers with different values, attitudes and beliefs. These factors naturally make them fearful of the possibility of having to administer rigid criteria for each particular circumstance if the courts or a higher tribunal began to impose binding decisions and in a recent lecture Donnison has intimated that the Commission should[41]

> abandon the aspirations to match the benefits we pay to the infinite variety of human needs we encounter — the aspiration for creative justice.

Conclusion

Views about the nature of society and social policy inevitably influence attitudes to the question of legalism and discretion.[42] Those who accept the consensus model of society where there are no fundamental structural conflicts of values and interests and where the powers of the state are not viewed as a menace to the individual, would believe that discretionary powers will be used to help those in need and disputes will be rare and resolved amicably within an accepted framework. In contrast, those who see society as a state of dichotomic conflict between those who have power, authority and wealth and those who do not, will view rights as meaningless. Benefits are a means of social control or a sop to help keep down unrest and any control over discretion exists to propagate a consensual view of society. Opponents of the system seek to change it by revolution and others despite what they see as its hypocrisy try to work the system for the benefit of the needy. Finally there is the open model:[43]

> that of a society which recognises a continuing multiple conflict of interests and values taking place within an over-arching structure of a more or less fluid or dynamic nature. In this society there are not just two sides but many conflicts.

Rights are essential in this society because they are the means of managing these conflicts.

The fullest discussion of the issue of legalism and discretion is in a book by an American lawyer, Kenneth Culp Davis.[44] He has argued that although discretion is inevitable and necessary for individualised justice, it is often much greater than it should be and it needs to be restricted.[45]

Discretion is a tool indispensable for the individualiization of justice. . . . Discretion is our principal source of creativeness in government and in law. Discretion is a tool only when properly used; perhaps nine-tenths of injustice in our legal system flows from discretion, and perhaps only one tenth from rules.

Let us not overemphasize either the need for discretion or its danger; let us emphasize both the need for discretion and its dangers.

In his book he goes on to outline a framework that could confine, structure and check discretionary power. More meaningful standards should be set out in statute, better and more elaborate and more open administrative rule making is required to confine and structure discretion, there is a need for improvements in the fairness and accessibility of tribunals, and finally for the elimination of barriers to judicial review.

References

1   R. M. Titmuss, 'Welfare rights, law and discretion', *Political Quarterly,* vol. 42, no. 2, 1971, p. 130.
2   R. M. Tawney, *Equality,* Allen & Unwin, 1964, p. 217.
3   T. H. Marshall, *Sociology at the Crossroads,* Heinemann, 1963, pp. 67-127.
4   Universal Declaration of Human Rights, 1948, article 25.
5   A. V. Dicey, *Law of the Constitution* (8th edn), Macmillan, 1915, p. xliv.
6   W. A. Robson, *Justice and Administrative Law,* Macmillan, 1928.
7   S. and B. Webb, *English Local Government — The Parish and the County,* vol. 1, Longmans, 1906, p. 419.
8   Robson, op. cit., p. 33.
9   Op. cit., p. 37.
10 Quoted in Robson, op. cit., p. 229.
11 Titmuss, op. cit., p. 131.
12 O. Stevenson, *Claimant or Client,* Allen & Unwin, 1973, p. 27.
13 But see M. Phillips, 'Accountable social work', *New Society,* 15 April 1976, pp. 136-7.
14 R. Newnham, 'No benefits for evicted families', *Roof,* March 1977.
15 See A. Kahn, *Social Work,* vol. 26, no. 3, July 1969.

154   Legalism and Discretion

16 R. M. Titmuss, *Commitment to Welfare*, Allen & Unwin, 1968, p. 68.
17 C. A. Reich, 'Individual rights and social welfare: the emerging legal issues', *Yale Law Journal*, vol. 74, 1965, p. 1245.
18 J. D. B. Mitchell, *Constitutional Law* (2nd edn), Green, Edinburgh, 1968, p. 323.
19 Reich, op. cit., p. 1245.
20 DHSS Statistical and Research Report Series 1, *Families Receiving Supplementary Benefits*, R. Marshall, HMSO, 1972.
21 R v West London SBAT ex parte Clarke (1975) 3 All ER 513 (DC).
22 J. B. Cullingworth, *Council Housing: Purposes, Procedures and Priorities*, Central Housing Advisory Committee, HMSO, 1969.
23 J. Heywood and B. Allen, *Financial Help in Social Work*, Manchester University Press, 1971.
24 S. A. de Smith, *Judicial Review of Administrative Action*, Stevens, 1968, p. 3.
25 R. Brook, *Rights in the Welfare State*, CPAG Pamphlet 4. H. Rose, *Rights, Participation and Conflict*, CPAG Pamphlet 5.
26 K. Bell, *Research Study on Supplementary Benefit Appeal Tribunals*, DHSS, HMSO, 1975. R. Lister, *Justice for the Claimant*, CPAG, 1974.
27 B. Wootton, *Social Science and Social Pathology*, Allen & Unwin, 1959.
28 A. Sinfield, *Which Way for Social Work?*, Fabian Society, 1969.
29 A. Lynes, *Welfare Rights*, Fabian Society, 1969.
30 For a fuller discussion of these see 'Which Way Welfare Rights', CPAG, November 1975.
31 F. F. Piven and R. Cloward, *Regulating the Poor*, Pantheon, 1971, p. 321.
32 'Which Way Welfare Rights?', p. 21.
33 J. Bradshaw, 'For your clients' benefit', *Social Work Today*, vol. 5, no. 8, 1974, p. 232.
34 *Poverty*, no. 28, 1973, p. 32.
35 Law Commission, *Remedies in Administrative Law*, Published working paper no. 40, 1971.
36 R v Sheffield SBAT ex parte Shine (1975) 2 All ER 807 (CA).
37 D. V. Donnison, 'Supplementary benefits: dilemmas and priorities', *Journal of Social Policy*, vol. 5, no. 4, pp. 337-59.
38 R. M. Titmuss, 'Welfare Rights, Law and Discretion', p. 127.
39 DHSS, *Cohabitation*, HMSO, 1971. Supplementary Benefits Commission, *Living Together as Husband and Wife*, HMSO, 1976.
40 R. Lister, *As Man and Wife, A Study of the Cohabitation Rule*, CPAG, 1973.
41 D. V. Donnison, 'How much discretion', *SBC Notes and News*, 7 April 1977.
42 R. White, 'Lawyers and the Enforcement of Rights' in P. Morris *et al.*, *Social Need and Legal Action*, Martin Robertson, 1973.
43 Op. cit., p. 17.
44 K. C. Davis, *Discretionary Justice*, University of Illinois, 1971.
45 Op. cit., p. 25.

Chapter ten

The Redress of Grievances

As we have built up the structure of the health and social services, the sheer size of the administrative machinery involved has led to the replacement of many individual decisions by the formulation of general rules of procedure. This kind of routinisation seems to be an inevitable consequence of administrative growth, but it does not always adequately meet the needs of individuals. Sometimes the rules are interpreted too inflexibly by junior staff, and a considerable sense of frustration or injustice can be built up at counter level by a clerk or porter who 'goes by the book' in inappropriate circumstances. Sometimes the rules, which may be very complex, are not fully implemented — as in the case of a claimant to Supplementary Benefit who receives less than he is entitled to. Sometimes the rules do not give adequate coverage to the situation. Sometimes there is plain incompetence or an honest mistake, as where the wrong limb is removed in an operation.

No administrative system is perfect. No administrative system is proof against all possibilities of error all the time. The health and social services are particularly vulnerable to complaints, for two reasons. First, however large and complex the services themselves become, they are concerned primarily with individual human needs, and it is the well-being of the individual which is the acid test of their efficiency. Second, the consumer (that is, the patient, claimant or client) is also the tax-payer, and in democratic theory at least the ultimate controller of the service. It is important therefore that there should be means for the redress of grievances, and that these should be well known and available to all.

Traditional modes of complaint

There are time-honoured approaches to complaints against the system, and these too have become increasingly sophisticated with the passage of time. One can approach a Member of Parliament, and a study of the subjects brought up at Question Time in the House of Commons will show the variety of subjects which are still aired in this way. Though

Question Time is limited, Members of Parliament are often able to do a great deal behind the scenes at Westminster, either by a direct approach to a minister or civil servant, or by letter. Many hold 'surgeries' in their constituencies, so that constituents can bring their problems to be dealt with, and a number of local councillors now do the same.

One can approach the mass media. Letters to the *Daily Mirror* and the *News of the World* probably stand as good a chance of securing redress today as the traditional 'letter to *The Times*'. Radio and television now offer many opportunities for expressing grievances, from a two-minute spot on local radio to a fully-prepared appearance on *Panorama* or *This Week*. In policy terms, documentaries like Jeremy Sandford's *Cathy, Come Home* or *Edna the Inebriate Woman* have had a powerfull effect.

One can simply protest publicly. The strike, the sit-in, the march, the demonstration, the public petition are all possible means of action which have developed in the last twenty years (perhaps originating in the 'Ban the Bomb' campaigns of the 1950s) and no longer have left-wing associations. Farmers and doctors (not noticeably left-wing groups) threaten to strike, and ladies in twin-sets and pearls have sat elegantly in the streets of well-to-do London suburbs.

One can sometimes proceed through the courts, and it is important that the extent of the powers of the judiciary should be recognised in this context. Professor S. A. de Smith has summarized them as follows:[1]

> Judicial review of administrative action may be invoked for a wide range of purposes by a person claiming to be aggrieved.
> 1. To obtain damages or another private law remedy (for example, an injuction) for a civil wrong such as a breach of contract or a tort.
> 2. To have an order, act or decision of a public body quashed or declared invalid on the ground that it is *ultra vires* or outside jurisdiction.
> 3. To procure, on appeal, the reversal or variation of an order or determination for error of law. . . .
> 4. To restrain the performance or continuance of unlawful action. . . .
> 5. To obtain release from unlawful detention. . . .
> 6. To secure an authoritative statement of the law governing a specific legal dispute by means of a binding declaration awarded by the courts.
> 7. To secure the performance of a public duty (for example, to make reimbursement; to exercise a discretion according to law; to hear an application or appeal within a tribunal's jurisdiction). . . .

8. To defend oneself in proceedings which rely on the validity of an administrative act or order.

He goes on to point out that public authorities can appear in court for other reasons: as defendants, for example, in actions arising out of the requirements of the Public Health Acts, or as applicants for permission to exercise powers such as those to abate public nuisances.

Matters arising from the administration of the social services can and do come before the ordinary courts of law under the above heads. Action taken by a central government ministry or a local government department to implement policy in the field of health, housing, or education, for example, might be challenged in the courts as being *ultra vires*. A local authority might find itself defending a civil action for damages where personal injury is alleged to have resulted from negligence in the running of a residential institution.

Individual employees of social service organisations may in certain circumstances be personally answerable for their actions in carrying out their duties. The nurse who physically ill-treats hospital patients may face criminal charges.[2]

However, though the courts remain the basic constitutional means of redress, legal procedures involving court action are slow, often expensive, and frequently uncertain in outcome. So cumbersome are the powers for obtaining redress in administrative law that the Law Commission has been searching for ways of easing access to the courts.[3] However the courts are already overburdened and since the late 1950s, we have seen the development of a number of other means of redress.

Internal monitoring

Grievances and complaints can be seen as an administrative problem to be dealt with by the organisation itself. Many large organisations have developed systems of internal monitoring which should counteract the bureaucratic tendency to compartmentalise inefficiency. Under such a system, a complaint against any part of the organisation should automatically set in train a review procedure located elsewhere in the organisation. For instance, the Davies Committee reporting on Hospital Complaints Procedures commented:[4]

> In the Hospital Service, the investigation and satisfaction of complaints is primarily a function of management. To deal initially with complaints in any other manner would in our view be unnecessary, cumbersome and unrealistic.

Organisations administering the health and social services in fact employ a wide variety of internal methods. Minor matters may be referred to the member of staff next in seniority to the officer involved in the original action or decision which has led to dispute. Routinised arrangements may be in operation for a special 'designated officer' to handle particular types of complaints – this now happens in the initial handling of appeals in relation to supplementary benefits. Standing committees may exist to deal with other issues, and special reviews and internal inquiries may be constituted on an *ad hoc* basis to investigate particular incidents. For instance, in the National Health Service, section 70 of the National Health Service Act 1946 gives the Minister (i.e. the Secretary of State) power to set up a public inquiry where serious failures occur. This section was invoked for the Farleigh and Whittingham Inquiries.[5] Under Circulars HM(66)15 and HM(61)112, Regional Health Authorities and Area Health Authorities may similarly set up inquiries of their own; but these two circulars give general guidance only, and have been seriously criticised as inadequate.

According to the Davies Report (1973), between 8,000 and 9,000 enquiries are set afoot each year by authorities under the circular, while between 1,500 and 2,000 enquiries go direct from members of parliament to DHSS.[6] According to R. J. Coleman,[7] in a twelve-month period some 26,000 'determinations' or first decisions on Supplementary Benefit were challenged by claimants. About a third of these were resolved by administrative review, and thus never reached the stage of a formal appeal to a Supplementary Benefit Appeals Tribunal.

It can be argued that in the health and social services in particular it is important that complaints and grievances should be dealt with quickly and routinely, and as close to the point of origin as possible. Questions of immediate need may be involved, or special considerations relating to the vulnerability of the client. A 'model' code for procedures in the Personal Social Services recently offered for consideration is prefaced by the statement that:[8]

> A formal appeal can be very damaging to the client, and generally should be avoided. . . . Every effort should be made to satisfy complainants before they are referred for a formal appeal.

On the other hand, there are limitations to the usefulness of internal monitoring. Because it is internal, justice is not 'seen to be done', and one set of officials may see the viewpoint of another set of officials (with whom they have to work on a long-term basis) more readily than they see that of the flustered, inarticulate or over-vehement client. If there is genuine injustice, there is at least the possibility that it will be hushed up, and even compounded by further injustice in the way of reprisals and victimisation. There have been well-publicised cases in the Hospital Service, and these led the Davies Committee to draw up a suggested Code of Practice which would safeguard the complainant. So far, the recommendations have not been implemented. The need for similar safeguards in the Personal Social Services has recently been the subject of active debate.

Beyond the work of internal monitoring, however well organised and protected from abuse, there exists a need for independent adjudication and review.

Administrative tribunals

Rent Tribunals, National Insurance Tribunals, Supplementary Benefits Tribunals, Industrial Tribunals, Mental Health Review Tribunals and many others now exist to provide cheap, speedy and equitable arbitration. Administrative tribunals have been classified into more than 50 types, and there are more than 2,000 separate tribunals in existence.

The history of administrative tribunals goes back to the introduction of a state system for social insurance in the National Insurance Act of 1911. The scheme, which was gradually extended to a substantial proportion of the working population through the ensuing decade, gave substantive entitlement to cash benefits and health care. It was foreseen that disputes would arise over the extent and nature of these entitlements, and an appeals system was introduced from the beginning.[9] A similar model was used with pensions legislation after the First World War, and has subsequently been widely applied, not only because of the expense and delay of court actions, but because new and very technical areas of expertise were often involved.

Like internal monitoring procedures, administrative tribunals can often be criticised for being to close to the administration itself. They often meet on the premises of the service in question, and although members are not paid officials, their expenses are met by the service. The procedure — for instance in Mental Health Review Tribunals, where the patient has to face a panel consisting of a medical practitioner, a lawyer and a 'lay' member with experience in the social services — can put the appellant at a disadvantage.[10] However overtly fair the system, there are intangible issues of professional and class solidarity between the officials and the tribunal members which can influence the outcome, and tribunal chairmen have not always been sufficiently aware of these factors.

The Franks Committee[11] reported in 1957 after conducting the first thorough review of tribunal procedures. They accepted that tribunals were a necessary and 'permanent factor of our society' and predicted that the numbers of tribunals were likely to increase rather than to diminish. At the same time, they were critical of many existing tribunal procedures, and made recommendations for ensuring 'openness, fairness and impartiality'.

The recommendations of the Franks Committee were largely accepted and implemented. They included the setting up of the Council on Tribunals, under the Tribunals and Inquiries Act.[12] Members have wide powers to attend tribunals, investigate complaints and review tribunal proceedings. The Council of Tribunals may report direct to the Lord Chancellor. At the same time, direct administrative action was taken to remove the control of membership of tribunals from the Ministers responsible for departments, and to vest it instead in the Lord Chancellor. Procedural matters concerning the appellant's rights before, during and after the hearing were also dealt with. The use of legal aid to enable appellants to be formally represented was extended to some tribunals.

Schwartz and Wade have summarised the position as follows:[13]

it may be said that the work of tribunals has been improved by the Act of 1958 and the continuing effects which date from that statute. Tribunals are now seen to be an integral part of the machinery of justice, related directly to the Courts through the channels of appeal and judicial review, and arriving at the best practicable level of fairness in procedure. With something like 2,000 separate tribunals in operation, it cannot be expected that all will work equally well, or that there will be no complaints.

One kind of tribunal about which there has been considerable concern is the Supplementary Benefits Appeal Tribunal. It has been claimed that these tribunals do not meet the criteria of 'openness, fairness and impartiality' set for them by the Frank's Committee[14] and in response to research by Kathleen Bell confirming this[15] the government undertook to reform them by providing training for chairmen and giving easier access to the courts for the purposes of reviewing their decisions.

The 'ombudsman' principle

In 1961, *Justice* published the report of a committee which it had instituted under the chairmanship of Sir John Whyatt entitled 'The Citizen and the Administration'. Its main recommendation was that an officer analogous to that of the Scandinavian ombudsman should be introduced. He would receive individual complaints against maladministration by central government departments through MPs; he would conduct impartial and informal investigations and have access to departmental files; his proposed title would be 'Parliamentary Commissioner'. It was not foreseen that he would primarily be concerned with breaches of the law; he would have no power to prosecute public officials; and his enquiries would not be conducted in public with attendant publicity. These proposals attracted much popular support, but were rejected by the Conservative government of the day as being incompatible to parliament and calculated to impede the dispatch of public business. The Labour Party however incorporated a version of the ombudsman idea in their election manifesto in 1966, and having been returned to office published a White Paper proposing the appointment of a Parliamentary Commissioner on substantially the lines proposed in the Whyatt Report.[16] The Parliamentary Commissioner Act of 1967 was the outcome.

The commissioner is appointed by the Crown on the Prime Minister's advice. He can only be removed on addresses from both Houses of Parliament. He has his own office, and appoints his own staff, mostly drawn from the civil service. By 1970 he had a staff of about 70, not one of them a professional lawyer. His terms of reference are to investigate complaints by individuals and bodies corporate (other than local authorities and other public corporations) who claim to have 'sustained injustice in consequence of maladministration' while in the UK at the hands of scheduled central government departments or persons or bodies acting on their behalf, performing or failing to perform administrative functions (i.e. not legislative or judicial).

The Commissioner cannot act on his own initiative, nor can he be approached directly by a member of the public. His role was until recently restricted to acting on written complaints MPs forwarded with the consent of complainants. His constitutional position as an adjunct to parliament is reinforced by the fact that he is answerable to a Select Committee of the House of Commons and must make an annual Report to both Houses. (He may also issue special reports which similarly must be laid before Parliament.) His investigations must be conducted in private, and the official head of the departments concerned and any other official implicated in the complaint must be notified and given the opportunity to comment on the allegations. His powers to investigate are comprehensive: he can administer oaths, compel attendance of witnesses, and wilful obstruction of his enquiries is punishable as if it were a contempt of court. He must be allowed access to any relevant document other than one relating to Cabinet or Cabinet Committee proceedings. The Commissioner has, however, no power to alter or rescind decisions. Statute empowers him to make reports on his investigations, or give to the MP who referred a complaint his reasons for investigating. Reports go to the MP concerned, to the official against whom the allegations were made and his departmental head. If it appears to the Parliamentary Commissioner that an injustice has been caused by maladministration and not rectified, he may then make a special report to both Houses.

Although clearly of crucial importance, the terms 'injustice' and 'maladministration' were not defined. It seems that in this context 'injustice' means something wider than legally redressible damage; it includes hardship and a sense of grievance which ought not to have arisen. In defending the decision not to define 'maladministration' in the Act, Richard Crossman, then Lord President of the Council, declared in the House of Commons that 'it would be a wonderful exercise to try — the definition would encompass bias, neglect, inattention, delay, incompetence, ineptitude, perversity, turpitude, arbitrariness and so on.'[17] More specifically, Sir William Armstrong, Head of the Home Civil Service, offered to the Select Committee of the House of Commons which was reviewing the Act's first year of operation, a list of examples: failure to answer a letter; losing the papers or part of them; giving misleading statements to citizens about their legal position; delay in reaching a decision; exhibiting bias; giving incomplete or ambiguous instructions to the officer who is applying the rule; getting the facts of the case wrong; or failing to take facts into account which the department should have taken into account.[18]

The Parliamentary Commissioner has been given extensive statutory powers, and has consistently been urged to broaden his interpretation of them. Nevertheless the Act itself and its subsequent implementation have been subject to considerable criticism. Professor Harry Street commented[19] that 'our Act is a half-hearted affair hinged about with restrictions and exceptions'.

The 'Ombudsman' principle has been widened more recently by the appointment of the Health Service Commissioner and of the Commission for Local Administration. The office of the Health Service Commissioner is administratively combined with that of the Parliamentary Commissioner: one official holds both titles, though there are separate secretariats. It was set up under the National Health Service Reorganisation Act of 1973, and covers all aspects of the National Health Service at all levels, though with some significant exceptions: the Health Service Commissioner may not investigate the exercise of clinical judgment by doctors, dentists, pharmacists or opticians; matters of staff appointment, pay or promotion; or any issue which may properly be dealt with by a Family Practitioner Committee, an administrative tribunal, the courts or a section 70 enquiry.[20]

The Health Service Commissioner's terms of reference are wider than those of the Parliamentary Commissioner, and the Davies Committee took the view that there were 'important differences' that should characterise the working of the two offices.[21] In addition to 'maladministration', the Health Services Commissioner may investigate a failure to provide a service which it was an authority's duty to provide, and a failure in a service provided. He may be approached directly by complainants — the MP is not involved — but the complainant or his representative must first have brought the issue to the notice of the organisation concerned. This gives an opportunity for internal monitoring and review procedures to provide a solution at an early stage.

The Commission for Local Administration, set up in 1974, consists in England of three Local Commissioners, one for London, one for the North and one for the South, each with his or her own secretariat.[22] They deal with complaints against local authorities on the grounds of 'maladministration' only. Complaints have to go to the local authority member concerned with a request for transmission to the Local Commissioner. Only where this is not complied with may a member of the public approach the Local Commissioner direct. Certain matters, including teaching and the internal organisation of schools and colleges, the general level of rates and water charges and job grievances are exempt from enquiry.

The Personal Social Services Council has published a useful guide to complaints procedures in the social services, both statutory and voluntary, which includes notes on the work of the Health Service Commission and the Commissioner for Local Administration.

Consumer protection

Recent developments in the evolution of a policy to protect consumers also have a relevance to social policy, since they deal with such matters as land, housing, private insurance, public utilities, consumer goods and professional services. The creation of a government Department of Prices and Consumer Protection in 1974 was a major step away from the traditional *laissez-faire* view that the best safeguard for the public is free competition and free consumer choice. Labour Party documents have pointed to the dangers of price-fixing associations, deceptive advertising and unduly high credit rates which are not always apparent to the purchaser at the time of purchase.[23]

The Director-General of Fair Trading, whose office was set up in 1973, has a general responsibility to investigate practices which 'adversely affect the interests' of consumers. One of the first actions of the Office of Fair Trading was to analyse consumer complaints to various organisations over a nine-month period (over 142,000 complaints were collected). The Office of Fair Trading attempts to set up voluntary codes of practice for various classes of traders, but may under certain conditions seek undertakings from individual traders who are judged to be persistently trading on unfair terms. If such an undertaking is broken, the case may be taken before the Restrictive Practices Court. The Director-General also has the power to initiate proposals for legislation on matters of unfair trading, these being subject to the scrutiny of the Consumer Protection Advisory Service and the Secretary of State for Prices and Consumer Protection.

Since the late 1960s, the work of the Consumers' Association in pioneering consumer advice centres has mushroomed, and the Local Government Act 1972 empowered local authorities to grant-aid these centres. In 1975, a central government grant of £1.4 million was made to set up another forty centres. These tend to be concentrated in working-class areas, where shoppers are thought to be most vulnerable to commercial pressures.[24]

The National Consumer Council, set up in 1975, has a broad remit to cover many kinds of consumer interests, including those in the health and social services and public utilities. A Government White Paper stated[25]

It is the inarticulate and disadvantaged who most need a body to speak for them and ensure that they are protected, and it is they whose needs have least been met by the consumer activities of the last decade. The government believes that the new body proposed will be in a position to insist that the interests of all consumers, including the least articulate, should be taken into account.

Conclusion

Other kinds of complaints machinery, such as the Community Health Councils and the machinery against discrimination on grounds of sex or race, have been outlined in earlier chapters. The nature of material in the field of 'redress of grievances' is such that at present we can do little more than to describe what exists, and to provide some sort of map of the ground which it covers. Development has been fragmentary, and procedures do not add up to one coherent system based on a set of clear and universally agreed administrative principles. Machinery has developed on an *ad hoc* basis, often in response to immediate social or political pressure.

Some bodies which have been described here exist purely for dealing with complaints. Others, like the Office of Fair Trading or Community Health Councils, have what might be termed a preventive function — they deal with classes of complaint rather than with individual complaints, though it may be the individual complaint which alerts their interest in the question.

The most obvious problem of this mass of machinery is its lack of comprehensibility to ordinary people. It involves a maze of procedural problems. There are major variations in the status of the organisations set up, the scope of their powers, and the nature of their work.

The very complexity and sophistication of the machinery may be used to defeat or stifle complaints, and it is difficult to believe that this is altogether unintended. There has been some anxiety in official circles as to whether the development of complaints procedures would lead to a mass of frivolous and tendentious complaints likely to overwhelm the machinery; and whether, on the other hand, the provision of complaints machinery would not unduly raise public expectations of the services. In times of severe constraints and manpower shortage, it is easy to see that there are limits to the scope which can be given to complaints procedures if the services themselves are not to be brought to a standstill, and their workers unduly harassed. The problem is to devise systems which operate easily and well for the legitimate complaint, but which deter the merely troublesome.

It must be stressed that the development of complaints machinery is still comparatively new, and it may take some years of experience to get it working properly. There is a considerable need for research into such matters as who gets appointed to the new bodies, and the kinds of knowledge and professional expertise which they bring to their tasks; the kinds of interpretations they adopt; the kinds of procedures and decisions which ensue. Basically, what we need to know is whether a set of fairly expensive and elaborate pieces of administrative machinery are operating fairly between the 'trading agencies' (including the health and social services) on one hand, and the aggrieved client, or patient or consumer on the other. It may be some time before the accumulation of case material and the weight of experience is sufficient to remove legal obscurantism and create a system which the ordinary citizen can use with ease and confidence for the redress of his genuine grievances.

References

1   S. A. de Smith, *Constitutional and Administrative Law,* Penguin, 1971, p. 546.
2   E.g. *Report of the Farleigh Hospital Committee of Inquiry,* Cmnd 4557, HMSO, April 1971. The events concerned took place in 1967/8, but the Report was held up pending criminal prosecutions.
3   Law Commission Remedies in Administrative Law, Published Working Paper no. 40, 1971.
4   *Report of the Committee on Hospital Complaints Procedures,* HMSO, 1973, para. 1.7.
5   Farleigh Report, op. cit. *Report of the Committee of Inquiry into Whittingham Hospital,* Cmnd 4861, HMSO, February 1972.
6   *Report of the Committee on Hospital Complaints Procedures,* paras 2.2 and 2.8.
7   R. J. Coleman, 'Supplementary benefits and the administrative review of administrative action', *Poverty* (no. 7), CPAG, 1970.
8   *Complaints procedures in the Personal Social Services,* A Discussion Paper, Personal Social Services Council, 1976, appendix B, p. 8.
9   National Insurance Act, 1911, section 90 (unemployment insurance).
10 L. Gostin, *A Human Condition,* vol. I, Mind Report 1976, chapter 7, passim.
11 *Report of Committee on Administrative Tribunals and Enquiries,* Cmnd 218, HMSO, 1957.
12 Tribunals and Inquiries Act, 1958. For an account of the Franks Report and the Act, see K. Bell, *Tribunals in the Social Services,* Routledge & Kegan Paul, 1959, chapter 3.
13 B. Schwartz and H. W. R. Wade, *Legal Control of Government,* Clarendon Press, 1972, p. 162.
14 M. Adler and A. Bradley (eds), *Justice, Discretion and Poverty,* Professional Books, 1975.
15 K. Bell, *Research Study of Supplementary Benefits Appeal Tribunals,* HMSO, 1975.
16 Justice Educational and Research Trust, *The Citizen and the Administration,* Stevens, 1961.
17 Hansard, *House of Commons Debates,* 18 October 1966, vol. 734, col. 51.

18 *Parliamentary Papers*, House of Commons, no. 350 of 1967–8,
    HMSO, 1968, pp. 100–1, question 643.
19 Harry Street, *Justice in the Welfare State*, Stevens, 1975, p. 115.
20 *Health Service Commissioner for England*, pamphlet issued by the
    Office of the Health Services Commissioner, Church House, Great
    Smith Street, London SW1P 3BW, July 1973.
21 *Report of the Committee on Hospital Complaints Procedures*,
    para. 10.19.
22 See M. R. Hyde, 'The Commissioner for Local Administration', in
    K. Jones, M. Brown and S. Baldwin (eds), *The Year Book of Social
    Policy in Britain 1976*, Routledge & Kegan Paul, 1977.
23 'Help for the Consumer', *Labour Party Discussion Notes*, Labour
    Party, Transport House, London, 1958.
24 For a discussion of the work of the OFT and the DPCP, see
    E. Freudenheim, 'Consumer Protection in the Market-place', in
    K. Jones and S. Baldwin (eds), *The Year Book of Social Policy in
    Britain 1975*, Routledge & Kegan Paul, 1976.
25 Department of Prices and Consumer Protection, National Con-
    sumers' Agency, Cmnd 5726, HMSO, 1974. For an account of the
    work of the National Consumer Council, see Mark Goyder, 'The
    National Consumer Council: speaking for whom?' in K. Jones and
    S. Baldwin (eds), op. cit.

Index

172   Index